Complex Cases in Peripheral Vascular Interventions

Complex Cases in Peripheral Vascular Interventions

Edited by

Martin Schillinger
Medical University of Vienna
General Hospital
Vienna, Austria

Erich Minar
Medical University of Vienna
General Hospital
Vienna, Austria

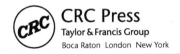

CRC Press
Taylor & Francis Group
Boca Raton London New York

CRC Press is an imprint of the
Taylor & Francis Group, an **informa** business

First published 2010 by Informa Healthcare
This edition published in 2010 by Informa Healthcare

Published 2019 by CRC Press
Taylor & Francis Group
6000 Broken Sound Parkway NW, Suite 300
Boca Raton, FL 33487-2742

First issued in paperback 2019

No claim to original U.S. Government works

ISBN 13: 978-0-367-44599-7 (pbk)
ISBN 13: 978-1-84184-731-3 (hbk)

This book contains information obtained from authentic and highly regarded sources. While all reasonable efforts have been made to publish reliable data and information, neither the author[s] nor the publisher can accept any legal responsibility or liability for any errors or omissions that may be made. The publishers wish to make clear that any views or opinions expressed in this book by individual editors, authors or contributors are personal to them and do not necessarily reflect the views/opinions of the publishers. The information or guidance contained in this book is intended for use by medical, scientific or health-care professionals and is provided strictly as a supplement to the medical or other professional's own judgement, their knowledge of the patient's medical history, relevant manufacturer's instructions and the appropriate best practice guidelines. Because of the rapid advances in medical science, any information or advice on dosages, procedures or diagnoses should be independently verified. The reader is strongly urged to consult the relevant national drug formulary and the drug companies' and device or material manufacturers' printed instructions, and their websites, before administering or utilizing any of the drugs, devices or materials mentioned in this book. This book does not indicate whether a particular treatment is appropriate or suitable for a particular individual. Ultimately it is the sole responsibility of the medical professional to make his or her own professional judgements, so as to advise and treat patients appropriately. The authors and publishers have also attempted to trace the copyright holders of all material reproduced in this publication and apologize to copyright holders if permission to publish in this form has not been obtained. If any copyright material has not been acknowledged please write and let us know so we may rectify in any future reprint.

**Visit the Taylor & Francis Web site at
http://www.taylorandfrancis.com**

**and the CRC Press Web site at
http://www.crcpress.com**

A CIP record for this book is available from the British Library.

Library of Congress Cataloging-in-Publication Data available on application

Typeset by Aptara, Delhi, India

Foreword

Vascular intervention represents a unique corner of medical care. While the potentially analogous field of coronary intervention is practiced by a single, nonsurgical specialty and has progressed in a fairly orderly fashion with a reasonably standardized set of techniques and produced a wealth of randomized data, vascular intervention has followed a decidedly different path. It is practiced by physicians from at least four different medical, surgical, and radiologic specialty training backgrounds with variable skill sets that nevertheless converge on a significant overlap of procedures, but which cover a myriad of vascular territories, both visceral and peripheral. And the techniques and tools in vascular intervention have evolved quickly in spite of the challenges of diverse practitioners, and in concert with industry partners working to improve its tools. As a result, over the past several years, endovascular intervention has evolved as the preferred first approach in many vascular territories, supplanting decades-old surgical approaches. This progress, however, has not produced nearly the same volume or quality of data, nor standardization of technique, largely as a result of a lack of a regulatory impetus but it had been related to an overall smaller volume of activity than that of coronary work.

Owing to the rapid pace of the prior and current evolution in this field, the lack of a singular specialty training "track," the many interventionalists who "grandfathered" into this field, the paucity of data to support decision-making in the vascular patient vis-à-vis medical or surgical options, and fractured training programs often split between endovascular skills and other specialty training needs (interventional cardiology, vascular surgery, nonvascular interventional radiology, etc.), the operator practicing endovascular intervention may have limited exposure to the variety of techniques and approaches available for the care of the vascular patient.

On this background, we are fortunate to have two world-renowned interventionalists who between them have more than 35 years of experience and nearly 600 publications in this field, which in addition to covering intervention in almost every conceivable vascular territory, but also nondevice intervention ranging from the pharmacology through brachytherapy. In a word, Drs. Minar and Schillinger have been at the forefront and instrumental in shaping this field through their tireless research and investigation. Here they have assembled an all-star group of multidisciplinary interventionalists, and they employ a unique and effective method of transferring those experts' knowledge to the reader. While the case-based style of teaching is not new, the editors here have the experts' focus not only on the specific case at hand but also the broader aspects of the vascular territory; so often the contextual facet of the potential intervention is either unclear or not fully considered, which makes this formatting even more vital. In addition, more practical information such as the choice of tools and variety of approaches are detailed. Finally, the authors perform a critique of the case and discuss alternate approaches to complete the case successfully.

The editors have sectioned the book into vascular territories, which help highlight the distinctive aspects of each intervention. Some will be more sensitive to embolization, others aggressive to interventional techniques, and some in which residual stenosis may not be considered a critical determinant of success. The tool sets, imaging, access, as well as the frequency and consequences of adverse outcomes for each are unique and require a nuanced understanding. Save for intracranial interventions, this book should enable most operators to approach the significant majority of vascular syndromes requiring intervention.

Publications like this are important in the field of intervention practiced by such a disparate group of physicians in order to maximize the transfer of knowledge from among our ranks. Eleanor Roosevelt, herself an interventionalist of sorts, once advised, "Learn from the mistakes of others. You can't live long enough to make them all yourself." In this book, the reader will find that Drs. Minar and Schillinger have assembled a wealth of accumulated knowledge intended to minimize the interventionalist's need for discovery at the bedside, and enable them to be more effective interventionalists with greater options at their disposal. I believe Eleanor would have heartily approved.

William A. Gray, MD

Preface

Indications for endovascular treatment of peripheral arterial diseases are dramatically expanding during the recent years, and peripheral vascular interventions (PVI) today are a well-accepted therapeutic approach for virtually all vessel areas. Rapidly advancing technologies enable treatment of more and more complex lesions. The minimal invasive approach offers the advantage of a reduced risk for complications compared to conventional surgery and enables treatment even of severely diseased patients who otherwise would have been considered unfit for surgical procedures.

With increasing numbers of heavily diseased patients treated in the cath lab, several centers have gained an exceptional expertise in treatment of complex morphologies. Sophisticated interventional strategies and meticulous techniques have been developed to handle morphologies that would have been considered not feasible for PVI in earlier years. Furthermore, industry has recognized the utmost importance of PVI and meanwhile offers a multitude of technical solutions dedicated to specific peripheral vessel areas and specific vascular morphologies. Today, particularly for complex scenarios, the concept of "one fits all" has been abandoned and has been replaced by a patient- and lesion-tailored treatment strategy.

The present book aims to systematically review complex cases in PVI. Typical and atypical complex cases are described for all peripheral vessel areas, and methods how to successfully and safely handle these interventions are outlined.

The book is divided in two sections:

Section I—General considerations: This section briefly reviews general aspects on managing complex patients in PVI.

Section II—Complex Cases in Specific Vessel Areas: Section II covers the interventions from puncture to closure, from the head to the toe. Each of the chapters on the specific vessel areas is divided into three parts:

(Part 1) The *Introduction* to each vessel area addresses the following questions:

(a) What makes a lesion "complex" in this vessel area?
(b) What are the clinical indications for endovascular treatment of complex lesions in this vessel area?
(c) What are the potential hazards of treating complex lesions in this vessel area?
(d) Which specific interventional strategies can be considered for this vessel area?
(e) Which specific interventional tools are available to handle complex lesions in this vessel area?
(f) Summary on technical success rates, acute and long-term outcomes after endovascular treatment of complex lesions in this vessel area.
(g) Checklist for the authors' recommended equipment for complex interventions in this specific vessel area.

(Part 2) Selected teaching cases in the specific vessel area are then described step-by-step from puncture to closure addressing the same issues as listed above for the specific cases:

(a) What made the lesion "complex" in this specific case?
(b) What was the clinical indication for treatment of this specific case?
(c) What were the potential hazards of treating this specific patient and this lesion?
(d) Which interventional strategies were considered for this lesion?
(e) Which interventional tools were used to handle this lesion?

(f) Summary: How was the case managed, is there anything that could have been improved, what was the immediate and long-term outcome?

(g) List of equipment used in this case.

(h) Key learning issues of this specific case.

(*Part 3*) Authors' summary of key issues for successful and safe treatment of complex lesions in this vessel area.

In summary, the book intends to focus on practical tips for the interventionist in the cath lab, to review complex cases and outline the different strategies theoretically and in real-life cases, thus to share the experience of high-volume interventionists with the reader.

Martin Schillinger, MD
Erich Minar, MD

Contents

Contributors

I. Baumgartner Swiss Cardiovascular Center, Clinical and Interventional Angiology, Inselspital, University Hospital Bern, Bern, Switzerland

Marc Bosiers Department of Vascular Surgery, A.Z. Sint-Blasius, Dendermonde, Belgium

Anthony J. Comerota Jobst Vascular Center, Toledo, Ohio, U.S.A.

Martin Czerny Department of Cardiothoracic Surgery, University of Vienna Medical School, Vienna, Austria

Koen Deloose Department of Vascular Surgery, A.Z. Sint-Blasius, Dendermonde, Belgium

N. Diehm Swiss Cardiovascular Center, Clinical and Interventional Angiology, Inselspital, University Hospital Bern, Bern, Switzerland

Edward B. Diethrich Arizona Heart Institute and Arizona Heart Hospital, Phoenix, Arizona, U.S.A.

D. D. Do Swiss Cardiovascular Center, Clinical and Interventional Angiology, Inselspital, University Hospital Bern, Bern, Switzerland

Johanna T. Fifi Department of Radiology, St. Luke's-Roosevelt Hospital, New York, New York, U.S.A.

Jennifer Franke CardioVascular Center Frankfurt Sankt Katharinen, Frankfurt, Germany

Marilyn H. Gravett Jobst Vascular Center, Toledo, Ohio, U.S.A.

Lanfroi Graziani Invasive Cardiology Unit, Istituto Clinico Città di Brescia, Brescia, Italy

Michael Grimm Department of Cardiothoracic Surgery, University of Vienna Medical School, Vienna, Austria

Patrick Haage Department of Diagnostic and Interventional Radiology, HELIOS Klinikum Wuppertal, University Hospital Witten/Herdecke, Wuppertal, Germany

Michael R. Jaff Section of Vascular Medicine, Division of Cardiology, Massachusetts General Hospital, Boston, and The Vascular Center, Massachusetts General Hospital, Boston, Massachusetts, U.S.A.

J. Stephen Jenkins Interventional Cardiology Research, Ochsner Heart and Vascular Institute, New Orleans, Louisiana, U.S.A.

Yuji Kanaoka Department of Surgery, Jikei University School of Medicine, Nishishimbashi, Minatoku, Tokyo, Japan

Barry Katzen Baptist Cardiac and Vascular Institute, Miami, Florida, U.S.A.

Thomas J. Kiernan Section of Vascular Medicine, Division of Cardiology, Massachusetts General Hospital, Boston, Massachusetts, U.S.A.

Hans Krankenberg Medical Care Center, Prof. Mathey, Prof. Schofer, Hamburg, Germany

Klaus Mathias   Department of Radiology, Klinikum Dortmund, Academic Teaching Hospital of the University of Muenster, Dortmund, Germany

Philip M. Meyers   Departments of Radiology and Neurological Surgery, Columbia University, College of Physicians and Surgeons, Neurological Institute of New York, New York, New York, U.S.A.

Erich Minar   Department of Internal Medicine II, Division of Angiology, Medical University Vienna, General Hospital, Vienna, Austria

Takao Ohki   Department of Surgery, Jikei University School of Medicine, Nishishimbashi, Minatoku, Tokyo, Japan

Rajan A. G. Patel   Department of Cardiology, Ochsner Heart and Vascular Institute, Ochsner Clinic Foundation, New Orleans, Louisiana, U.S.A.

Patrick Peeters   Department of Cardiovascular and Thoracic Surgery, Imelda Hospital, Bonheiden, Belgium

Céline Rahman   Department of Neurology, Columbia University College of Physicians and Surgeons, New York, New York, U.S.A.

Stephen R. Ramee   Department of Cardiology, Ochsner Heart and Vascular Institute, Ochsner Clinic Foundation, New Orleans, Louisiana, U.S.A.

Dierk Scheinert   Parkkrankenhaus Leipzig, Medizinische Klinik I, Angiologie, Kardiologie, Herzzentrum Leipzig, Abteilung für Angiologie, Leipzig, Germany

Martin Schillinger   Department of Internal Medicine II, Division of Angiology, Medical University Vienna, General Hospital, Vienna, Austria

Michael Schlüter   Medical Care Center, Prof. Mathey, Prof. Schofer, Hamburg, Germany

Andrej Schmidt   Parkkrankenhaus Leipzig, Medizinische Klinik I, Angiologie, Kardiologie, Herzzentrum Leipzig, Abteilung für Angiologie, Leipzig, Germany

Horst Sievert   CardioVascular Center Frankfurt Sankt Katharinen, Frankfurt, Germany

Thilo Tübler   Medical Care Center, Prof. Mathey, Prof. Schofer, Hamburg, Germany

Frank J. Veith   The Cleveland Clinic, Cleveland, Ohio, and New York University, New York, New York, U.S.A.

Jürgen Verbist   Department of Cardiovascular and Thoracic Surgery, Imelda Hospital, Bonheiden, Belgium

Dierk Vorwerk   Department of Diagnostic and Interventional Radiology, Klinikum Ingolstadt, Ingolstadt, Germany

Hubert Wallner   Kardinal Schwarzenberg´sches Krankenhaus, Schwarzach, Salzburg, Austria

Christopher J. White   Department of Cardiology, Ochsner Heart and Vascular Institute, Ochsner Clinic Foundation, New Orleans, Louisiana, U.S.A.

Bryan P. Yan   Section of Vascular Medicine, Division of Cardiology, Massachusetts General Hospital, Boston, Massachusetts, U.S.A.

Thomas Zeller   Department of Angiology, Herz-Zentrum Bad Krozingen, Bad Krozingen, Germany

1 | Why Should We Tackle Complex Lesions by Endovascular Techniques?

Martin Schillinger

Department of Internal Medicine II, Division of Angiology, Medical University Vienna, General Hospital, Vienna, Austria

INTRODUCTION

Minimally invasive endovascular treatment of peripheral arteries is one of the most rapidly evolving techniques in interventional therapies. In the early days of endovascular therapy, when it mainly consisted of plain balloon angioplasty, treatment was offered exclusively for short and easy lesions, whereas more complex and longer lesions generally were considered indications for open vascular surgery. This concept is still reflected by the guidelines of the Transatlantic inter-society consensus (TASC) I document published in the year 2000 (1). However, with increasing experience and confidence in the minimally invasive approach and upcoming advanced technologies, treatment of more complex lesions was becoming clinical routine. Seven years after publication of the first Transatlantic guidelines for treatment of patients with peripheral artery disease, the second version of the TASC document (2) defined more widespread indications for endovascular therapy. Meanwhile clinical practice has further advanced, and in many centers TASC II surgical indications are routinely and successfully treated by endovascular means. However, with lesions getting more complex, interventionists are also confronted with more diseased patients and thus there is an increased risk for complications. Nevertheless, increasing evidence suggests that particularly in heavily diseased high-risk patients, endovascular solutions may offer substantial advantages compared to vascular surgical procedures. Proper physician training, education of complex scenarios, and awareness of potential complications are key issues for running a peripheral interventions program, which offers the full range of what is technically possible today.

WHY ENDOVASCULAR FIRST?

Primarily, all vascular conditions are amenable for two treatment options: conservative medical treatment and revascularization. The first and the most important clinical question for each patient is whether revascularization is necessary. Discussing the specific indications for revascularization of each vessel area exceeds the scope of this book, but each chapter provides a brief overview on clinical indications for the respective procedures. If revascularisation is indicated, we have to decide between open vascular surgery or endovascular therapy. Most high volume centers have adopted an "endovascular-first" approach whenever technically possible. Importantly, interventionists always have to keep the clinical indication in mind, particularly when treating complex patients. An example for clinical decision-making and its impact on revascularization strategy is given in Figure 1. The patient presented with an occlusion of the superficial femoral artery (SFA) and an occlusion of all three tibioperoneal vessels [Fig. 1(A)]. First, because of a flow-limiting dissection, the SFA was successfully recanalized, dilated, and stented [Fig. 1(B)]. In earlier days, interventions were stopped at this stage, which is today considered adequate only in patients with intermittent claudication. However, since this was a patient with critical limb ischemia, complete revascularization was anticipated and two of the three occluded tibioperoneal arteries were re-opened by long-segment balloon angioplasty [Fig. 1(C)].

In general, three major factors determine the decision for endovascular therapy or open vascular surgery: technical success, procedural complications, and patency rates. Targeting complex lesions and complex patients by endovascular techniques, major advances have been made in recent years in the improvement of technical success and avoidance of complications. In general, technical success rates even in complex anatomies exceed 90% in all vessel areas

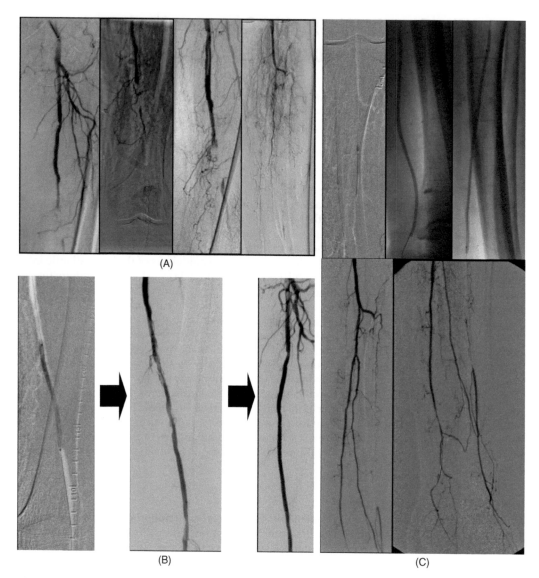

Figure 1   (A) Occlusion of the superficial femoral artery (SFA) and all tibioperoneal arteries in a patient with critical limb ischemia. (B) Successful recanalization, balloon angioplasty, and stenting of the SFA lesions. (C) Recanalization and long-segment balloon angioplasty of the posterior tibial and fibular arteries.

(3–11). Tailored strategies for chronic total occlusions like re-entry devices enable successful recanalization of long-segment and heavily calcified lesions. Adoption of coronary chronic total occlusion technology has significantly advanced success rates particularly in below-the-knee interventions (Fig. 2).

Addressing the issue of complications, endovascular therapy traditionally is considered a minimally invasive and safe approach with respect to morbidity and mortality (12–16). The reduction of device diameters and sheath sizes, introduction of monorail technology, and the more careful application of anticoagulant substances, have certainly contributed to safety of endovascular therapy. A negligible mortality risk, no relevant immobilization, a shorter hospital stay, and a significantly lower risk for in-hospital complications compared to open vascular surgery, remain the major arguments for the "endovascular-first" approach. Unfortunately, scientifically hard data comparing technical success and complication rates between endovascular and surgical approaches are scarce. In the field of carotid revascularization, comparative data

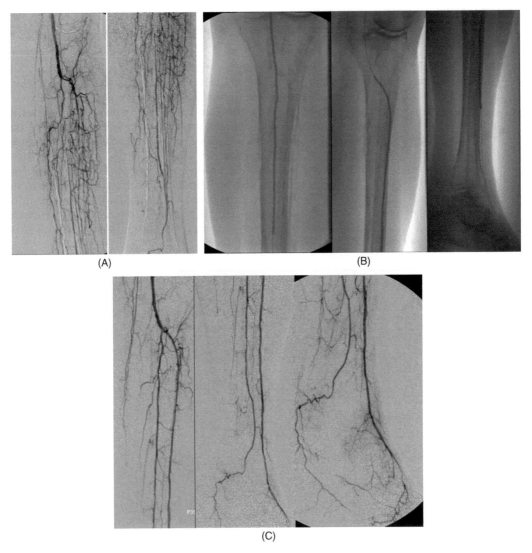

(A) (B)

(C)

Figure 2 (A) Total occlusion of the anterior and posterior tibial arteries and proximal occlusion of the fibular artery in a patient with ischemic ulcers of the toes. (B) Long-segment balloon angioplasty of the fibular artery, the anterior tibial artery, and the dorsalis pedis artery. (C) Angiographic outcome after balloon angioplasty of the fibular artery, the anterior tibial artery, and the dorsalis pedis artery.

from the SAPPHIRE, SPACE, and EVA-3S studies (17–19) are available but these studies mainly focus on neurological outcomes, and admittedly these data do not unequivocally support the hypothesis "endovascular-first" with respect to early results. In the peripheral field, the BASIL trial (20) revealed comparable survival rates after lower limb interventions or surgery and equivalent leg outcomes until three years.

Finally, addressing the issue of patency of endovascular and surgical approaches, restenosis still has to be considered the Achilles heel of endovascular procedures (21–29). Restenosis rates particularly after infrainguinal interventions remain unfavorably high. If long-term outcome is the main therapeutic goal, surgery always has to be considered a good option.

In summary, an accurate revascularization strategy is "endovascular-first" but "primum est nihil nocere". However, endovascular therapies may not prohibit or complicate later vascular surgical procedures, if these are necessary due to failure of the endovascular approach.

WHAT MAKES A LESION "COMPLEX"?

Characteristics of complex lesions may vary in between different vessel areas, but some general considerations can be made.

- Length of the lesion. Usually, the longer the more complex. Very long lesions typically are encountered in the femoropopliteal and below-the-knee segments (Fig. 3). The most critical part of the revascularization process, irrespective of the length, remains the re-entry point.
- Occlusions across bifurcations. Re-entry to the true lumen can be complex in these usually long lesions when bifurcations are included. This may typically occur at the level of the tibioperoneal trifurcation (Fig. 3) or if a pelvic occlusion includes the femoral bifurcation (Fig. 4).
- Diseased re-entry segments. Recanalization of occlusions frequently is done (whether on purpose or not) by subintimal wire passage. This technique, as described by Bolia, is done with a loop in the wire. As soon as the loop has passed the lesion and enters a healthy vascular segment, re-entry in the true lumen usually is achieved. In patients with heavily disease landing zones (Fig. 5) re-entry can be very complex because the loop continues to dissect the artery instead of re-entering the true lumen.

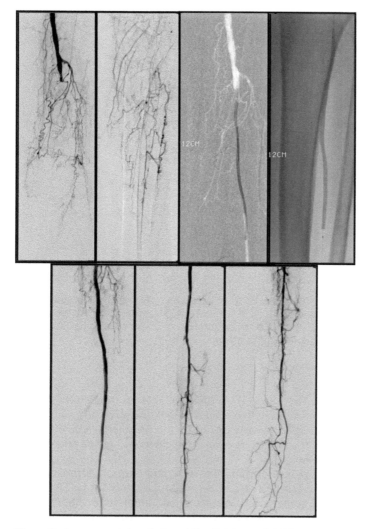

Figure 3 Long-segment occlusion of the distal superficial femoral artery, entire popliteal artery, and tibioperoneal trifurcation. Below the knee only the fibular artery can be detected. Successful recanalization and balloon angioplasty.

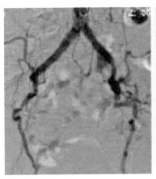
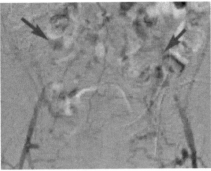
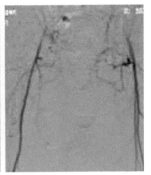

Figure 4 Occlusion of both external iliac and common femoral arteries.

- Heavy calcification. Calcium can cause problems both during the recanalization phase, inhibiting wire passage, as well as after successful wire passage when residual stenosis and even stent compression endanger a technical success (Fig. 6).
- Thrombus. Thrombotic lesions always have to be considered as potentially complex because of the evident risk of embolization. Particularly in carotid interventions (Fig. 7), thrombotic lesions have to be tackled extremely carefully, but also peripheral interventions can get complex following embolization (Fig. 8).
- Bifurcated lesions. Unlike in coronary arteries, recommendations of how to handle bifurcation lesions are missing (Fig. 9). Plaque shift and side-branch occlusion can have serious negative long-term effects, particularly if the "side branch" is a vessel of major importance, like the deep femoral artery.
- Flush ostial occlusions or strong collaterals originating at the beginning of the occlusion. Particularly in cases when the occlusion has a hard fibrous or calcified cap, inserting the wire into the occlusion can be tricky because the wire likely will take the way of less resistance to the collateral.
- Dissections. If dissection (spontaneous or due to a prior revascularization attempt) is present, re-entry to the true lumen may be difficult, especially when the false lumen expands because of contrast injections.

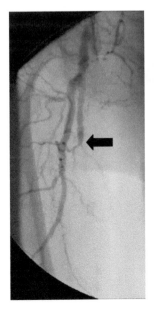
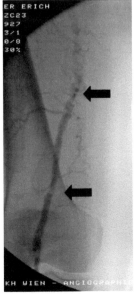

Figure 5 Long-segment occlusion of the superficial femoral artery with heavily disease and stenosed landing zone for re-entry.

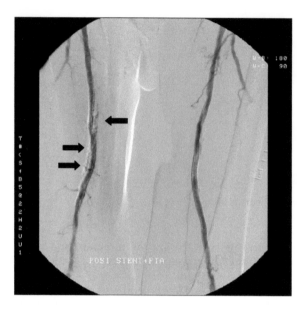

Figure 6 Suboptimal expansion of self-expanding stents in the superficial femoral artery due to heavy calcification.

WHAT ARE THE CLINICAL INDICATIONS FOR ENDOVASCULAR TREATMENT OF COMPLEX LESIONS?

As stated above, interventionalists always have to keep in mind the clinical indication for revascularization. Complex lesions mean lower technical success rates, higher complication rates, and higher risk for recurrence. In this context, the indication for endovascular treatment is not only driven by patients' symptoms and need for revascularization, but also by the interventional expertise in the treating center.

WHAT ARE THE POTENTIAL HAZARDS OF TREATING COMPLEX LESIONS?

Two major hazards of failed interventions in complex lesions have to be discussed. One is the obvious risk for complications, which include systemic risks, like renal failure due to contrast overload or heart failure due to fluid overload, and vascular complications, which are mentioned in more detail in the respective chapters. The other and less obvious risk is that further endovascular or surgical revascularization attempts are complicated or prohibited by an inadequate first attempt.

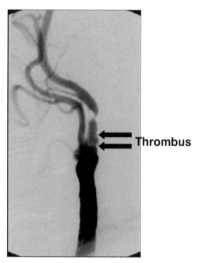

Figure 7 Thrombotic particles in a high-grade carotid stenosis.

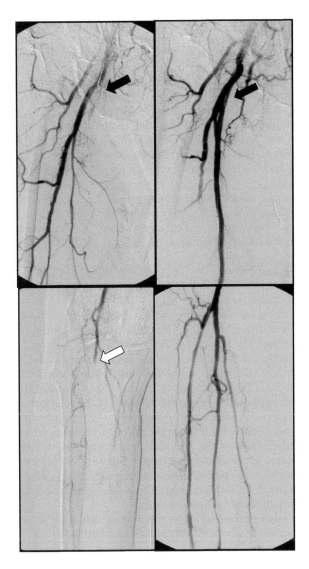

Figure 8 Thrombotic occlusion of the ostium of the superficial femoral artery (SFA) with distal embolization and occlusion of the crural trifurcation. Successful stenting of the SFA and aspiration thrombectomy of the tibioperoneal arteries.

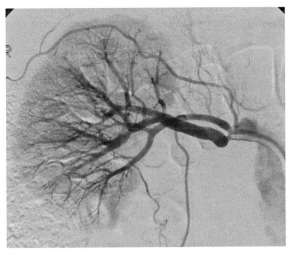

Figure 9 Example of a bifurcated renal artery stenosis with two major segmental branches.

WHICH SPECIFIC INTERVENTIONAL STRATEGIES AND TOOLS CAN BE CONSIDERED FOR TREATMENT OF COMPLEX LESIONS?

- Long lesions. Intraluminal or subintimal techniques can be applied, but especially in long occlusions, these approaches frequently cannot be differentiated. Re-entry devices like the Outback catheter or the Pioneer catheter can be helpful in gaining access to the true lumen.
- Occlusions across bifurcations. Trying different choices of wires, re-entry devices, and retrograde recanalization techniques are most frequently applied for this problem.
- Diseased re-entry segments. This clearly is the domain of the above-mentioned re-entry devices. Alternatively, the "bad end" of the Terumo glidewire or a denuded tip of a V18-Control Wire can be used to have a needle-like device, which enables puncture of the prohibitive membrane between the false and the true lumen. Again, if these techniques fail, retrograde recanalization can be considered.
- Heavy calcification. In terms of wire passage, subintimal passage around the calcium most frequently is the only way to overcome "rocky" segments. Before stenting, these segments should be pretreated with atherectomy, and balloon-expanding stents clearly are superior in this indication. But especially in the SFA, the risks and benefits of a balloon-expanding stent have to be carefully weighed.
- Thrombus. Small thrombi should be aspirated before any other manipulation is anticipated. In cases with a high thrombus burden, pretreatment with thrombolysis has to be considered depending on the clinical indication and vessel area treated.
- Bifurcated lesions. The strategy mainly depends on the sizing or the vessels, plaque burden, and angle of the vessel. Preservation of both branches with wires and kissing balloon technique is frequently applied in all vessel areas. Placing a stent in the main vessel, across the side branch, is defined as provisional stenting. Several two-stent techniques are available, with various levels of complexity—the culotte technique, the T technique, the Y technique, the V or simultaneous kissing stents, and the crush technique and its variations (reverse and step). The decision of which technique to apply will also be determined by the territory of treatment. In carotids, the side branch (external carotid artery) is ignored. A different situation is faced when treating the subclavian–vertebral bifurcation or a renal bifurcation, where two stent techniques frequently seem adequate. For the aortoiliac bifurcation, the kissing stent technique also is a routine procedure, whereas overstenting the femoral bifurcation remains a "don't". The tibioperoneal bifurcation is open to all above-mentioned approaches. However, when using two stents it is important to notice that the above-mentioned coronary techniques make sense only when balloon-expanding stents are used.
- Flush ostial occlusions or strong collaterals originating at the beginning of the occlusion. Entry through the cap of the occlusion usually can be achieved by the use of different curves of diagnostic catheters to support the direction of the tip of a stiff guidewire.
- Dissections. This also is the domain of a re-entry device. Again, alternatively the "bad end" of the Terumo glidewire or a denuded tip of a V18-Control Wire can be used to have a needle-like device which enables puncture of the prohibitive membrane between the false and the true lumen and retrograde recanalization can be considered.

KEY ISSUES FOR ENDOVASCULAR TREATMENT OF COMPLEX LESIONS

Three main issues have to be considered when treating complex lesions and complex patients. First, the clinical indication has to justify the risk of a complex intervention. Second, preprocedural noninvasive diagnostic methods should adequately identify complex morphologies to allow precise planning of the procedure. Third, physician training and expertise and awareness for potential hazards and their solutions are crucial to guarantee good outcomes and low complication rates.

REFERENCES

1. Dormandy JA, Rutherford RB. Management of peripheral arterial disease (PAD). TASC Working Group. Transatlantic inter-society consensus (TASC). J Vasc Surg 2000; 31:S1–S296.
2. Norgren L, Hiatt WR, Dormandy JA, et al. TASC II Working Group. Inter-society consensus for the management of peripheral arterial disease (TASC II). J Vasc Surg 2007; 26:S5–S67.

3. Standards of Practice Committee of the Society of Cardiovascular and Interventional Radiology. Standards for interventional radiology. J Vasc Interv Radiol 1991; 2:59–65.
4. Sherif C, Dick P, Sabeti S, et al. Neurological outcome after carotid artery stenting compared to medical therapy in patients with asymptomatic high grade carotid artery stenosis. J Endovasc Ther 2005; 12:145–155.
5. Sabeti S, Schillinger M, Mlekusch W, et al. Contralateral high grade carotid artery stenosis or occlusion is not associated with an increased risk for poor neurological outcome after carotid stenting. Radiology 2004; 230:70–76.
6. Schillinger M, Haumer M, Schillinger S, et al. Outcome of conservative vs. interventional treatment of subclavian artery stenosis. J Endovasc Ther 2002; 9:139–146.
7. Schillinger M, Exner M, Mlekusch W, et al. Fibrinogen and restenosis after endovascular treatment of the iliac arteries: a marker of inflammation or coagulation? Thromb Haemost 2002; 87:959–965.
8. Ahmadi R, Ugurluoglu A, Schillinger M, et al. Duplex-Ultrasound guided femoropopliteal PTA: Initial and 12 months results – a case control study. J Endovasc Ther 2002; 9:873–881.
9. Dick P, Mlekusch W, Sabeti S, et al. Outcome after endovascular treatment of deep femoral artery stenosis: results in a consecutive patient series and systematic review of the literature. J Endovasc Ther 2006; 13:221–228.
10. Ahmadi R, Willfort A, Lang W, et al. Carotid artery stenting: effect of learning and intermediate term morphological outcome. J Endovasc Ther 2001; 8:539–549.
11. Ahmadi R, Schillinger M, Sabeti S, et al. Renal Artery PTA and Stent Implantation: Immediate and Late Clinical and Morphological Outcome. Wien Klin Wochenschr 2002; 114:21–27.
12. Mlekusch W, Schillinger M, Sabeti S, et al. Frequency and risk factors for hemodynamic instability due to hypotension and bradycardia after elective carotid stenting. J Endovasc Ther 2003; 10:851–859.
13. Amighi J, Sabeti S, Dick P, et al. Impact of rapid exchange vs. over-the-wire technique on procedure complications of renal artery angioplasty. J Endovasc Ther 2005; 12:233–239.
14. Sabeti S, Schillinger M, Mlekusch W, et al. Contrast induced acute renal failure in patients undergoing renal artery angiography vs. renal artery PTA. Eur J Vasc Endovasc Surg 2002; 24:156–160.
15. Schillinger M, Haumer M, Mlekusch W, et al. Predicting renal failure after peripheral percutaneous transluminal angioplasty in high risk patients. J Endovasc Ther 2001; 8:609–614.
16. Boltuch J, Sabeti S, Amighi J, et al. Procedure-related complications and neurological adverse events after protected vs. unprotected carotid stenting. J Endovasc Ther 2005; 12:538–547.
17. SPACE Collaborative group. 30 day results from the SPACE trial of stent-protected angioplasty versus carotid endarterectomy in symptomatic patients: a randomised non-inferiority trial. Lancet 2006; 368:1239–1247.
18. Mas JL, Chatellier G, Beyssen B, et al. EVA 3S Investigators. N Engl J Med 2006; 355:1660–1671.
19. Yadav J, Wholey MH, Kuntz RE, et al. Protected carotid-artery stenting versus endarterectomy in high-risk patients. N Engl J Med 2004; 351:1565–1567.
20. Adam DJ, Beard JD, Cleveland T, et al. BASIL trial participants. Bypass versus angioplasty in severe ischemia of the leg (BASIL): multicentre, randomized controlled trial. Lancet 2005; 366:1925–1934.
21. Schillinger M, Haumer M, Schillinger S, et al. Risk stratification after subclavian artery PTA: increased rate of restenosis after stent implantation. J Endovasc Ther 2001; 8:550–557.
22. Sabeti S, Schillinger M, Amighi J, et al. Patency of nitinol vs. Wallstents in the superficial femoral artery – a propensity score adjusted analysis. Radiology 2004; 232:516–521.
23. Schillinger M, Haumer M, Schlerka G, et al. Restenosis after percutaneous transluminal angioplasty in patients with peripheral artery disease: the role of inflammation. J Endovasc Ther 2001; 8:477–483.
24. Amighi J, Sabeti S, Schlager O, et al. Outcome of conservative vs. interventional treatment of patients with intermittent claudication. Eur J Vasc Endovasc Surg 2004; 27:254–258.
25. Sabeti S, Amighi J, Ahmadi R, et al. Outcome of long-segment femoropopliteal stent implantation using self-expanding nitinol stents. J Endovasc Ther 2005; 12:6–12.
26. Schlager O, Dick P, Sabeti S, et al. Stenting of the superficial femoral artery – the dark sides: restenosis, clinical deterioration and fractures. J Endovasc Ther 2005; 12:676–684.
27. Schillinger M, Mlekusch W, Haumer M, et al. One year follow up after percutaneous transluminal angioplasty and elective stent implantation in de-novo versus recurrent femoropopliteal lesions. J Endovasc Ther 2003:10:288–297.
28. Schillinger M, Sabeti S, Loewe C, et al. Balloon angioplasty versus implantation of nitinol stents in the superficial femoral artery. N Engl J Med 2006; 354:1879–1888.
29. Schillinger M, Exner M, Mlekusch W, et al. Endovascular revascularization below the knee: 6-months results and predictive value of C-reactive protein level. Radiology 2003; 227:419–425.

2 | Pharmacological Prerequisites for Treatment of Complex Patients with Peripheral Artery Disease

Erich Minar

Department of Internal Medicine II, Division of Angiology, Medical University Vienna, General Hospital, Vienna, Austria

INTRODUCTION

A patient can be characterized as a "complex" patient either by the complex morphology of his vascular disease, as described in the different chapters of this book, or by the different unfavorable medical comorbidities. Both factors are responsible for an increased complication rate in such complex patients. Complex morphological features often lead to a longer duration of an intervention, even with an experienced interventionist, and each prolonged intervention can be associated with adverse events. Otherwise, vascular or nonvascular comorbidities can in most cases be identified easily by history and preinterventional examination of the patient, and this enables effective risk evaluation. The main goal should then be to reduce the overall peri- and postinterventional risk of the patient by adequate treatment, which is most often pharmacological.

While revascularization and in some cases also additional pharmacologic therapy with vasoactive drugs are used for improvement of symptoms and quality of life, the main goal of improvement of overall prognosis and survival of these patients (by reducing cardiovascular morbidity and mortality) can mainly be achieved by different pharmacologic treatment. Because of the presence of mostly multiple risk factors and because of the systemic nature of atherosclerosis and the high risk of ischemic events, patients with peripheral artery disease (PAD) should be candidates for aggressive secondary prevention strategies including antiplatelet therapy and aggressive risk factor modification, e.g., with lipid-lowering and antihypertensive treatment.

ANTIPLATELET THERAPY

PAD is a serious medical problem and an indicator of systemic atherosclerosis. Concerning development and manifestation of PAD, atherosclerosis and in further consequence atherothrombosis are the main etiopathogenic factors. In patients with primary diagnosis of PAD, the prevalence of atherosclerotic manifestations in other vessel areas is higher than in patients with a primary diagnosis of cardio- or cerebrovascular disease. The diagnosis of PAD is therefore a marker for mostly generalized and severe atherosclerosis (1). Many studies such as the recent REACH (Reduction of Atherothrombosis for Continued Health) Registry, which included 55,814 patients with known atherosclerotic disease (coronary artery disease (CAD), PAD, and cerebrovascular disease), have clearly demonstrated that patients with polyvascular disease have a significant worse outcome as compared to patients with only CAD (2).

Patients with intermittent claudication (IC) have a relatively good prognosis concerning amputation-free survival with only 1% to 2% of them needing major amputation over a five-year period. Otherwise, the prognosis concerning overall survival is poor. The 5-, 10-, and 15-year morbidity and mortality rates from all causes are approximately 30%, 50%, and 70%, respectively, with CAD being by far the most common cause of death (1). Patients with chronic critical limb ischemia (CLI) have an even much worse prognosis with 20% mortality in the first year after presentation.

The main reason to administer antiplatelet therapy to patients with PAD is to prevent severe vascular events such as myocardial infarction, stroke, or vascular death. The Antithrombotic Trialists' Collaboration meta-analysis in 42 trials found that among 9214 patients with PAD, there was a 23% reduction in serious vascular events ($P = 0.004$) in patients treated with antiplatelet therapy (3).

The CAPRIE trial (Clopidogrel versus Aspirin in Patients at Risk of Ischemic Events) demonstrated that the combined risk of death from vascular causes, myocardial infarction, and stroke was significantly, albeit moderately, lower with clopidogrel (75 mg/day) compared with aspirin (325 mg q.d.) (4). Despite this difference, in the recently published recommendations of the eighth ACCP Conference on Antithrombotic and Thrombolytic Therapy it was recommended, by placing a relatively high value on avoiding large expenditures to achieve small reductions in vascular events, that aspirin be used instead of clopidogrel (5). Unfortunately, the recent Transatlantic inter-society consensus (TASC) II paper does not give clear recommendations concerning this point.

In the past few years, "resistance" to antiplatelet drugs has become a major point of interest. Interpatient variability in drug response has been shown to be, at least partially, the result of polymorphisms in genes encoding drug targets, such as receptors or enzymes (6). Many tests of platelet function are now available for clinical use, and some of these tests have shown that hyporesponsiveness to antiplatelet drugs in the laboratory (i.e., resistance) is associated with adverse clinical events in different patient populations (7).

However, in most of these studies, the number of major adverse clinical events was low. Furthermore, uniform definitions and standardized assays are not yet available, and there are also no published studies addressing the clinical effectiveness of altering therapy based on the results of monitoring antiplatelet therapy. Therefore, monitoring of antiplatelet therapy in patients with vascular disease cannot be generally recommended currently for clinical routine.

Dual Antiplatelet Therapy

The routine use of dual antiplatelet therapy of aspirin and clopidogrel seems not justified in the routine patient with PAD without planned intervention. The CHARISMA trial (Clopidogrel for High Atherothrombotic Risk and Ischemic Stabilization, Management, and Avoidance) compared the effects of such a dual antiplatelet therapy with clopidogrel plus low-dose aspirin versus aspirin alone (75 to 162 mg/day) on the incidence of cardiovascular events in 15,603 patients at high risk for atherothrombotic events followed up for a median of 28 months (8). The primary efficacy end point, a composite of MI, stroke, or death from cardiovascular causes, was not significantly different between the two treatment arms. However, in a subset of 9478 patients with previous MI, ischemic stroke, or symptomatic PAD, combination therapy with clopidogrel plus aspirin showed a significant reduction in the rate of cardiovascular death, MI, or stroke (7.3% vs. 8.8%) but with a significantly higher risk of transfusion-requiring bleeding (8). Therefore, some specialists argue that the risk–benefit of dual antiplatelet therapy with aspirin and clopidogrel may be justified in high-risk symptomatic patients but definitely not in asymptomatic patients. Otherwise, according to most vascular specialists working in this field, the slight additive benefit is not justified by the increased economic cost and hemorrhagic risk.

Dual Antiplatelet Therapy in Patients with Planned Intervention

In contrast to the coronary field, there are nearly no sufficient studies dealing with the question of optimal peri- and postinterventional treatment in noncoronary vessels. While it is generally accepted that dual antiplatelet therapy should be prescribed for at least one month—better, however, for three months—in patients with stent implantation in the carotid arteries, this question is not clarified at all in patients with PAD. Unfortunately also TASC II as consensus paper does not give any clear recommendations. It is only stated that antiplatelet therapy should be started preoperatively and continued as adjuvant pharmacotherapy after an endovascular or surgical procedure. In our department we prescribe dual antiplatelet therapy after stent implantation in the infrainguinal region for three months. However, as already mentioned, this recommendation is not evidence based on hard scientific data. Patients treated by angioplasty alone are not prescribed dual antiplatelet therapy on a regular basis.

In the near future, drug-eluting stents may help to improve the long-term patency after intervention in the lower limb arteries. However, as yet, trials evaluating DES in the peripheral arteries were underpowered and demonstrated no improved patency compared to bare metal stents. Otherwise, the concept of combining the advantages of the mechanical scaffolding properties of nitinol stents with the antiproliferative action of drugs seems appealing, and some groups reported promising results especially in the infrapopliteal vessels. Because of the experiences in the coronary field we recommend (despite lack of data) also prolonged dual antiplatelet therapy after peripheral DES implantation, especially in the smaller lower leg arteries, for at least six months.

To guarantee an optimal antiaggregatory effect already at the time of the intervention, antiplatelet pretreatment should start at least seven days before the planned intervention. Otherwise, a loading dose has to be given at the beginning of the intervention: 500 mg of aspirin and 300 mg (or according to newer data from the cardiologists, even 600 mg) of clopidogrel, respectively.

Until now it has not been demonstrated that antiplatelet therapy with aspirin and/or clopidogrel has any positive influence concerning reduction of restenosis after angioplasty or stent implantation in patients with PAD. Therefore, it is interesting that a recent randomized study from a Japanese group demonstrated a significant reduction of re-stenosis after femoropopliteal endovascular therapy, by a combined therapy of aspirin with cilostazol (this is a vasoactive drug with also antiplatelet effects) compared to a combination of aspirin with ticlopidine (a thienopyridine replaced by clopidogrel in most centers) (9).

Combined Anticoagulant and Antiplatelet Therapy

Because the results of previous randomized trials evaluating oral anticoagulants in patients with PAD—who represent a group at a high risk for thrombotic events—have been inconclusive, recently a large international, randomized clinical trial has been performed to determine if moderate levels of oral anticoagulation (OAC) (with an INR of 2–3) improve upon antiplatelet therapy alone (10). In this Warfarin Antiplatelet Vascular Evaluation (WAVE) trial, after a mean follow-up time of 35 months the combination of an oral anticoagulant and antiplatelet therapy was not more effective than antiplatelet therapy alone in preventing major cardiovascular complications and was associated with an increase in life-threatening bleeding. The outcome of myocardial infarction, stroke, or death from cardiovascular causes occurred in 12.2% of patients receiving combination therapy and in 13.3% of patients receiving antiplatelet therapy alone. Otherwise, life-threatening bleeding occurred in 4% of patients receiving combination therapy as compared to 1.2% in the antiplatelet therapy alone group.

PERI-INTERVENTIONAL ANTITHROMBOTIC THERAPY (TABLE 1)

Because of the rapid advances in technology concerning endovascular procedures, more and more complex interventions are carried out nearly on a routine basis. Otherwise, we are faced with an increased thrombotic risk with treatment of such patients. Therefore, it is also necessary to prescribe intensive supplementary antithrombotic therapy for prophylaxis of acute thrombotic occlusion.

Heparin

Unfractionated heparin (UFH) is the classic anticoagulant agent administered during endovascular interventions to prevent embolization or new thrombus formation. Its efficacy is only limited by the fact that it does not resolve already existing thrombi. The half-life is prolonged in patients with renal insufficiency. Despite its widespread use, there are no clear recommendations concerning the optimal dose, because the benefit of any antithrombotic drug or regimen during peripheral endovascular interventions has not been demonstrated in any randomized study (in contrast to coronary interventions). UFH is commonly administered with a bolus of about 5000 IU following vascular access, and further doses—sometimes dependent on activated clotting time measurements—are given during procedures with longer duration. Otherwise, some experienced investigators administer less than 5000 IU in less complex interventions with expected short (e.g., < 30 minutes) duration. The main complications are of course bleeding—the risk is especially increased in combination with GP IIb/IIIa inhibitors—and an immune-mediated platelet activation causing heparin-induced thrombocytopenia with potentially severe thromboembolic complications in the arterial and/or venous system (11). *Low molecular weight heparin* has a more favorable benefit/risk ratio and superior pharmacokinetic properties compared to UFH. Because there are nearly no data for their routine use in peripheral vascular interventions, the use of UFH is preferred currently in most vascular centers performing peripheral interventions. One of the main advantages of UFH in this situation is the possibility to neutralize the anticoagulant activity by protamine in case of severe bleeding complications.

Table 1 Peri-interventional Pharmacotherapy

Antiplatelet therapy: starting $\geq$ 7 days before intervention, otherwise loading dose

– *Low-dose aspirin* (about 100 mg/day; loading dose: 500 mg); all patients
– *Clopidogrel:* (75 mg/day; loading dose 300–600 mg; duration: 3–6 months); in special situations (see text)

Anticoagulant therapy:

– *Heparin*
  ● Unfractionated heparin: Bolus of 5000 IU; with longer duration interventions: further dose according to ACT measurement
  ● Less complex intervention with short duration: 3000 IU (Low molecular weight heparin: no sufficient data)
– *Bivalirudin:* Bolus of 0.75 mg/kg; then infusion of 1.75 mg/kg/hr during intervention (dose recommendation from Cardiology)

Glycoprotein IIb/IIIa receptor inhibitors:

– *Abciximab:* Bolus of 0.25 mg/kg; then infusion of 0.125 µg/kg/min for 12 hr

Thrombolytic agents: dosage "as high as necessary and as low as possible"

– Classical drugs
  ● *Streptokinase*
  ● *Urokinase:* recommended maximal dose: 500,000 IU
  ● *rt-PA:* recommended maximal dose: 10 mg
– Newer drugs:
  ● *Reteplase*
  ● *Tenecteplase*
  ● *Alfimeprase*

Vasodilating drugs:

– *Prostanoids:*
  ● Iloprost: intra-arterial bolus of 3000 ng (according to surgical data, no experience after endovascular interventions)
  ● Alprostadil: intra-arterial infusion of 10 µg/30–60 min
– *Nitroglycerin:* Repeated intra-arterial bolus of 0.1–0.2 mg/10 mL solution
– *Papaverine:* 30–60 mg intra-arterial
– *Tolazoline:* 12.5 mg intra-arterial
– *Nifedipine:* 10 mg orally

Abbreviations: ACT, activated clotting time; rt-PA, recombinant tissue plasminogen activator.

Bivalirudin

This drug belongs to the group of direct thrombin inhibitors, which bind directly to thrombin. According to a lot of recent data from coronary trials, the main benefit of bivalirudin over heparin is a significant reduction in the incidence of major bleeding complications (12).

Unfortunately until now, sufficient data are not available concerning the use of bivalirudin in peripheral interventions so as to evaluate the safety and feasibility of using this drug as the procedural anticoagulant in patients undergoing peripheral interventions. Only recently have some interventionists started using this agent as the sole anticoagulant for peripheral interventions. Observational results reported from single centers are promising (13). Ischemic and bleeding events are low and, compared with those reported in the literature, suggest that bivalirudin is safe to be used in this population.

Glycoprotein IIb/IIIa Receptor Inhibitors

Intravenous platelet glycoprotein (GP) IIb/IIIa receptor inhibitors have shown convincing clinical efficacy in percutaneous coronary interventions. In the past few years, there is increasing evidence that GP IIb/IIIa receptor blockade might also have an important role in peripheral arterial intervention (14). However, because the use of adjunctive therapy with GP IIb/IIIa receptor blockade in noncoronary interventions is rather new, the reported data of controlled, randomized, and prospective trials are mainly limited to cardiovascular disease. Otherwise, although peripheral arterial occlusions differ from coronary occlusions with respect to the size and age of the occluding thrombus, the success of GP IIb/IIIa inhibition in the setting of acute coronary occlusion might translate to the peripheral vessels. However, indication for "off-label" use in peripheral interventions should be strictly restrictive, since its application has to be balanced against bleeding complications and the rather high costs. The theory behind the use of GP IIb/IIIa antagonists during peripheral arterial interventions in chronic lesions is to prevent early thrombosis in lesions at high risk for such an occurrence. The phenomenon of "de-thrombosis," that is the dissolution of thrombus by GP IIb/IIIa inhibitors without concomitant plasminogen activators, further increased the interest in peripheral arterial application of these agents.

Abciximab, the most widely studied of all GP IIb/IIIa inhibitors, is a monoclonal antibody, while eptifibatide and tirofiban are small-molecule antagonists. The drugs are given intravenously starting with a bolus followed by intravenous infusion for 12 to 36 hours. Although there are extensive data for all three GP IIb/IIIa receptor antagonists available for coronary indication, in PAD the literature is mainly limited to the use of abciximab. It was demonstrated in the PROMPT trial (15) that the speed of thrombolysis could be enhanced by adjunctive GP IIb/IIIa blockade with abciximab. A further study demonstrated a favorable effect of abciximab on patency and clinical outcome in patients undergoing endovascular revascularization of long-segment femoropopliteal occlusions not hampered by serious bleeding complications (16). Very recently, Keo et al. (17) reported favorable results of provisional abciximab therapy in complex peripheral catheter interventions with imminent risk of early re-thrombosis. This risk was defined by revascularization of arterial occlusions in association with one or more of the following circumstances: time-consuming intervention >3 hours; compromised contrast flow not solved by stenting; distal embolization not solved by mechanical thromboembolectomy; peri-interventional notice of thrombus evolution despite adequate heparin adjustment. In the RELAX trial (18), a multicenter prospective comparison of reteplase alone versus reteplase with abciximab, the GP IIb/IIIa inhibitor reduced the incidence of distal embolization during thrombolysis from 31% to 5% ($P = 0.01$).

In our laboratory, at present, abciximab is used during peripheral interventions only in patients at high risk of early re-occlusion, such as patients with treated long-segment occlusions and poor run-off or residual intraluminal thrombus. Tepe et al. (14) have recently recommended that until data from larger prospective clinical trials are available, adjunct GP IIb/IIIa inhibitors should be used only in selected patients with a higher risk of failure during thrombolysis or re-thrombosis during time-consuming and technically complicated vascular interventions, i.e., the complex patients.

Thrombolytic Agents

Different thrombolytic agents are currently available for patients with acute limb ischemia, and various techniques of intra-arterial thrombolysis are used for application of these agents (19). The efficacy of several fibrinolytic drugs, such as urokinase, streptokinase, and recombinant tissue plasminogen activator, has been reviewed in a recent meta-analysis (20). Alfimeprase is a newer direct-acting fibrinolytic agent that does not require activation of plasminogen, and this mechanism may potentially reduce the frequency of bleeding complications. However, clinical data with this new drug are limited until now (21).

While data show that intrathrombus delivery of thrombolytic agents is more effective than nonselective intra-arterial catheter-directed infusion, no particular thrombolytic regime has yet been proven to be clearly superior. Because thrombolysis in general is limited by a relatively high rate of bleeding complications as well as long infusion times, many interventionists try to reduce the overall amount of applied thrombolytic drug and to decrease the procedural time. This goal can be reached by advanced endovascular methods such as selective catheter-directed thrombolysis with intra-arterial application of the agent with the so-called pulse-spray technique or by combination of mechanical thrombectomy with low-dose thrombolysis. These techniques have substantial benefits concerning efficacy with quicker recanalization and safety with less bleeding complications compared to former studies. Therefore, a combination of aspiration thromboembolectomy or any kind of mechanical thromboembolectomy with selective intra-arterial low-dose local thrombolysis—in contrast to nonselective catheter-directed thrombolysis alone—can be recommended today as the preferred treatment option in these patients.

PERI- AND POSTINTERVENTIONAL MANAGEMENT OF ANTITHROMBOTIC THERAPY IN PATIENTS WITH ATRIAL FIBRILLATION

Atrial fibrillation (AF) is the most common clinically relevant arrhythmia among adults, affecting over 1 in 25 adults, 60 years or older and 1 in 10 persons, 80 years or older (22). Furthermore, AF is the most potent common risk factor for ischemic stroke.

Numerous clinical trials performed over the past several decades have focused on testing the efficacy and safety of OAC with vitamin K antagonists (i.e., warfarin and other coumarins) or antiplatelet drugs, especially aspirin, for the prevention of stroke and other systemic embolism in persons with AF. With recent advances in our understanding of the coagulation process and drug development, new therapeutic strategies that intervene in different parts of the coagulation pathways (such as tissue factor/factor VIIa, factor VIIIa, factor Xa, and thrombin/factor IIa) are being evaluated as alternative antithrombotic therapies. Across all primary prevention trials and despite variation in anticoagulation intensity target ranges, participants randomly assigned to OAC therapy experienced large consistent reductions in the risk of ischemic stroke compared with control subjects, with relative risk reductions of stroke ranging from about 50% to as high as 85% (23). Otherwise, randomized trials have provided much weaker support for the efficacy of aspirin compared with oral vitamin K antagonists. Therefore, OAC is strongly recommended in all high-risk AF patients (defined as having one or more risk factors including diabetes mellitus, congestive heart failure or left ventricular systolic dysfunction, coronary artery disease, a history of stroke/transient ischemic attack or systemic embolism, hypertension, the female gender, and advancing age). Current evidence supports an international normalized ratio (INR) target of 2.0 to 3.0 (23).

It has also been demonstrated that OAC therapy was superior to dual antiplatelet therapy with clopidogrel and aspirin for prevention of vascular events in patients with AF at high risk of stroke, especially in those already on OAC therapy (24). Therefore, it is often a difficult problem to handle peri- and postinterventional antithrombotic treatment in patients on long-term OAC, such as patients with AF or after venous thromboembolism with further need for antiplatelet therapy after an endovascular intervention.

There is lack of published evidence on the optimal peri- and postinterventional antithrombotic management strategy in anticoagulated AF patients. There are only available expert committee reports or opinions and/or clinical experiences of respected authorities mainly concerning coronary interventions (25). A delicate balance between the risk of thromboembolic complications or thrombotic re-occlusion and the risk of major bleeding is needed (26).

After angioplasty without stent implantation or after stent implantation in the aortoiliac vessels, antiplatelet therapy with aspirin alone is the current practice. Otherwise, dual antiplatelet therapy, for at least one month, is the current practice in most centers for the prevention of in-stent thrombosis after infrainguinal stent implantation. Unfortunately, such dual antiplatelet therapy does not adequately protect against thromboembolic complications caused by AF (24). Otherwise, not all patients requiring chronic anticoagulation have a similar risk of thromboembolic complications. Therefore, it appears to be reasonable to adjust the need or extent of anticoagulation, in case of antithrombotic triple therapy with dual antiplatelet therapy, to the perceived thromboembolic risk in patients after infrainguinal stenting. More frequent laboratory analyses might also be helpful to ensure INR values are well within the recommended evidence-based ranges.

According to data from the cardiologists, the recommended duration of dual antiplatelet therapy varies, ranging from four weeks following bare-metal stent implantation during elective angioplasty to at least 6 to 12 months with drug-eluting stents, in view of the risk of late stent thrombosis. The 2006 American College of Cardiology/American Heart Association/European Society of Cardiology guidelines on AF management suggest that the maintenance regimen should be a combination of clopidogrel and coumarin derivatives for 9 to 12 months, after which the coumarin may be continued as monotherapy (25).

PERI-INTERVENTIONAL APPLICATION OF VASODILATORS

During and/or after complex peripheral endovascular interventions, a slow flow can be observed sometimes, causing suspicion of severe spasm. This problem can be observed especially during intervention of infrapopliteal arteries, and it can also be a severe problem during stent angioplasty of the carotid arteries mainly caused by the embolic protection device. In the carotid arteries, an intra-arterial bolus application of 0.1–0.2 mg nitroglycerin is mainly used as an antispasmodic agent, while different vasodilating agents are used in the peripheral circulation. However, there are no widespread recommendations in the literature mainly because of the lack of any study data.

A strong vasodilation can be induced after intra-arterial administration of prostanoids such as iloprost or alprostadil. These drugs are mainly used for treatment of chronic CLI, and because of their pharmacological profile, prostanoids also represent an interesting group of drugs for adjuvant treatment of patients with acute limb ischemia. Furthermore, small studies with prostanoids in distal bypass surgery have shown that intragraft injection at the end of the bypass procedure can reduce the distal resistance and produce a sustained increase in blood flow through femorodistal vein grafts in the early postoperative period (27,28). We use these drugs mainly peri- and post-interventionally in patients with CLI. Otherwise they can, in accordance with the above-mentioned surgical data, also be given as bolus intra-arterially to reduce the peripheral resistance in patients with slow flow and suspicion of vasospasm. Positive effects can also be expected by an antiplatelet effect of these substances.

Other antispasmodic agents are intravenous papaverine or tolazoline and oral nifedipine.

RISK FACTOR MODIFICATION

PAD is considered a CAD equivalent, and the American Heart Association (AHA), National Heart, Lung and Blood Institute, and the National Cholesterol Education Program (NCEP) recommend identical atherosclerotic risk-reduction strategies for PAD and CAD patients (29). From studies of patients with PAD, and also generalizing from other trials in patients with atherosclerotic diseases, there is good evidence that by addressing the key risk factors—smoking, dyslipidemia, and hypertension—the mortality and morbidity of cardiovascular ischemic events can be definitely reduced.

Otherwise, there is also a growing body of evidence that treatment of these modifiable risk factors is often neglected in PAD patients compared to cohorts of patients presenting with CAD or stroke. The above-mentioned REACH registry has also clearly demonstrated that despite their well-known adverse effects, the classic cardiovascular risk factors have been still largely undertreated and undercontrolled in patients with PAD in many regions of the world, also during the past few years (30).

Despite a demonstrated positive effect of exercise and diet on many of the risk factors, most patients will require additive pharmacotherapy to achieve the therapeutic goals.

Statins

Multiple epidemiological studies have persuasively correlated chronic statin use with a favorable decrease in cardiovascular events. The relative risk reduction is 20% to 30% in all subgroups for the primary outcome of the combined incidence of coronary death and MI over a three- to six-year follow-up period.

The Heart Protection Study was the first large study that demonstrated the positive effects of statins also for the subgroup ($N = 6748$) of patients with PAD. In the PAD subgroup, there was a 25% risk reduction over five years (31).

Dietary modification and pharmacological therapy with regard to dyslipidemia should be tailored to meet the current guidelines for high-risk patients. Concerning low-density lipoprotein (LDL) cholesterol, a value of less than 100 mg/dL or even less than 70 mg/dL for those at very high risk should be the goal. The ACC/AHA guidelines define "very high-risk" PAD patients as those with multiple risk factors (especially diabetes), severe or poorly controlled risk factors (especially smoking), and risk factors of the metabolic syndrome (especially elevated triglycerides in the face of an elevated non-HDL cholesterol). A recent prospective observational cohort study of nearly 1400 PAD patients showed that intensive therapy with statins targeting an LDL ≤70 mg/dL improved overall as well as cardiac mortality at a mean follow-up of 6 years

(32). For the patient who fails to achieve LDL goals, options include switching to a more potent statin or adding ezetimibe at 10 mg/day. A fasting lipid profile should be obtained six weeks after changes in medication or dose are made.

A recent meta-analysis of postoperative mortality and morbidity in patients on preoperative statin therapy gives a 1.2% and 4.4% absolute reduction in 30-day mortality for cardiac and vascular surgery, respectively (33). The positive effects observed perioperatively may also be expected in patients treated by an endovascular method.

Statins are also promoted as an important perioperative risk reduction strategy because of their so-called pleiotropic effects. Among many others, possible mechanisms for the so-called pleiotropic effects include improvement of vasomotor regulation of blood flow [LDL-C worsens endothelial function and bioavailability of nitric oxide (NO)], neoangiogenesis (collateral circulation), reduction in thrombus formation and platelet activation, antioxidant properties, reduction of the inflammatory burden with better plaque stability, or even a reduction of plaque size (34,35). Statin therapy was especially associated with improved survival and event-free survival rates in patients with severe PAD in states of high inflammatory activity (36). Statins therefore should be rigorously prescribed in these patients. The observed interaction with inflammation supports the view that statins exert their beneficial effects in patients with advanced atherosclerosis partly via an anti-inflammatory pathway or, alternatively, by attenuating the deleterious effects of inflammation.

Furthermore, a protective effect of statins on renal function has been reported in patients with CAD and PAD.

In patients with PAD, statins seem also to favorably influence leg function (37), in addition to reducing cardiovascular events and improving survival rates.

Antihypertensive Treatment

In patients presenting with PAD, hypertension is a major associated cardiovascular risk factor. Hypertension also increases the risk of cardiovascular disease complications and mortality in patients with established PAD. Unfortunately, blood pressure management in PAD tends to be poor. In the PARTNERS (The PAD Awareness, Risk, and Treatment: New Resources for Survival) program, hypertension was less often treated in new (84%) and prior (88%) PAD patients compared to treatment of hypertension in subjects with cardiovascular disease (95%) (38). Furthermore, underdiagnosis of PAD in primary care practice may also be a barrier to effective secondary prevention of the high ischemic cardiovascular risk associated with PAD.

It is also important to identify possible underlying causes for secondary hypertension so that specific treatment may be targeted against causes of hypertension. Atheromatous renal artery stenosis is one of these important common underlying causes of hypertension in PAD.

Current evidence supports a low threshold for blood pressure treatment in PAD and intensive blood pressure control to reduce the high risk of cardiovascular disease and death in patients with PAD. Optimal treatment targets should be <140/85 mmHg, with the lower target of <130/80 mmHg in the presence of diabetes mellitus or chronic renal disease. The importance of intensive blood pressure control for reduction of cardiovascular events has especially been demonstrated in PAD patients with diabetes (39).

An important goal to be reached in hypertensive patients with PAD is to make an appropriate choice among the available antihypertensive drug classes.

According to recent guidelines, most drugs classes can be used to treat hypertension in symptomatic PAD. Class-specific selection of antihypertensive treatment in PAD should take into consideration indications and contraindications based on other significant comorbidity.

There has been some doubt whether β-blocking agents should be the first-line drugs in uncomplicated hypertensive patients with PAD. These drugs have until recently been considered relatively contraindicated in patients with PAD because of the perceived risk that these drugs could reduce the peripheral circulation by inhibition of β_2 receptors and thus worsen intermittent claudication. However, β-blockers are definitely not contraindicated in patients with intermittent claudication (40). On the contrary, because of their cardioprotective effect they are associated with improved survival in patients with PAD (41). Furthermore, β-blocking agents should be used in patients with PAD and further accepted indications for β-blocking agents such as angina pectoris, post infarction, chronic heart failure, and aortic dissection (where it is a cornerstone of medical approach). Otherwise, these drugs should be prescribed cautiously in patients with CLI.

If the indication is systolic hypertension in the elderly (which is frequently associated with PAD), diuretics and calcium channel blocking agents are often recommended. However, there is little published hard evidence for calcium antagonists in the specific setting of hypertension in patients with PAD. There are also no large outcome studies specifically addressing treatment with (low-dose) diuretics in PAD with hypertension, but there is little doubt that diuretics are effective antihypertensive agents both for lowering blood pressure and for the reduction of cardiovascular morbidity and mortality in uncomplicated hypertension.

Blockade of the renin-angiotensin system is an important approach to the prevention of cardiovascular events. In the Heart Outcomes Prevention Evaluation (HOPE) study, including patients with PAD, the risk of heart attack, stroke, and death from vascular causes was reduced by 22% for patients given the (ACE) inhibitor, ramipril (42). This effect was independent of its antihypertensive effect. In cases where ACE inhibitors are not well tolerated, angiotensin II receptor blockers may offer an alternative. In the largest angiotensin receptor blocker cardio-vascular outcome study to date, the ONTARGET trial compared the efficacy of therapy with the angiotensin II receptor blocker, telmisartan and the ACE inhibitor, ramipril as well as the combination of the two drugs in reducing cardiovascular events in patients at high risk (history of CAD, stroke or transient ischemic attack, PAD, or diabetes with evidence of end-organ damage) (43). Telmisartan was equivalent to ramipril in patients with vascular disease or high-risk diabetes and was associated with less angioedema. The combination of the two drugs was associated with more adverse events without an increase in benefit.

Diabetes

Many patients with PAD have diabetes. Epidemiologic studies have shown a relationship between glycated hemoglobin levels and cardiovascular events in patients with type 2 diabetes. Otherwise, previous randomized trials evaluating the effects of glycemic control in patients with diabetes have provided inconsistent evidence of effects on vascular disease. For example, the incidence of amputation for PAD was not reduced by tight glycemic control in the U.K. Prospective Diabetes Study (44). Therefore, there are little data to support that aggressive control of blood glucose levels improves risk of MI, stroke, vascular death, or amputation. Otherwise, according to the consensus paper, TASC II, patients with diabetes and PAD should have an aggressive control of blood glucose levels with a hemoglobin A_{1c} goal of <7.0% or as close to 6% as possible (1). In the new TASC paper this recommendation is graded as C, meaning that it is based on evidence obtained from expert committee reports or opinions and/or clinical experiences of respected authorities, while there are no applicable studies of good quality.

The importance of strict diabetic control concerning major cardiovascular events was also questioned by the recently published ACCORD-study (45). About one-third of the patients in this study had a history of macrovascular disease. The findings of this study indicated that a comprehensive, customized, therapeutic strategy that targeted glycated hemoglobin levels below 6.0% increased the rate of death from any cause after a mean of 3.5 years, as compared with a strategy that targeted levels of 7.0% to 7.9% in patients with a median glycated hemoglobin level of 8.1%, and with either previous cardiovascular events or multiple cardiovascular risk factors. These findings identify a previously unrecognized harm of intensive glucose lowering in high-risk patients with type 2 diabetes.

In another similar, recently published large trial with more than 11,000 patients a strategy of intensive glucose control, involving gliclazide (modified release) and other drugs as required that lowered the glycated hemoglobin value to 6.5%, yielded a 10% relative reduction in the combined outcome of major macrovascular and microvascular events, primarily as a consequence of a 21% relative reduction in nephropathy (46).

It is beyond any doubt that in high-risk patients with type 2 diabetes, intensive intervention concerning therapy of risk factors, such as hypertension and hyperlipidemia, with multiple drug combinations and behavior modification has sustained beneficial effects with respect to vascular complications and on rates of death from cardiovascular causes (47).

PATIENTS WITH IMPAIRED KIDNEY FUNCTION

Patients with chronic kidney disease are at higher risk of cardiovascular morbidity and mortality because of higher prevalence of traditional cardiovascular risk factors, such as hypertension, diabetes mellitus, dyslipidemia, and ischemic heart disease. The level of kidney function is an independent predictor of short- and long-term, all-cause cardio- and cerebrovascular mortality (48). Renal insufficiency was reported to be a strong independent predictor of mortality in CLI patients, and mortality risk was highest among patients with a glomerular filtration rate <30 mL/min/1.73 m^2 (49). Renal insufficiency is also a risk factor for poor outcome (poorer postoperative survival and higher amputation rates) after infrainguinal bypass in patients with CLI, because dialysis-dependent patients usually have heavily calcified distal arteries. Furthermore, wound healing is poor due to anemia, malnutrition, impaired immunity, and tendency to infection. The increased risks of surgery in these mostly high-risk patients have lead—together with the improved technology—to a steadily increasing application of endovascular interventions as well as in patients with chronic kidney disease.

It is important to avoid contrast media–induced acute renal failure or deterioration of kidney function, since mortality is increased if patients with underlying chronic kidney disease develop contrast media–induced acute renal failure after coronary interventions (50). The most effective preventive measure is adequate hydration of the patient, mainly with electrolyte solutions. Alternatively, isotonic sodium bicarbonate solution may be used. Acetylcysteine (600 mg b.i.d. before and on the day of the intervention) may be used since there are some positive studies and it has almost no side effects. However, its efficacy is unclear to date (50).

Statin therapy also seems to be associated with improved outcomes in patients with renal impairment, as it was demonstrated in vascular surgery patients (51).

SUMMARY

Patients with PAD can mostly be judged as "complex" patients due to different medical comorbidities, mainly due to the underlying atherothrombotic disease. Therefore, these patients need intensive antithrombotic therapy, mostly by antiplatelet agents, and aggressive risk factor modification including especially lipid-lowering and antihypertensive treatment. Special care has to be taken considering peri-interventional antithrombotic management in patients on long-term OAC treatment, such as patients with AF.

REFERENCES

1. Norgren L, Hiatt WR, Dormandy JA, et al. TASC II Working Group. Inter-society consensus for the management of peripheral arterial disease (TASC II). Eur J Vasc Endovasc Surg 2007; 33(suppl 1): S1–S75.
2. Steg PG, Bhatt DL, Wilson PW, et al. One-year cardiovascular event rates in outpatients with atherothrombosis. JAMA 2007; 297:1197–1206.
3. Antithrombotic Trialists' Collaboration. Collaborative metaanalysis of randomised trials of antiplatelet therapy for prevention of death, myocardial infarction, and stroke in high risk patients. BMJ 2002; 324:71–86.
4. CAPRIE Steering Committee. A randomised, blinded, trial of clopidogrel versus aspirin in patients at risk of ischaemic events (CAPRIE). Lancet 1996; 348: 1329–1339.
5. Sobel M, Verhaeghe R. Antithrombotic therapy for peripheral artery occlusive disease: American College of Chest Physicians Evidence- Based Clinical Practice Guidelines (8th Edition). Chest 2008; 133:815S–843S.
6. Undas A, Brummel-Ziedins KE, Mann KG. Antithrombotic properties of aspirin and resistance to aspirin: beyond strictly antiplatelet actions. Blood 2007; 109:2285–9220.
7. Eikelboom JW, Hirsh J, Weitz JI. Aspirin-resistant thromboxane biosynthesis and the risk of myocardial infarction, stroke, or cardiovascular death in patients at high risk for cardiovascular events. Circulation 2002; 105:1650–1655.
8. Bhatt DL, Flather MD, Hacke W, et al. Patients with prior myocardial infarction, stroke, or symptomatic peripheral arterial disease in the CHARISMA trial. J Am Coll Cardiol 2007; 49:1982–1988.
9. Iida O, Nanto S, Uematsu M, et al. Cilostazol reduces restenosis after endovascular therapy in patients with femoropopliteal lesions. J Vasc Surg 2008; 48:144–149.
10. The Warfarin Antiplatelet Vascular Evaluation Trial Investigators. Oral anticoagulant and antiplatelet therapy and peripheral arterial disease. N Engl J Med 2007; 357:217–227.

11. Keo HH, Baumgartner I. Complications of pharmacologic interventions: antiplatelet, antithrombotic, and anticoagulant agents. In: Schillinger M, Minar E, eds. Complications in Peripheral Vascular Interventions. London: Informa Healthcare, 2007:71–80.

12. Kastrati A, Neumann FJ, Mehilli J, et al. Bivalirudin versus unfractionated heparin during percutaneous coronary intervention. N Engl J Med 2008; 359:688–696.

13. Katzen BT, Ardid MI, MacLean AA, et al. Bivalirudin as an anticoagulation agent: safety and efficacy in peripheral interventions. J Vasc Interv Radiol 2005; 16:1183–1187.

14. Tepe G, Wiskirchen J, Pereira P, et al. GP IIb/IIIa blockade during peripheral artery interventions. Cardiovasc Intervent Radiol 2008; 31:8–13.

15. Duda SH, Tepe G, Luz O, et al. Peripheral artery occlusion: treatment with abciximab plus urokinase versus with urokinase alone—a randomized pilot trial (the PROMPT Study). Platelet Receptor Antibodies in Order to Manage Peripheral Artery Thrombosis. Radiology 2001; 221:689–696.

16. Doerffler-Melly J, Mahler F, Do DD, et al. Adjunctive abciximab improves patency and functional outcome in endovascular treatment of femoropopliteal occlusions: initial experience. Radiology 2005; 237: 1103–1109.

17. Keo H, Diehm N, Baumgartner, et al. Single center experience with provisional abciximab therapy in complex lower limb interventions. VASA 2008; 37:257–264.

18. Ouriel K, Castaneda F, McNamara T, et al. Reteplase monotherapy and reteplase/abciximab combination therapy in peripheral arterial occlusive disease: Results from the RELAX trial. J Vasc Intervent Radiol 2004; 15:229–238.

19. Working Party on Thrombolysis in the Management of Limb Ischemia. Thrombolysis in the management of lower limb peripheral arterial occlusion–a consensus document. J Vasc Interv Radiol. 2003; 14:S337–S349.

20. Kessel D, Berridge D, Robertson I. Infusion techniques for peripheral arterial thrombolysis. Cochrane Database Syst Rev 2004; (1):CD000985.

21. Moise MA, Kashyap VS. Alfimeprase for the treatment of acute peripheral arterial occlusion. Expert Opin Biol Ther 2008; 8: 683–689.

22. Go AS, Hylek EM, Phillips JA, et al. Prevalence of diagnosed atrial fibrillation in adults: national implications for rhythm management and stroke prevention: The AnTicoagulation and Risk Factors in Atrial Fibrillation (ATRIA) study. JAMA 2001; 285:2370–2375.

23. Singer DE, Albers GW, Dalen JE. Antithrombotic therapy in atrial fibrillation: American College of Chest Physicians Evidence-Based Clinical Practice Guidelines (8th Edition). Chest 2008; 133; S546–S592.

24. The ACTIVE Writing Group of the ACTIVE Investigators. Clopidogrel plus aspirin versus oral anticoagulation for atrial fibrillation in the Atrial fibrillation Clopidogrel Trial with Irbesartan for prevention of Vascular Events (ACTIVE W): a randomised controlled trial. Lancet 2006; 367:1903–1912.

25. Fuster V, Rydén LE, Cannom DS, et al. ACC/AHA/ESC 2006 Guidelines for the management of patients with atrial fibrillation—executive summary: a report of the American College of Cardiology/American Heart Association Task Force and the European Society of Cardiology Committee for Practice Guidelines (Writing Committee to Revise the 2001 Guidelines for the management of patients with atrial fibrillation). J Am Coll Cardiol 2006; 48:854–906.

26. Sinnaeve PR. The good, the bad, and the ugly: triple therapy after PCI in patients requiring chronic anticoagulation. Eur Heart J 2007; 28:657–658.

27. Hickey NC, Shearman, CP, Crowson MC, et al. Iloprost improves femoro-distal graft flow after a single bolus injection. Eur J Vasc Surg 1991; 5:19–22.

28. Thul R, Heckenkamp J, Gawenda M, et al. The role of intra-operative prostavasin application during crural bypass surgery. Zentralbl Chir 2007; 132:485–490.

29. Smith SC Jr, Allen J, Blair SN, et al. AHA/ACC guidelines for secondary prevention for patients with coronary and other atherosclerotic vascular disease: 2006 update: endorsed by the National Heart, Lung, and Blood Institute. Circulation 2006; 113:2363–2372.

30. Bhatt DL, Steg PG, Ohman EM, et al. International prevalence, recognition, and treatment of cardiovascular risk factors in outpatients with atherothrombosis. JAMA 2006; 295:180–189.

31. Heart Protection Study Collaborative Group. MRC/BHF Heart Protection Study of cholesterol lowering with simvastatin in 20.536 high-risk individuals: a randomized placebo-controlled trial. Lancet 2002; 360:7–22.

32. Feringa HH, Karagiannis SE, van Waning VH, et al. The effect of intensified lipid-lowering therapy on long term prognosis in patients with peripheral arterial disease. J Vasc Surg 2007; 45:936–943.

33. Hindler K, Shaw AD, Samuels J, et al. Improved postoperative outcomes associated with preoperative statin therapy. Anesthesiology 2006; 105:1260–1272.

34. Paraskevas KI, Mikhailidis DP, Athyros VG. Additional effects of statins in surgical patients. Ann Surg 2008; 248:140–141.

35. Williams TM, Harken AH. Statins for surgical patients. Ann Surg 2008; 247:30–37.
36. Schillinger M, Exner M, Mlekusch W, et al. Statin therapy improves cardiovascular outcome of patients with peripheral artery disease. Eur Heart J 2004; 25:742–748.
37. McDermott MM, Guralnik JM, Greenland P, et al. Statin use and leg functioning in patients with and without lower-extremity peripheral artery disease. Circulation 2003; 107:757–761.
38. Hirsch AT, Criqui MH, Treat-Jacobson D, et al. Peripheral arterial disease detection, awareness, and treatment in primary care. JAMA 2001; 286:1317–1324.
39. Mehler PS, Coll JR, Estacio R, et al. Intensive blood pressure control reduces the risk of cardiovascular events in patients with peripheral arterial disease and type 2 diabetes. Circulation 2003; 107:753–756.
40. Radack K, Deck C. ß-Adrenergic blocker therapy does not worsen intermittent claudication in subjects with peripheral arterial disease: a meta-analysis of randomized controlled trials. Arch Intern Med 1991; 151:1769–1776.
41. Feringa HH, van Waning VH, Bax JJ, et al. Cardioprotective medication is associated with improved survival in patients with peripheral arterial disease. J Am Coll Cardiol 2006; 47: 1182–1187.
42. Yusuf S, Sleight P, Pogue J, et al. Effects of an angiotensin-converting-enzyme inhibitor, ramipril, on cardiovascular events in high-risk patients. N Engl J Med 2000; 342:145–153.
43. The ONTARGET Investigators. Telmisartan, ramipril, or both in patients at high risk for vascular events. N Engl J Med 2008; 358:1547–1559.
44. UK Prospective Diabetes Study (UKPDS) Group. Intensive blood-glucose control with sulphonylureas or insulin compared with conventional treatment and risk of complications in patients with type 2 diabetes (UKPDS 33). Lancet 1998; 352:837–853.
45. The Action to Control Cardiovascular Risk in Diabetes Study Group. Effects of intensive glucose lowering in type 2 diabetes. N Engl J Med 2008; 358:2545–2559.
46. The ADVANCE Collaborative Group. Intensive Blood Glucose Control and Vascular Outcomes in Patients with Type 2 Diabetes. N Engl J Med 2008; 358:2560–2572.
47. Gaede P, Lund-Andersen H, Parving HH, et al. Effect of a multifactorial intervention on mortality in type 2 diabetes. N Engl J Med 2008; 358:580–591.
48. O'Hare AM, Berthenthal D, Shlipak MG, et al. Impact of renal insufficiency on mortality in advanced lower extremity peripheral arterial disease. J Am Soc Nephrol 2005; 16:514–519.
49. Dangas G, Iakovou O, Nikolsky E, et al. Contrast-induced nephropathy after percutaneous coronary interventions in relation to chronic kidney disease and hemodynamic variables. Am J Cardiol 2005; 95:13–19.
50. Oberbauer R. Contrast media associated complications. In: Schillinger M, Minar E, eds. Complications in Peripheral Vascular Interventions. London: Informa Healthcare, 2007:27–38.
51. Welten GM, Chonchol M, Hoeks SE, et al. Statin therapy is associated with improved outcomes in vascular surgery patients with renal impairment. Am Heart J. 2007; 154: 954–961.

3 | Preprocedural Imaging in Peripheral Arterial Disease

Thomas J. Kiernan and Bryan P. Yan

Section of Vascular Medicine, Division of Cardiology, Massachusetts General Hospital, Boston, Massachusetts, U.S.A.

Michael R. Jaff

Section of Vascular Medicine, Division of Cardiology, Massachusetts General Hospital, Boston, and The Vascular Center, Massachusetts General Hospital, Boston, Massachusetts, U.S.A.

INTRODUCTION

Endovascular therapy for peripheral vascular disease has become the mainstay for the majority of revascularization procedures. This is largely due to dramatic advances in device technology, as well as increasing skills of interventionists. Multiple specialists are committed to advancing this aspect of the care of patients with peripheral vascular disease. However, in order to determine the appropriate therapy for patients with vascular disease, accurate diagnostic testing must be available before invasive procedures are attempted. This chapter highlights current strategies for the diagnosis of peripheral artery disease (PAD) of the lower extremities, renal and extracranial carotid arteries.

IMAGING FOR PERIPHERAL ARTERIAL DISEASE OF THE LOWER EXTREMITIES

There are two components for the diagnosis of PAD: physiologic testing to determine the presence, severity, and function impact of PAD, and anatomic assessment to determine optimal revascularization options.

Noninvasive Vascular Testing

Ankle–Brachial Index

The ankle–brachial index (ABI) is the basis for the diagnosis of PAD. This safe, simple, and highly accurate test should follow the performance of a comprehensive history and physical examination. The ABI is performed by determining the ratio of systolic blood pressure of the ankle arteries relative to that of the brachial arteries using a hand-held, continuous wave Doppler device with a 5- to 10-MHz transducer. This test requires a blood pressure cuff and acoustic gel. Measurements for the ABI should be obtained after the patient has been supine for 5 to 10 minutes. The test requires that the systolic blood pressure be recorded in both brachial arteries and in both the dorsalis pedis and posterior tibial arteries of each limb. The ABI is calculated for each leg by dividing the highest ankle systolic pressure by the highest brachial systolic pressure, recording the value to two decimal places. In general, the ankle pressure will exceed the brachial pressure by 10 to 15 mm Hg in healthy individuals as a result of higher peripheral resistance at the ankles. The ABI is interpreted according to recent practice guidelines for PAD management from the American College of Cardiology and the American Heart Association (ACC/AHA) (1) (Table 1).

An ABI of 0.90 or less has a sensitivity of 95% and a specificity of 100%, relative to the gold standard, contrast angiography, for detecting a stenosis of at least 50% in the lower extremity arteries. Significant medial artery calcification will prevent arterial compression and result in elevated ABI values. This finding is most commonly seen in diabetic patients but may also be present in elderly individuals, patients with chronic kidney disease who require dialysis, and patients receiving chronic steroid therapy. An ABI >1.30 suggests medial artery calcification and has been shown to be associated with increased mortality similar to a low ABI (2).

Table 1   Index of ABI Values

ABI	Interpretation
>1.3	Noncompressible
0.91–1.29	Normal
0.41–0.90	Mild-to-moderate PAD
0–0.40	Severe PAD

The ABI correlates with cardiovascular outcomes. Epidemiologic studies have shown an association between the ABI and cardiovascular morbidity and mortality as well as an association between a low ABI and reduced limb function. In a cohort study of 154 patients with an ABI less than 0.90, Sikkink et al. (3) reported the following five-year cumulative survival rates, according to patients' resting ABIs:

- 63% for those with an ABI less than 0.50,
- 71% for those with an ABI of 0.50 to 0.69, and
- 91% for those with an ABI of 0.70 to 0.89.

A normal ABI in the face of symptoms suggestive of intermittent claudication should not discourage the clinician from pursuing the diagnosis of PAD. Physicians should then pursue exercise testing, including waveform and pressure measurements at rest and after formal treadmill exercise testing. This phenomenon of a normal resting ABI, which deteriorates following treadmill exercise testing, is most often found among patients with aortoiliac atherosclerosis.

Pulse Volume Recordings

The ABI only provides information suggesting artery disease between the arm and the ankle. If the clinician requires more specific information describing the segment of artery(ies) involved, other noninvasive tests should be performed.

The location and extent of PAD can be further defined by segmental limb systolic blood pressure measurements, recorded with a Doppler instrument while plethysmographic cuffs are placed at various points on the lower limb, including the upper thigh, the lower thigh, the upper calf just below the knee, the ankle, metatarsal, and digit (Fig. 1). The high thigh pressure is normally >30 mm Hg higher than the brachial pressure, largely due to the relationship between cuff and thigh sizes, as well as increasing peripheral arterial resistance. Moving distally along the limb, a drop in pressure >20 mm Hg between sequential cuff levels indicates arterial disease of the segment proximal to the lower cuff. For example, a segmental limb pressure of 120 mm Hg at the lower thigh and 80 mm Hg at the upper calf would suggest distal superficial femoral artery or popliteal artery disease. In addition, comparison of the same cuff pressure between limbs can be helpful as a confirmatory diagnostic tool.

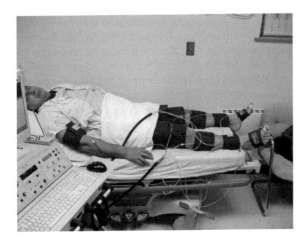

Figure 1   Patient scheduled to undergo physiologic noninvasive vascular testing for peripheral artery disease.

Segmental limb pressure measurements have the same limitation as the ABI with regard to noncompressible vessels. Although segmental limb pressures can be measured alone, they are commonly obtained with pulse volume recordings; the combination of the two measures has a reported diagnostic accuracy of 97% (4). Pulse volume recordings are obtained with a cuff system that incorporates a pneumoplethysmograph to detect volume changes in the limb throughout the cardiac cycle. Changes in pulse contour and amplitude can be analyzed, providing additional information on the status of the limb arteries. Cuffs are inflated to ~65 mm Hg, and with each volume of arterial blood passing beneath the cuff, the change in size of the artery is detected and recorded. A normal waveform has a steep upstroke, a sharp systolic peak, a narrow pulse width, a dicrotic notch, and a downslope bowing to the baseline (5) [Fig. 2(A)]. In the presence of PAD, the slope of the upstroke flattens, the peak becomes more rounded and has a wider pulse width, the dicrotic notch disappears, and the downslope bows away from the baseline [Fig. 2(B)].

Exercise Stress Testing

Exercise treadmill testing with the measurement of pre- and postexercise ABIs and waveforms are used to determine whether one's lower extremity symptoms are due to PAD (claudication) or due to an alternate cause (pseudoclaudication) as well as to assess the functional status of an individual with PAD. It is also an important method of noninvasively detecting PAD when the ABI is normal, but there is a high clinical suspicion for arterial disease. Finally, treadmill testing may be the first opportunity to diagnose occult coronary artery disease using electrocardiographic tracings. Once a baseline ABI is obtained, the patient is placed on a treadmill using a preset speed and grade (commonly 2 mph at 12% grade). The patient's leg symptoms, their intensity, and their location should be recorded at symptom-onset, with changes during the examination, and at the time of maximal discomfort when the patient must stop ambulating. When the patient has walked until maximal discomfort or the test has reached a prespecified endpoint (e.g., 5 minutes), the ABI is remeasured; a reduction in ankle pressure >20 mm Hg or a decrease in the postexercise ABI >0.15 suggests hemodynamically significant arterial disease. Some laboratories also repeat ankle pressures at one minute intervals until reaching the preexercise baseline, suggesting that the longer the time to normalization (pulse reappearance time), the worse the arterial ischemia. Exercising produces significant peripheral vasodilatation, which, in the presence of arterial stenosis, results in a significant blood pressure gradient. A normal individual will have no change or a slight increase in the ABI; the ABI will drop in patients with PAD.

Duplex Ultrasonography

Arterial duplex ultrasonography (DUS) of the lower extremities is commonly used to diagnose PAD. It is especially helpful in determining the exact location of disease and in delineating between stenotic and occlusive lesions, an added benefit when preparing for an endovascular. DUS combines color Doppler imaging, Doppler spectral waveform analysis, and Doppler-derived systolic and diastolic flow velocities. A normal peripheral arterial Doppler waveform is triphasic [Fig. 3(A)]. Cardiac systole results in initial forward flow of blood, followed by a brief period of flow reversal in early diastole and subsequent forward flow in late diastole. The flow-reversal component, a result of high peripheral vascular resistance, is absent in the presence of hemodynamically significant stenosis due to damping of pulse wave reflection, along with a marked increase in systolic flow velocities [Fig. 3(B)]. Doppler waveform analysis can be used to identify other indicators of disease, including the presence of turbulence.

Koelemay et al. performed a meta-analysis of studies on the utility of DUS for detecting occlusion or stenosis greater than or equal to 50% of peripheral arteries (6). The sensitivity and specificity rates were 86% and 97%, respectively, for aortoiliac arteries; 80% and 96% for the femoropopliteal arteries; and 83% and 84% for the infragenicular arteries. DUS is widely accepted and recommended for surveillance of surgical vein grafts despite mixed results in published studies of its clinical utility (1). Although ultrasound surveillance of synthetic grafts or arteries after angioplasty are often performed, their value remains unproven. Despite accuracy, some limitations exist. Although DUS is an accurate noninvasive test for PAD, it requires technical expertise that may be lacking in many centers. Other limitations are diminished

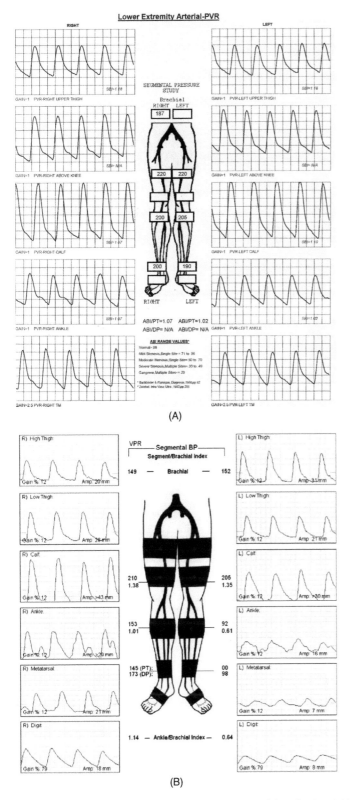

(A)

(B)

Figure 2 (**A**) Normal physiologic lower extremity arterial study at rest. Note the normal pulse volume recordings (see text), segmental pressures, and ankle–brachial indices (Right: 1.07; Left 1.02). (**B**) Pulse volume recordings suggest left femoropopliteal artery disease. Note the absence of augmentation of the left calf PVR compared to the right. The left ABI is 0.64.

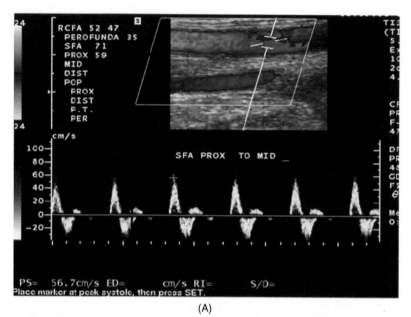

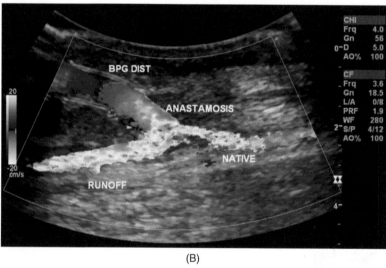

Figure 3 (**A**) (*see color insert*) Normal triphasic Doppler waveform performed during Duplex ultrasonography. However, note the incorrect Doppler angle, demonstrating lack of parallel placement compared to the direction of arterial blood flow. (**B**) Arterial duplex ultrasonography demonstrating a severe (>75%) stenosis of the distal anastomosis of a left lower extremity arterial bypass graft. Peak systolic velocity 484.5 cm/sec. Note the correct Doppler angle orientation.

accuracy in assessing the aortoiliac vessels due to body habitus and bowel gas, signal "dropout" in heavily calcified vessels, and reduced sensitivity for significant stenosis in the presence of multiple lesions within close proximity (tandem lesions).

Magnetic Resonance Angiography

Three-dimensional (3D) gadolinium-enhanced magnetic resonance angiography (MRA) facilitates noninvasive assessment of the peripheral arteries without sedation, catheterization, ionizing radiation, or potentially nephrotoxic iodinated contrast agents. Koelemay et al. published a meta-analysis of 34 studies (1090 patients) between January 1985 and May 2000, reporting high accuracy for the assessment of the lower extremity arteries using MRA (7). Furthermore, 3D gadolinium-enhanced MRA improved diagnostic performance compared with 2D MRA;

the estimated points of equal sensitivity and specificity were 94% and 90% for 3D gadolinium-enhanced MRA and 2D MRA, respectively.

MRA is a particularly useful imaging tool in PAD. It does not expose patients to ionizing radiation, and the addition of gadolinium contrast offers advantages in evaluating revascularization options for patients. Time of flight (2D-TOF) imaging can be performed but is time-consuming and is unreliable in imaging vessels out of axis of the magnetic pulse (such as the proximal anterior tibial artery). Many investigators routinely use gadolinium-enhanced MRA. The large field of view required to image the lower extremities requires three to four overlapping stations with separate contrast boluses. Alternatively, use of bolus chase techniques with floating tables is possible.

Contrast-enhanced MRA has replaced X-ray angiography for diagnosis and procedural planning at many institutions. Early experience comparing contrast-enhanced MRA with DUS showed MRA to be impressively accurate in planning peripheral arterial revascularization. A retrospective series of 100 patients who underwent both imaging methods found that MRA was more effective than DUS in planning revascularization (8). The ACC/AHA guidelines on PAD suggest that MRA may be useful in determining the location and severity of stenosis and may aid in decisions between endovascular and surgical revascularization (1) (Fig. 4).

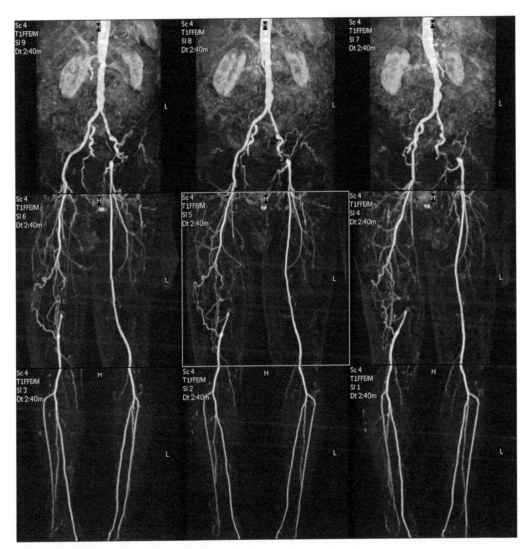

Figure 4 Gadolinium-enhanced magnetic resonance arteriogram, demonstrating diffuse aortic atherosclerosis, occlusion of the left common and external iliac arteries, and right superficial femoral artery.

From a technology standpoint, MR often classifies moderate stenoses as severe and severe stenoses as occlusions. This tendency to overestimate the extent of stenosis may be avoided by close postprocessing of images and by improved timing of contrast agent administration. When areas of stenoses are seen on 3D reconstructed images, cross-sectional source images should be examined, recognizing that the Fourier transformations required to construct 3D images degrade spatial resolution. In addition, MRA cannot reliably detect arterial calcification, which is a potential limitation when revascularization options are being considered. Finally, the metal alloys used in current endovascular stents result in signal dropout, which precludes imaging of segments within stents, although MRA can reliably determine the presence of flow proximal and distal to the stent. With newer alloys, imaging within stents using MRA may become a reality.

The limits of MRA center on patient factors and technology issues. Patients with implantable defibrillators and permanent pacemakers may not undergo MR studies, for fear of causing these devices to malfunction. Patients with intracranial aneurysm clips also are deemed to be at high risk if exposed to the magnetic environment. Claustrophobia is also a major issue, precluding approximately 10% of patients from completing MR studies. It must be stated, however, that the U.S. Food and Drug Administration (FDA) has issued a warning on the use of gadolinium in patients with renal impairment because it has been linked to the development of nephrogenic systemic fibrosis, also known as nephrogenic fibrosing dermopathy (9).

Computed Tomography Angiography

Computed tomography angiography (CTA) is increasingly attractive due to rapid technical developments. Shorter acquisition times, thinner slices, higher spatial resolution, and improvement of multidetector computed tomographic (CT) scanners enable scanning of the whole vascular tree in a limited period with a decreasing (but still substantial) amount of contrast medium. Recent studies on CTA report sensitivity and specificity rates of approximately 98% for detecting PAD (10,11). The diagnostic accuracy of CTA seems to compare well with MRA (12), although studies directly comparing these imaging modalities are lacking.

A recent meta-analysis by Met et al. analyzed 957 patients with symptoms of peripheral arterial disease. Overall, the sensitivity of CTA for detecting more than 50% stenosis or occlusion was 95% [95% confidence interval (CI), 92–97%) and specificity was 96% (95% CI, 93%–97%) when compared with digital subtraction angiography (DSA). CAT correctly identified occlusions in 94% of segments, the presence of more than 50% stenosis in 87% of segments, and the absence of significant stenosis in 96% of segments. Overstaging occurred in 8% of segments and understaging in 15% (13).

Venous opacification and asymmetric filling of the arteries in the legs may degrade vessel detail. Evaluation of peripheral arterial stents can be performed with CTA, as there is no signal dropout during CTA scanning. However, the true degree of instent stenosis has not been adequately quantified with current technology and scanning algorithms (Fig. 5).

Because of the need for large volumes of iodinated contrast media administered via a peripheral intravenous cannula, CTA cannot be performed in patients with azotemia or in individuals at increased risk of contrast-induced acute tubular necrosis. In addition, repetitive CTA studies are not recommended, because patients will receive considerable exposure to ionizing radiation. Furthermore, CTA has its limitations in patients with heavily calcified arteries. Particularly, evaluation of below the knee arteries of diabetic patient with excessive mediasclerosis is problematic.

INDICATIONS FOR ARTERIOGRAPHY AND INTERVENTION IN PERIPHERAL ARTERIAL DISEASE OF THE LOWER EXTREMITIES

Diagnostic DSA is currently reserved for patients in whom revascularization is planned or for those situations in which the results from noninvasive imaging are ambiguous. Digital subtraction angiography is preferred for its enhanced imaging capabilities compared with unsubtracted imaging techniques. Technically, DSA imaging of the abdominal aorta with bilateral lower-extremity runoff angiography requires an image intensifier large enough to include both legs in the same field (≥15 in.) and has road-mapping capability and stepping-table acquisition.

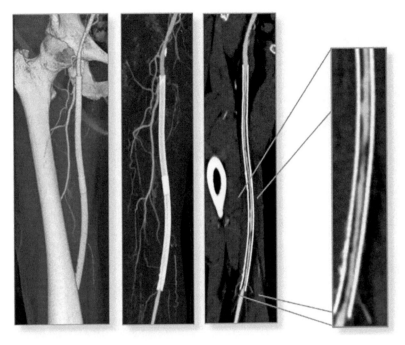

Figure 5 Computed tomographic arteriogram of the right lower extremity, demonstrating long superficial femoral artery stent. Note the "cut through" image demonstrating in-stent restenosis.

Imaging for Renal Artery Disease

Atherosclerotic renal artery stenosis is common in patients with coronary and peripheral artery disease. However, once identified, the true benefits of revascularization for renal artery disease (RAS) remain uncertain (14). Before proceeding to revascularization, an accurate diagnosis of RAS must be made.

DUS

Renal artery DUS is a safe and accurate test to determine the presence and severity of RAS (Fig. 6). However, this is a technically challenging examination, which requires skill and perseverance by the technologist and supervising physician.

Several investigators have demonstrated the validity of renal artery DUS to diagnose renal artery stenosis. In one prospective series, 29 patients (58 renal arteries) underwent DUS and contrast arteriography. The sensitivity of renal artery DUS was 84%, specificity of 97%, and positive predictive value of 94% for a detection of >60% stenosis (15). Utilizing criteria of peak systolic velocity within the renal artery >180 cm/sec, duplex scanning was able to discern between normal and diseased renal arteries with sensitivity of 95% and specificity of 90% (16). The ratio of peak systolic velocity (PSV) in the area of renal artery stenosis compared to the PSV within the aorta [renal-to-aortic ratio [RAR]) of >3.5 predicts the presence of >60% renal artery stenosis. Using this criterion, renal artery duplex demonstrated a sensitivity of 92%.

In a prospective series of 102 consecutive patients who underwent both DUS and contrast arteriography, there was a higher sensitivity for detecting stenoses of <60% and 80–99% compared with a stenosis of 60–79% using DUS. Occluded renal arteries were correctly identified by ultrasonography in 22 of 23 cases. The overall sensitivity of DUS was 98%, specificity 99%, positive predictive value 99%, and negative predictive value 97% (17).

One of the greatest utilities of renal artery DUS is surveillance of renal artery stents. A recent publication identified excellent utility of this in following patency versus stenosis within stents in the renal arteries. Chi et al. studied 67 patients with renal stents and 55 patients without renal stents. In this study, a statistically significant correlation was found for both PSV and RAR

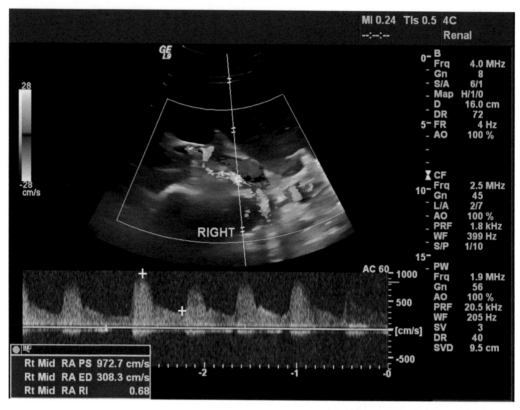

Figure 6 (*See color insert*) Renal artery duplex ultrasonography, demonstrating severe right renal artery stenosis. Note the dramatic elevation in peak systolic (972 cm/sec) and end-diastolic velocities (308 cm/sec).

in detecting renal instent restenosis (ISR) ($p = 0.02$). For any level of angiographic stenosis $\geq 50\%$, the ISR group had relatively higher PSV and RAR compared with the nonstented group. Receiver operating characteristic curves indicated that PSV ≥ 395 cm/sec or RAR ≥ 5.1 was the most predictive of angiographically significant ISR $\geq 70\%$ (18) (Fig. 7).

Limitations of direct visualization of the renal arteries include body habitus and overlying bowel gas obscuring identification of the renal arteries. Given that many patients have both main renal artery disease and parenchymal renal disease, the addition of resistive indices within the parenchyma may help predict which patients will benefit from revascularization (19). However, renal resistive indices have not been consistently identified as a reliable predictor of clinical outcomes following renal artery stent revascularization (20).

Magnetic Resonance Angiography
Although conventional DSA remains the gold standard for the diagnosis of renal artery stenosis, it is typically not used as a screening study because of the invasive nature and associated complication rate (21). Of the less-invasive alternatives, contrast-enhanced MR angiography (CE-MRA) has emerged as a promising technique for evaluating the renal arteries (22–24), with a meta-analysis (25) showing it performs significantly better than DUS, captopril renal scintigraphy, or the captopril test (Fig. 8). This same study showed CE-MRA and CT angiography (CTA) to be roughly equivalent, although CTA has the distinct disadvantages of ionizing radiation and administration of nephrotoxic contrast material. However, approximately 10% of patients cannot undergo MRA because of implanted metal (i.e., permanent pacemakers) or claustrophobia. Finally, in patients who have undergone renal revascularization with metallic endoluminal stents, MRA cannot be used to determine patency of the stent due to signal dropout from the metal.

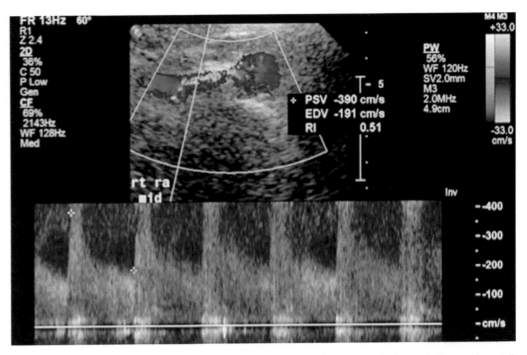

Figure 7 (*See color insert*) Duplex ultrasonography of right renal artery stent, demonstrating peak systolic velocity 390 cm/sec, suggestive of >60% in-stent restenosis.

Computerized Tomographic Angiography

CTA has recently gained attention as a less-invasive method of imaging the renal arteries. With improving technology, multidetector CTA images have demonstrated excellent sensitivity to determine renal artery stenosis (Fig. 9). This examination requires the administration of iodinated contrast via a peripheral intravenous catheter and significant external beam radiation. A normal CTA virtually excludes the presence of significant RAS (26).

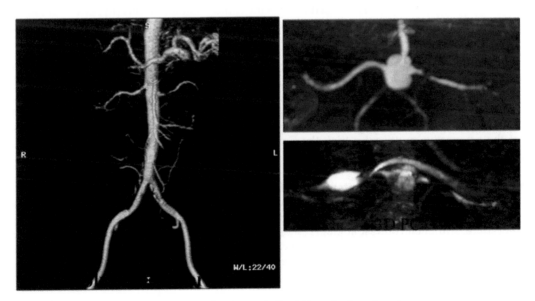

Figure 8 Magnetic resonance arteriography, demonstrating left renal artery stenosis.

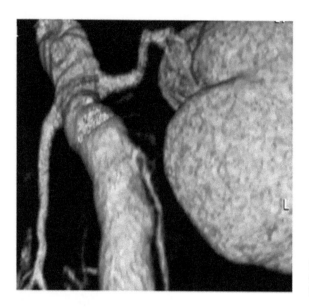

Figure 9 Computed tomographic arteriogram of the renal arteries, using surface-shaded technology.

In a recent prospective comparison trial of 356 patients who underwent CTA, MRA, and DSA because of high clinical suspicion for RAS, the sensitivity and specificity for MRA was 62% and 84%, and for CTA 64% and 92%, respectively (27).

The limitations of CT mainly concern the use of iodinated contrast agents that can increase the risk for contrast-induced nephropathy. Patients who are considered at highest risk are those with preexisting chronic kidney disease, especially elderly patients and those with diabetes mellitus. Other risk factors for contrast-induced nephropathy include multiple myeloma, proteinuria, concomitant nephrotoxic drug use, hypertension, congestive heart failure, hyperuricemia, and dehydration.

INDICATIONS FOR ARTERIOGRAPHY AND INTERVENTION IN RENAL ARTERY STENOSIS

Selective digital subtraction renal angiography is currently reserved for patients in whom revascularization is planned or for those situations in which the results from noninvasive imaging are uncertain. Intervention is only advised for specific clinical manifestations (hypertension, renal failure, and pulmonary edema) in which the patient has failed maximal medical therapy and the likelihood of clinical improvement is strong. Revascularization for "asymptomatic" renal artery stenosis is strongly discouraged (28). In some patients, severe renal artery stenosis may threaten renal function, particularly in those patients with global renal ischemia (bilateral renal artery stenosis or stenosis to a solitary functioning kidney). The level of hypertension and the severity of the baseline stenosis may predict progression from stenosis to occlusion. This risk approximates 50% over five years for lesions with baseline stenosis >60% at the time of initial detection (29). The future of percutaneous renal revascularization will depend on the results of the prospective multicenter trial, the Cardiovascular Outcomes for Renal Artery Lesions (CORAL) trial.

Preintervention Imaging for Internal Carotid Artery Revascularization

Extracranial carotid artery revascularization, with either surgical endarterectomy or percutaneous stenting, relies on accurate and safe imaging for diagnosis and assessment prior to the procedure. Although contrast angiography is still considered to be the reference standard for imaging the carotid artery, most patients evaluated for carotid disease today do not undergo angiography. DUS, MRA, and CTA have emerged as comparable, if not superior, imaging modalities for the assessment of the carotid artery disease in potential candidates for carotid revascularization.

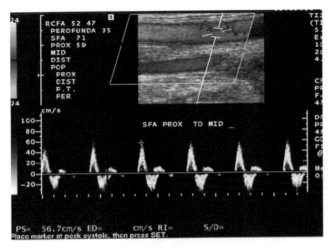

Figure 3.3A Normal triphasic Doppler waveform performed during Duplex ultrasonography. However, note the incorrect Doppler angle, demonstrating lack of parallel placement compared to the direction of arterial blood flow.

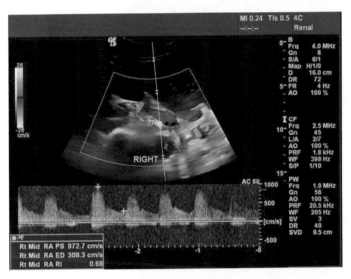

Figure 3.6 Renal artery duplex ultrasonography, demonstrating severe right renal artery stenosis. Note the dramatic elevation in peak systolic (972 cm/sec) and end-diastolic velocities (308 cm/sec).

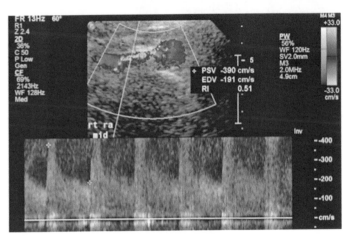

Figure 3.7 Duplex ultrasonography of right renal artery stent, demonstrating peak systolic velocity 390 cm/sec, suggestive of >60% in-stent restenosis.

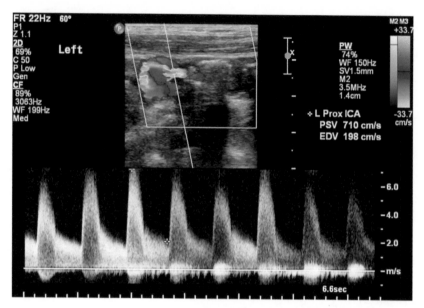

Figure 3.10 Carotid duplex ultrasonography, demonstrating critical (90–99%) left internal carotid artery stenosis. Note the peak systolic velocity elevation (710 cm/sec) and end-diastolic velocity (198 cm/sec).

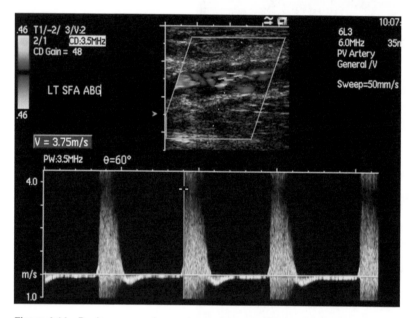

Figure 4.14 Duplex sonography one day postprocedurally showing a tight stenoses at the origin of the superficial femoral artery.

Severity of Stenosis

DUS

Carotid DUS is the initial diagnostic test for evaluating extracranial carotid artery disease. It is a safe, noninvasive, and inexpensive imaging test. Meta-analyses of published criteria for carotid DUS have demonstrated sensitivities of 98% and specificities of 88% for detecting ≥50% internal carotid artery (ICA) stenosis, and 94% and 90%, respectively, for detecting ≥70% ICA stenosis (30).

Spectral and color Doppler imaging are ideally recorded with an angle of insonation of ≤60°. The spectral Doppler waveform provides measurements of peak systolic and end-diastolic velocities, as well as ratios of the systolic velocities, to quantify degree of stenosis (Fig. 10). Abnormal flow patterns evident at sites of arterial narrowing are shown by changes (i.e., aliasing or reversal of flow) in color Doppler signal.

Limitations of carotid DUS include acoustic shadowing from calcific atherosclerotic plaque, compensatory elevation in peak systolic velocity with contralateral ICA occlusion, and increased peak systolic velocities in tortuous vessels without stenosis. The inability to visualize intracranial lesions, distal tortuosity, proximal disease, and arch type may hamper decision making prior to carotid artery stenting (CAS). A stenosis of greater than 95% can cause the flow and the peak systolic velocity at the site of the stenosis to decrease. Low velocities consistent with a narrowed lumen assessed by color Doppler are referred to as the "string sign." This trickle of flow is consistent with subtotal occlusion.

Accuracy of diagnostic criteria may vary between laboratories and technicians. Therefore, it is essential for individual vascular laboratories to maintain a strict quality-assurance program and proper accreditation (www.icavl.org).

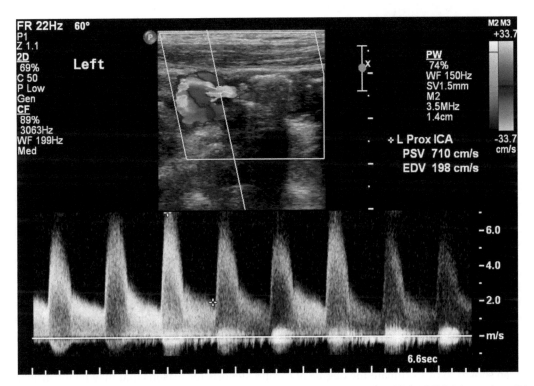

Figure 10 (*See color insert*) Carotid duplex ultrasonography, demonstrating critical (90–99%) left internal carotid artery stenosis. Note the peak systolic velocity elevation (710 cm/sec) and end-diastolic velocity (198 cm/sec).

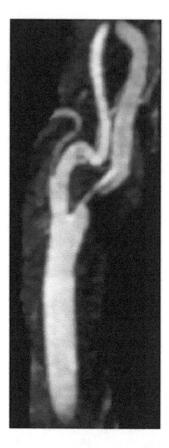

Figure 11 Magnetic resonance arteriography of the right carotid bifurcation, demonstrating a severe right internal carotid artery stenosis.

MRA

MRA of the cervical carotid arteries yields a 3D rendition of the entire carotid artery and offers the possibility of additional imaging of thoracic aorta and arch, intracranial circulation, and evaluation of cerebral parenchyma and other soft tissue (Fig. 11).

The accuracy of MRA in assessing severity of carotid artery stenosis has been shown to be comparable to that of other noninvasive imaging modalities. Using DSA as the gold standard, contrast-enhanced MRA (CE-MRA) showed sensitivity of 87% to 95% and specificity of 46% to 88%, 3D Time-of-flight MRA (TOF-MRA) showed sensitivity of 86% to 94% and specificity of 73% to 100%, and 2D TOF-MRA showed sensitivity of 84% to 94% and specificity of 94% to 97% (31–36). Recently developed 3D gradient echo CE-MRA sequences, which use k-space segmentation and temporal interpolation of k-space views, such as TRICKS (time-resolved imaging of contrast kinetics), allow imaging to be done in a fraction of the time required for conventional CE-MRA, and also permit time-resolved images showing distinct arterial and venous phases (37).

Disadvantages of MRA include cost, well-documented contraindications, administration of intravenous gadolinium in patients with renal impairment, and certain technical limitations. In all MR imaging, patient motion (including swallowing and vessel pulsation) can degrade image quality. Although the presence of signal dropout roughly corresponds to severe stenosis according to NASCET criteria (38), this relationship is inconsistent. Moreover, signal dropout occurs both with true complete occlusion and with slow flow distal to a severe stenosis so that TOF-MRA is unreliable for distinguishing these two conditions. CE-MRA is significantly less sensitive than TOF-MRA to flow artifacts but can still reduce its accuracy (39,40). CE-MRA has been shown to overestimate the degree of carotid stenosis for reasons that may be intrinsic to the technique (41), although the rate of misclassification of stenosis is low (42). CE-MRA may also be inaccurate in the presence of metallic surgical clips that introduce susceptibility artifacts (43), although this occurs with TOF imaging as well.

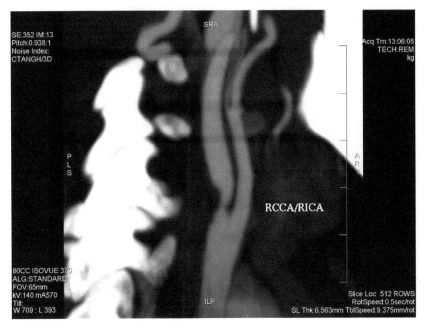

Figure 12 Computed tomographic arteriography of the right carotid bifurcation, suggesting ~70% internal carotid artery stenosis.

CTA

Although CTA exposes a patient to ionizing radiation and iodinated contrast, it has several advantages over DUS and MRA for carotid imaging. First, CTA has better overall spatial resolution than MRA, with smaller pixels providing more exquisite detailed vascular anatomy. A recent meta-analysis of the diagnostic accuracy of CTA for the assessment of carotid stenosis reviewed 28 studies that compared CTA with DSA (44). CTA was found to be highly accurate for diagnosing degree of carotid occlusion, with an overall sensitivity of 97% and specificity of 99%. For severe stenoses (70–99% range), CTA was found to be reliable, with sensitivity of 85% and specificity of 93%. Measurement of residual lumen diameter by CTA compares favorably to DSA, MRA, and ultrasonography (45–49) (Fig. 12).

There are several limitations of CTA for evaluation of ICA stenosis. Heavy, circumferential calcification of the ICA can cause beam-hardening artifact that can result in overestimation of stenosis (50). This may represent an advantage to CE-MRA, where dense calcification does not cause image degradation to the same extent as that seen with CTA. There are well-established risks associated with the use of iodinated CT contrast agents, as well as radiation exposure to such potentially radiosensitive tissues as the lenses and thyroid gland. For these reasons, CTA is not typically suggested as a first-line screening examination for asymptomatic or outpatient cohorts, but rather as a "problem-solving" tool when the results of screening DUS and MRA are discordant or when tandem lesions or other confounding factors that may influence surgery are suspected.

Plaque Characterization

Although the degree of carotid stenosis is the most widely accepted predictor of stroke risk, plaque morphology and ulceration are becoming recognized as significant risk factors for stroke (51) (Fig. 13). Intraplaque hemorrhage, commonly found in unstable plaques, has been associated with higher likelihood of recurrent ischemic events (hazard ratio = 4.8; 95% confidence interval, 1.1–20.9; $p < 0.05$) in patients with high-grade symptomatic carotid stenosis (52).

Ultrasound, MRA, and CTA have all shown some efficacy in detecting and characterizing plaque morphology (53). A study of 44 carotid arteries found both CTA (100% sensitive and specific) and CE-MRA (93% sensitive and 100% specific) to be highly accurate in detecting

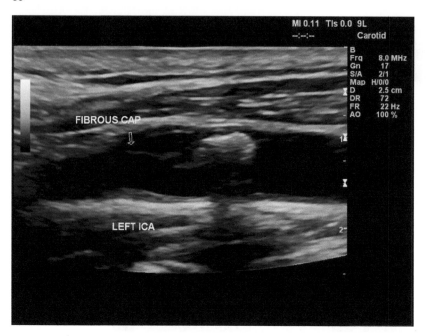

Figure 13   Gray scale carotid duplex ultrasonography, demonstrating lipid-laden plaque with a thin fibrous cap.

ulcerated plaques (54). DUS was less sensitive (38%) and specific (92%) in differentiating plaque composition and ulceration (53).

Knowledge of plaque morphology may influence the choice of stent and embolic protection systems used in CAS. A closed-cell stent may be preferable for the friable high-risk plaque, whereas an open-cell stent design would be acceptable for a more stale plaque with tortuous ICA anatomy. Furthermore, a "vulnerable" lipid-laden plaque may be more suited for proximal brain protection rather than a distal embolic filter, which involves crossing the lesion.

Anatomic Consideration

Unfavorable anatomy and significant contralateral stenosis (≥50%) are among some of the factors associated with increased complication risk during CAS. Aortic arch type (type 2 and 3), vascular anomalies (e.g., bovine anatomy), proximal and distal tortuosity, as well as occult tandem lesions, all increases the degree of difficulty for CAS and may be under-appreciated if DUS is used as the sole preoperative imaging test. By contrast, CE-MRA and CTA provide detailed images of arch, cervical, and intracranial anatomy. The identification of distal ICA tortuosity may preclude safe positioning of a distal neuroprotection device and a flow reversal system may be more appropriate. Assessment of intracranial circulation may be useful to predict patients with incomplete isolated hemispheres who are intolerant of reversal of flow and thus are not good candidates for this type of cerebral protection.

Complete signal dropout can occur on MRA with severe proximal ICA stenosis, despite the presence of a hairline residual lumen ("pseudo-occlusion"). Distinguishing between pseudo-occlusion and true complete occlusion has important prognostic implications. CTA is the most appropriate noninvasive method for differentiating these two entities because CT has higher spatial resolution and is unaffected by slow flow (55). A delayed CTA scan immediately following the arterial phase bolus administration is often helpful for the detection of hairline lumen when pseudo-occlusion is indeterminate secondary to very slow flow in the presence of a critical focal proximal ICA stenosis.

INDICATIONS FOR ARTERIOGRAPHY AND INTERVENTION IN CAROTID ARTERY STENOSIS

Conventional contrast angiography has long been considered the standard reference for imaging the cerebrovascular system. Single-plane angiography may underestimate the tortuosity of the

Table 2 High-Risk Anatomic Features for Carotid Artery Stenting and Endarterectomy

Carotid artery stenting	Carotid endarterectomy
Severe tortuosity of aortic arch	Lesion at C-2 or higher
Severe tortuosity of CCA or ICA	Lesion below clavicle
Intracranial aneurysm or AVM requiring treatment	Prior radical neck surgery or external beam radiation
Dense lesion calcification	Contralateral carotid occlusion
Visible thrombus in lesion	Prior ipsilateral carotid endarterectomy
Total occlusion	Contralateral laryngeal nerve palsy
Long subtotal occlusion (string sign)	Tracheostoma

great vessels, so orthogonal views, biplane angiography, or rotational acquisition is preferred. Although angiography is highly accurate in determining the degree of stenosis, it is less helpful in assessing plaque morphology. One study showed a sensitivity of 46% and specificity of 74% in detecting ulcerated plaques (56,57). There are inherent risks associated with invasive angiography, such as access site bleeding, contrast-induced nephropathy, and atheroembolism. The risk of neurologic deficits following cerebral angiography has been reported to range from 0.3% to 5.7% (58). In most cases, noninvasive imaging has come to replace conventional angiography in guiding treatment for carotid artery disease.

Cerebral angiography defines the aortic arch type, the configuration of the great vessels, the presence of tortuosity and atherosclerotic disease in the arch and great vessels, and the condition of the intracranial circulation, particularly with respect to intracranial stenosis, aneurysm, arteriovenous malformations, and patterns of collateral blood flow. Such information will influence choice of therapy and the interventional strategy. Anatomic high-risk features for carotid artery stenting and endarterectomy are shown in Table 2. Although decisions about the need for carotid endarterectomy are often made based on noninvasive imaging without carotid angiography, all patients being considered for carotid artery stenting must undergo angiography.

CONCLUSIONS

Imaging for peripheral artery disease has become sophisticated, safe, and accurate. For each of the three vascular beds discussed, we suggest that all imaging begin in the vascular diagnostic laboratory, utilizing physiologic testing (in the case of lower extremity artery disease), DUS, and if needed, axial imaging with either MRA or CTA. The choice of specific imaging strategies is largely based on the expertise by the technologists and physicians who perform and interpret the examinations.

DUS is the first line of diagnostic investigations *following* endovascular revascularization, as it is a reliable and useful tool and is able to image within metallic stents. MRA is hindered by metal artifact within stents, and although CTA may ultimately become the ideal test for stent surveillance, data is currently lacking for this indication. Organized surveillance of vascular stents may be clinically helpful in predicting adverse clinical outcomes in the face of in-stent restenosis.

REFERENCES

1. Hirsch AT, Haskal ZJ, Hertzer NR, et al. ACC/AHA 2005 guidelines for the management of patients with peripheral arterial disease (lower extremity, renal, mesenteric, and abdominal aortic): executive summary. J Am Coll Cardiol 2006; 47:1239–1312.
2. Ankle Brachial Index Collaboration. Ankle brachial index combined with Framingham risk score to predict cardiovascular events and mortality: a meta-analysis. JAMA 2008; 300(2):197–208.
3. Sikkink CJ, van Asten WN, van't Hof MA, et al. Decreased ankle/brachial indices in relation to morbidity and mortality in patients with peripheral arterial disease. Vasc Med 1997; 2:169–173.
4. Rutherford RB, Lowenstein DH, Klein MF. Combining segmental systolic pressures and plethysmography to diagnose arterial occlusive d of the legs. Am J Surg 1979; 138:211–218.

5. Darling RC, Raines JK, Brener BJ, et al. Quantitative segmental pulse volume recorder: a clinical tool. Surgery 1972; 72:873–877.

6. Koelemay MJ, den Hartog D, Prins MH, et al. Diagnosis of arterial disease of the lower extremities with duplex ultrasonography. Br J Surg 1996; 83:404–409.

7. Koelemay M, Lijmer J, Stoker J, et al. Magnetic resonance angiography for the evaluation of lower extremity arterial disease: a meta-analysis. JAMA 2001; 285:1338–1345.

8. Leiner T, Tordoir JH, Kessels AG, et al. Comparison of treatment plans for peripheral arterial disease made with multi-station contrast medium-enhanced magnetic resonance angiography and duplex ultrasound scanning. J Vasc Surg 2003; 37:1255–1262.

9. US Food and Drug Administration CfDEaR, Public Health Advisory. Gadolinium-Containing Contrast Agents for Magnetic Resonance Imaging (MRI): Omniscan, OptiMARK, Magnevist, ProHance, and MultiHance. http://www.fda.gov/cder/drug/advisory/gadolinium_agents.htm. Accessed December 2006.

10. Laswed T, Rizzo E, Guntern D, et al. Assessment of occlusive arterial disease of abdominal aorta and lower extremities arteries: value of multidetector CT angiography using an adaptive acquisition method. Eur Radiol 2008; 18(2):263–272.

11. Schernthaner R, Stadler A, Lomoschitz F, et al. Multidetector CT angiography in the assessment of peripheral arterial occlusive disease: accuracy in detecting the severity, number, and length of stenoses. Eur Radiol 2008; 18(4):665–671.

12. Nelemans PJ, Leiner T, de Vet HCW, et al. Peripheral arterial disease: meta-analysis of the diagnostic performance of MR angiography. Radiology 2000; 217(1):105–114.

13. Met R. Bipat S. Legemate DA. et al. Diagnostic performance of computed tomography angiography in peripheral arterial disease: a systematic review and meta-analysis. JAMA 2009; 301(4):415–424.

14. Mukherjee D. Renal artery revascularization: is there a rationale to perform? J Am Coll Cardiol Intv 2009; 2:183–184.

15. Taylor DC, Kettler MD, Moneta GL, et al. Duplex ultrasound scanning in the diagnosis of renal artery stenosis: a prospective evaluation. J VascSurg 1988; 7:363–269.

16. Strandness DE. Duplex imaging for the detection of renal artery stenosis. Am J Kid Dis 1994; 24:674–678.

17. Olin JW, Piedmonte MR, Young JR, et al. The utility of duplex ultrasound scanning of the renal arteries for diagnosing significant renal artery stenosis. Ann Intern Med 1995; 122:833–838.

18. Chi YW, White CJ, Thornton S, et al. Ultrasound velocity criteria for renal instent restenosis. J Vasc Surg 2009; 50(1):119–123.

19. Cohn EJ, Benjamin ME, Sandager GP, et al. Can intrarenal duplex waveform analysis predict successful renal artery revascularization? J VascSurg 1998; 28:471–481.

20. Zeller T, Bonvini RF, Sixt S. Color-coded duplex ultrasound for diagnosis of renal artery stenosis and as follow-up examination after revascularization. Catheter Cardiovasc Interv 2008; 71(7):995–999.

21. Young N, Chi K, Ajaka J, et al. Complications with outpatient angiography and interventional procedures. Cardiovasc Intervent Radiol 2002; 25:123–126.

22. Schoenberg S, Rieger J, Weber C, et al. High-spatial-resolution MR angiography of renal arteries with integrated parallel acquisitions: comparison with digital subtraction angiography and US. Radiology 2005; 235:687–698.

23. Schoenberg S, Knopp M, Londy F, et al. Morphologic and functional magnetic resonance imaging of renal artery stenosis: a multireader tricenter study. J Am Soc Nephrol 2002; 13:158–169.

24. Mittal T, Evans C, Perkins T, et al. Renal arteriography using gadolinium-enhanced 3D MR angiography: clinical experience with the technique, its limitations and pitfalls. Br J Radiol 2001; 74:495–502.

25. Gilfeather M, Yoon H, Siegelman E, et al. Renal artery stenosis: evaluation with conventional angiography versus gadolinium-enhanced MR angiography. Radiology 1999; 210:367–372.

26. Fleischmann D. Multiple detector row CT angiography of the renal and mesenteric vessels. Eur J Radiol 2003; 45(suppl 1):S79–S87.

27. Vasbinder GBC, Nelemans PJ, Kessels AGH, et al. Accuracy of computed tomographic angiography and magnetic resonance angiography for diagnosing renal artery stenosis. Ann Intern Med 2004; 141:674–682.

28. Creager MA, White CJ, Hiatt WR, et al.; American Heart Association. Atherosclerotic Peripheral Vascular Disease Symposium II: executive summary. Circulation 2008; 118(25):2811–2825.

29. Textor S. Ischemic nephropathy: where are we now? J Am Soc Nephrol 2004; 15:1974–1982.

30. Jahromi AS, Cina CS, Liu Y, et al. Sensitivity and specificity of color duplex ultrasound measurement in the estimation of internal carotid artery stenosis: a systematic review and meta-analysis. J Vasc Surg 2005; 41(6):962–972.

31. Anzalone N, Scomazzoni F, Castellano R, et al. Carotid artery stenosis: intraindividual correlations of 3D time-of-flight MR angiography, contrast-enhanced MR angiography, conventional DSA, and rotational angiography for detection and grading. Radiology 2005; 236(1):204–213.

32. DeMarco JK, Huston J III, Bernstein MA. Evaluation of classic 2D time-of-flight MR angiography in the depiction of severe carotid stenosis. AJR Am J Roentgenol 2004; 183(3):787–793.

33. JM UK-I, Trivedi RA, Cross JJ, et al. Measuring carotid stenosis on contrast-enhanced magnetic resonance angiography: diagnostic performance and reproducibility of 3 different methods. Stroke 2004; 35(9):2083–2088.

34. Johnston DC, Eastwood JD, Nguyen T, et al. Contrast-enhanced magnetic resonance angiography of carotid arteries: utility in routine clinical practice. Stroke 2002; 33(12):2834–2838.

35. Nederkoorn PJ, Elgersma OE, van der Graaf Y, et al. Carotid artery stenosis: accuracy of contrast-enhanced MR angiography for diagnosis. Radiology 2003; 228(3):677–682.

36. Scarabino T, Carriero A, Magarelli N, et al. MR angiography in carotid stenosis: a comparison of three techniques. Eur J Radiol 1998; 28(2):117–125.

37. Korosec FR, Frayne R, Grist TM, et al. Time-resolved contrast-enhanced 3D MR angiography. Magn Reson Med 1996; 36(3):345–351.

38. Huston J III, Lewis BD, Wiebers DO, et al. Carotid artery: prospective blinded comparison of two-dimensional time-of-flight MR angiography with conventional angiography and duplex US. Radiology 1993; 186(2):339–344.

39. Cloft HJ, Murphy KJ, Prince MR, et al. 3D gadolinium-enhanced MR angiography of the carotid arteries. Magn Reson Imaging 1996; 14(6):593–600.

40. Muhs BE, Gagne P, Wagener J, et al. Gadolinium-enhanced versus time-of-flight magnetic resonance angiography: what is the benefit of contrast enhancement in evaluating carotid stenosis? Ann Vasc Surg 2005; 19(6):823–828.

41. JM UK-I, Trivedi RA, Graves MJ, et al. Contrast-enhanced MR angiography for carotid disease: diagnostic and potential clinical impact. Neurology 2004; 62(8):1282–1290.

42. Patel SG, Collie DA, Wardlaw JM, et al. Outcome, observer reliability, and patient preferences if CTA, MRA, or Doppler ultrasound were used, individually or together, instead of digital subtraction angiography before carotid endarterectomy. J Neurol Neurosurg Psychiatry 2002; 73(1):21–28.

43. Phan T, Huston J III, Bernstein MA, et al. Contrast-enhanced magnetic resonance angiography of the cervical vessels: experience with 422 patients. Stroke 2001; 32(10):2282–2286.

44. Koelemay MJ, Nederkoorn PJ, Reitsma JB, et al. Systematic review of computed tomographic angiography for assessment of carotid artery disease. Stroke 2004; 35(10):2306–2312.

45. Anderson GB, Ashforth R, Steinke DE, et al. CT angiography for the detection and characterization of carotid artery bifurcation disease. Stroke 2000; 31(9):2168–2174.

46. Berg M, Zhang Z, Ikonen A, et al. Multi-detector row CT angiography in the assessment of carotid artery disease in symptomatic patients: comparison with rotational angiography and digital subtraction angiography. AJNR Am J Neuroradiol 2005; 26(5):1022–1034.

47. Josephson SA, Bryant SO, Mak HK, et al. Evaluation of carotid stenosis using CT angiography in the initial evaluation of stroke and TIA. Neurology 2004; 63(3):457–460.

48. Link J, Brossmann J, Grabener M, et al. Spiral CT angiography and selective digital subtraction angiography of internal carotid artery stenosis. AJNR Am J Neuroradiol 1996; 17(1):89–94.

49. Schwartz RB, Tice HM, Hooten SM, et al. Evaluation of cerebral aneurysms with helical CT: correlation with conventional angiography and MR angiography. Radiology 1994; 192(3):717–722.

50. Dix JE, Evans AJ, Kallmes DF, et al. Accuracy and precision of CT angiography in a model of carotid artery bifurcation stenosis. AJNR Am J Neuroradiol 1997; 18(3):409–415.

51. Wechsler LR. Ulceration and carotid artery disease. Stroke 1988; 19(5):650–653.

52. Altaf N, MacSweeney ST, Gladman J, et al. Carotid intraplaque hemorrhage predicts recurrent symptoms in patients with high-grade carotid stenosis. Stroke 2007; 38:1633–1635.

53. Saba L, Caddeo G, Sanfilippo R, et al. CT and ultrasound in the study of ulcerated carotid plaque compared with surgical results: potentialities and advantages of multidetector row CT angiography. AJNR Am J Neuroradiol 2007; 28(6):1061–1066.

54. Randoux B, Marro B, Koskas F, et al. Carotid artery stenosis: prospective comparison of CT, three-dimensional gadolinium-enhanced MR, and conventional angiography. Radiology 2001; 220: 179–185.

55. Lev MH, Romero JM, Goodman DN, et al. Total occlusion versus hairline residual lumen of the internal carotid arteries: accuracy of single section helical CT angiography. AJNR Am J Neuroradiol 2003; 24(6):1123–1129.

56. Streifler JY, Eliasziw M, Fox AJ, et al. Angiographic detection of carotid plaque ulceration. Comparison with surgical observations in a multicenter study. North American Symptomatic Carotid Endarterectomy Trial. Stroke 1994; 25:1130–1132.

57. American College of Cardiology Foundation, American Society of Interventional and Therapeutic Neuroradiology, et al. ACCF/SCAI/ SVMB/SIR/ASITN 2007 clinical expert consensus document on carotid stenting: A report of the American College of Cardiology Foundation Task Force on Clinical Expert Consensus Documents (ACCF/SCAI/ SVMB/SIR/ASITN Clinical Expert Consensus Document Committee on Carotid Stenting). J Am Coll Cardiol 2007; 49:126–170.

58. Connors JJ III, Sacks D, Furlan AJ, et al. Training, competency, and credentialing standards for diagnostic cervicocerebral angiography, carotid stenting, and cerebrovascular intervention: a joint statement from the American Academy of Neurology, American Association of Neurological Surgeons, American Society of Interventional and Therapeutic Radiology, American Society of Neuroradiology, Congress of Neurological Surgeons, AANS/CNS Cerebrovascular Section, and Society of Interventional Radiology. Radiology 2005; 234:26–34.

4 | Complex Vascular Access and Vessel Closure

I. Baumgartner, N. Diehm, and D. D. Do

Swiss Cardiovascular Center, Clinical and Interventional Angiology, Inselspital, University Hospital Bern, Bern, Switzerland

INTRODUCTION TO COMPLEX VASCULAR ACCESS AND VESSEL CLOSURE

The most convenient access route for peripheral arterial interventions is the common femoral artery. The femoral artery is a continuation of the external iliac artery. Its name changes as it passes deep into the inguinal ligament. The femoral artery is found at the midpoint of the inguinal ligament. The relationship of the femoral artery to other neurovascular structures passing deep into the inguinal ligament is expressed by the phrase *NAVEL*, useful to direct proper arterial access (Fig. 1). An arterial access without palpable pulse should not be performed because this is associated with increased complications such as bleeding, arteriovenous fistulas (AVF), or vasovagal reactions when repetitive punctures are needed.

The **retrograde femoral access** is the easiest and safest for peripheral arterial diagnostic and interventional procedures. The retrograde access becomes complex, with heavy calcifications of the femoral bifurcation, because of the risk of distal embolization or vessel occlusion due to plaque rupture. Moreover, heavy calcifications of the aortoiliac axis and an undersized or hairpin bending of the aortic bifurcation also makes crossover positioning of a sheath troublesome (see interventional strategies). The **ipsilateral antegrade access** has been advocated by many authorities as the best access site in patients with critical limb ischemia, especially when there is extensive atherosclerotic involvement of infragenicular vessels (1). The approach is technically more demanding, fraught by an increased risk of access site failure or complications (e.g., bleeding, dissection), and is associated with a steep learning curve as compared with the retrograde access (Fig. 2) (2). The antegrade access is challenging in obese patients or in patients with a high femoral bifurcation (direct puncture of superficial femoral artery [SFA] with increased risk of bleeding due to poor hemostasis; Fig. 3), as well as in patients with low body weight and with atherosclerotic lesions at the ostium of the SFA (compromised inflow with wedge position of sheath). Besides the risk of access failure and local angiographic complications, antegrade femoral access has other drawbacks, which include the inability to detect or treat proximal ipsilateral inflow lesions and contralateral or aortorenal lesions. Finally, while not substantial, manual compression on the femoral artery might be associated with an increased risk of ipsilateral vessel thrombosis, especially in those with extensive atherosclerotic disease and poor run-in or run-off.

The **transpopliteal retrograde approach** is a safe and efficient alternative after failed antegrade recanalization of the SFA or the use of re-entry devices (3). The **antegrade popliteal access** is described in rare instances with previous long-standing SFA occlusion and well-developed collateral reconstitution to approach infrapopliteal culprit lesions (4). The antegrade popliteal approach to obtain access to tibial arteries challenges the traditional tenets that critical limb ischemia can only be treated by establishing continuous in-line femorotibial flow. Below-knee lesions that could not be crossed by either of these techniques can also be approached via the tibial arteries. Even more technically demanding, and given the risk of iatrogenic vessel occlusion hampering bypass surgery, the **retrograde tibial access** should be limited to experienced operators. Perfusion of either the anterior or posterior tibial artery by collaterals at the level of the ankle is necessary, and these vessels have to be of sufficient caliber for percutaneous access (5).

The **brachial approach** is currently regarded as one of the most valuable low-risk alternative to avoid groin puncture, equivalent and sometimes superior to the femoral access in patients with absent femoral pulses, recent graft surgery, bilateral lesions of the common femoral artery, or occlusion of the iliac axis that does not allow for retrograde access of fragile femoral arteries (6). This approach gives high comfort to most patients and allows early ambulation. The brachial artery is found anteromedial to the upper arm. Access should be located about 1 to 2 cm above

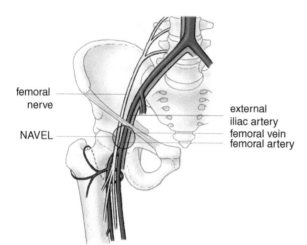

Figure 1 Relationship of femoral nerve, artery, and vein in the groin (NAVEL).

the antecubital fossa. In close vicinity there are the median nerves below the aponeurosis of the biceps brachii muscle and the radial nerve above the tendon of the biceps brachii muscle. Potential limitations are the long distance from the puncture site to that of intervention and that damage to the brachial artery can result in upper limb ischemia. To minimize, at least theoretically, the risk of cerebral complications, the left-sided approach should be preferred and heparin should be administered routinely.

HAZARDS AND COMPLICATIONS

The risk of complications for diagnostic catheterization is low (0.1%–1.1%), while in patients undergoing therapeutic procedures, with larger, up to 8-F (French) access sheaths and/or anticoagulation, this rate increases to 1.3% to 3.4%. The highest rate of complications 5.8% to 13.2% is seen in patients receiving a combination of heparin and multiple antiplatelet agents (7,8). Risk factors for vascular complications are patient-, procedure-, and drug related as given in Table 2. In a large, single-center, contemporary observational study, the female gender was the

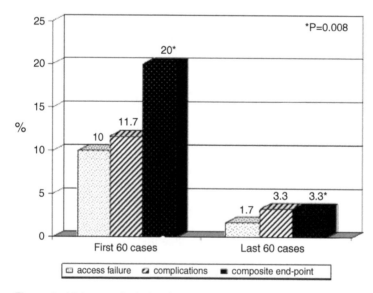

Figure 2 Histogram displaying the occurrence of in-training operator access failure, complications, and the composite endpoint of failure or complications, according to the caseload. All complications were adjudicated as minor and self-limiting angiographic complications, were conservatively and successfully managed, and did not cause interruption of the diagnostic or interventional procedure (28).

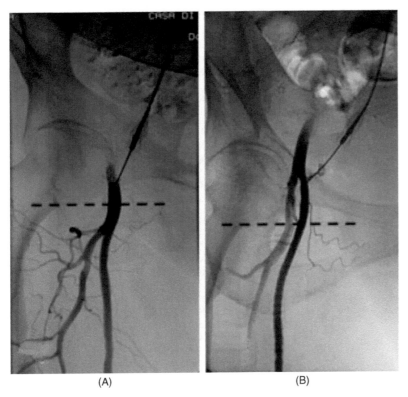

(A)   (B)

Figure 3   Panel A shows a case of low bifurcation. In such cases, the CFA can be easily punctured and cannulated even in obese patients. Panel B shows a case of high bifurcation. In these cases the CFA is more challenging. It may be acceptable to selectively puncture the SFA if this appears without significant atherosclerotic disease and of adequate size.

strongest independent predictor of any vascular complications with a risk-adjusted odds ratio for any vascular complication comparing women to men between 1.4 to 2.2

Most commonly observed and reported complications are access site bleedings, AVF, and pseudoaneurysm (Table 3). Most dangerous and lethal in 2% to 18% of patients is the occurrence of a retroperitoneal bleeding with an overall incidence reported to be 0.15% to 0.74%. Features of retroperitoneal bleeding include abdominal pain (42%), groin pain (46%), back pain (23%), diaphoresis (58%), bradycardia (31%), and hypotension (92%). The incidence of retroperitoneal bleeding is higher in patients with a low body surface area and in cases where the femoral puncture site is relatively high, that is, close to the inguinal ligament (9). The operator should always take measures to assure that the arterial puncture site is below the inguinal ligament (Fig. 4). Anatomy of the inferior epigastric artery has been pointed out to be an important predictor of femoral access site complications. The inferior epigastric artery is the last major branch of the external iliac artery before it crosses the inguinal ligament. Bleeding from the inferior epigastric artery can result from unintentional laceration of the artery during femoral access, high antegrade femoral artery puncture, or retrograde femoral artery access (10).

The transpopliteal access site is particularly prone to hematoma and AVF after sheath removal with manual compression. The overall complication rate ranges between 4% and 10%, with formation of an AVF in up to 4% of cases, which seems to be higher as compared with the femoral access. In a more recent series, complication rates were reported to be lower. Noory et al. reported 2.5% to 5.2% after manual compression (11). Yilmaz et al. reported an overall and puncture-related complication rate of 6.4% and 4.3% with 234 procedures in 174 consecutive patients with ultrasound-guided retrograde popliteal artery catheterization (12).

Major brachial access site complications are reported to be rare, with ≤0.6% in most studies using 6-F or smaller sized, armed sheaths (Table 4). In an earlier retrospective series, Heenan

Table 1 Clinical Indications for Available Access Routes and Closure Techniques

Access route	Closure technique	Indication
Retrograde femoral	Manual compression; plug-, clip- and suture-mediated closure devices approved	Standard access for diagnostic angiography and peripheral arterial interventions
Antegrade femoral	Manual compression; plug-mediated and clip-mediated closure devices safe in single-center case series (off-label use)	Enables access to very distal vessels (e.g., plantar or pedal arteries) remarks: – careful techniques to be employed – learning curve (access site failure, minor angiographic complications)
Brachial	Manual compression recommended, immediate ambulation; closure devices used in single-center series (off-label use), rather challenging with short subcutaneous access tunnel, questionable advantages	Most valuable low-risk alternative to transfemoral arterial access remarks: – intra-arterial administration of nitroglycerine to prevent arterial spasm – heparin administration to prevent thromboembolic complications – left-sides access preferred
Transpopliteal	Manual compression; closure devices (off-label use)	Retrograde popliteal access as alternative after failed antegrade recanalization of the SFA or to the use of re-entry devices antegrade popliteal access in rare instances with previous long-standing SFA occlusion and well-developed collateral reconstitution to approach infrapopliteal culprit lesions
Tibial	Manual compression	Experienced operators only remark: – interventional procedure from femoral access site to prevent larger sized tibial access and vessel trauma

Abbreviation: SFA, superficial femoral artery.

et al. reported on 62 brachial artery punctures in 53 patients over a five-year period. Catheter size ranged from 3-F to 8-F, 82% of the procedures were diagnostic and 18% were interventional. Glyceryl trinitrate was routinely administered. The overall incidence of complications was 8% and included hematoma and arterial spasm. However, none required surgical intervention, and all resolved without permanent sequelae (6).

In patients treated with oral anticoagulants the INR should be 1.5 if there is no urgent indication for treatment. Low molecular heparin should be stopped six hours and unfractionated heparin two hours before the intervention. In case of urgent need for treatment higher values up to an INR of 3 can be accepted if patients are not extremely obese. In these cases the crossover approach should be preferred as hemostasis is easier to be achieved.

Manual compression remains an unappealing, unpopular, and time-consuming part of the procedure. Noncompliance of the patient with lengthy immobilization may result in significant bleeding. Arterial puncture closing devices (PCD) have been developed to avoid manual compression and shorten bed rest (14). Relative risk of access site hematoma, local bleeding,

Table 2 Risk Factors for Vascular Complications

Patient related	Procedure related	Drug related
Female gender	Level of puncture site	Over anticoagulation
Advanced age	Larger arterial sheath diameter	GP IIb/IIIa antagonists
Hypertension	Prolonged sheath time	Thrombolysis
Obesity	Concomitant venous sheath	
Low weight	Need for repeat intervention	
Renal failure		
Low platelet count		

Table 3   Potential Vascular Access Complications

Complication	Frequency	Remarks
Hematoma	1.5%–12.7% – hematoma any size, isolated, and uneventful ≈10% – more severe with hemoglobin loss >2 g, need for blood transfusion or vascular repair ≈1%	High variability due to patient-, procedure, and drug related factors
Retroperitoneal bleeding	0.15%–0.74% (mortality 2%–18%)	Risk predictors: female gender, low body surface area, high femoral arterial puncture, ipsilateral antegrade femoral access, excessive anticoagulation
Pseudoaneurysm	0.8%–2.2%	Incidence lower with contemporary low-profile catheter systems Pseudoaneurysm repair: – ultrasound-guided compression (UGC) – duplex-guided thrombin injection (UGTI) – open operative repair UGTI minimally painful, can be done as outpatient procedure, anticoagulation therapy does not hinder success
Arteriovenous fistula (AVF)	Unknown	No systematic documentation in the literature
Dissection	0.42%–1.2%	Treatment: – not flow limiting → follow up – follow limiting → interventional treatment (long balloon inflation, stenting) – surgery rarely needed
Infection	Rare (< 0.3%) (related and nonrelated bacteremia 0.6%)	Septic complications, which included femoral artery mycotic aneurysm, septic arthritis, and septic thrombosis (0.24%). Risk predictors: duration of procedure, number of catheterizations at the same site, difficult vascular access, arterial sheath in place > 1 day, congestive heart failure
Neuropathy	Unknown	Direct access related injury of nerve or compression by large hematoma
Ischemia–thrombosis–emboli	0.1%–2%	High variability due to patient-, procedure-, and drug-related factors

AVF, and pseudoaneurysm using a percutaneous closure device (PCD) as compared to manual compression is not significantly different with 1.40, 1.48, 0.83, and 1.19, respectively. Relative risk of need for surgery, blood transfusion, and arterial leg ischemia after deployment of an arterial PCD was described to be 1.61, 1.21, and 2.10, respectively. From a large sized meta-analysis it was calculated that in a worst-case scenario for every 43 patients treated with a PCD, 1 patient will need surgery (15). Women show a significantly increased risk of developing severe complications secondary to the application of collagen-based arterial PCD, which is most probably related to the smaller arterial diameter at the puncture side (16). A serious complication with the use of PCD is infection of the puncture site, which is avoidable if meticulous techniques comprising resterilization of the access site and use of new draping and gloves are respected (17). Local infection, which can be fatal, has been described with the use of plug-mediated and suture-mediated systems (18). Embolization (of parts) of plug-related PCDs (19–21), and stenosis or occlusion occurring at the level of the puncture site have been described with the

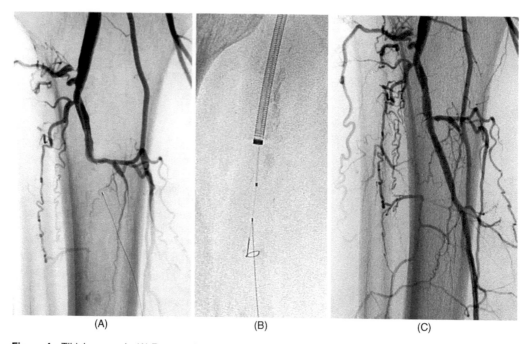

(A)   (B)   (C)

Figure 4 Tibial approach. (A) Retrograde wire passage through the vessel occlusion. (B) Snaring the retrograde wire from the femoral access. (C) Result after intervention (5).

use of suture- and plug-mediated PCDs. The presence of a severely diseased femoral artery seems to predispose to these complications (22,23). A femoral neuralgia syndrome caused by irritation of the anterior femoral cutaneous nerves is a rare condition that is related to the use of suture-mediated closure devices. Fascial closure, rather than arterial wall closure with use of the Perclose™ device has been described as leading to retroperitoneal hematoma.

Adverse events can be minimized by adherence to a few simple guidelines. PCDs should not be deployed if the arterial puncture is above the inguinal ligament or below the femoral bifurcation, if the vessel is diseased, or if the artery is less than 5 mm in diameter. Luminal compromise of 40% or more within 5 mm of the puncture site is an absolute contraindication for anchor systems such as the Angioseal™. Puncture should be restricted to the anterior vessel wall, as PCDs will not close the puncture of the posterior wall or multiple puncture sites. Relevant calcification that limits safe hemostasis using PCDs should be excluded by fluoroscopy. Some concerns have been raised about the possibility to re-puncture the access site after the use of PCD. This concern, especially directed towards collagen plug–mediated closure devices, seems not to hold true and re-puncturing can safely be performed.

Table 4 Complications After Brachial Puncture Observed at 30 Days (Consecutive Series of 88 Patients) (13)

Complication	No	(%)
Major complication	4	(4.5)
Hematoma > 4 cm in diameter or bleeding, requiring transfusion	3	(3.4)
Pseudoaneurysm	0	
Vessel occlusion or thrombosis	1	(1.1)
Minor complications	7	(8.0)
Hematoma < 4 cm or bleeding, not requiring transfusion	2	(2.3)
Oozing of blood	2	(2.3)
Arteriovenous fistula	1	(1.1)
Pain at the puncture site (up to 24 hr)	2	(2.3)
Overall complications	12	(12.5)

Table 5 Currently Commercially Available Devices

Closure device	Type	Puncture size (F)	Manufacturer
AngioLink EVS	Staple	6–8	Medtronic
Angioseal	Plug-wire	6–8	St. Jude Medical
Boomerang	Patch	5–6	Cardiva Medical
Chito-Seal	Patch	All	Abbott Vascular
Clo-Sur PAD	Patch	All	Medtronic
D-Stat	Patch	All	Vascular Solutions
Duett	Plug	5–9	Vascular Solutions
Elite	Plug	5–8	Datascope
Matrix VSG	Plug	5–7	AccessClosure
Neptune	Patch	All	Biotronik
Perclose	Suture	5–10	Abbott Vascular
QuickSeal	Plug	6–8	Sub-Q
Starclose	Staple	6	Abbott Vascular
StasysPatch	Patch	All	St. Jude Medical
SuperStitch	Suture	6–8	Sutura
Syvek Patch	Patch	All	Marine Polymer Technologies
Vasoseal	Plug	4–8	Datascope
X-site	Suture	6	Datascope

No superiority of any specific device has been demonstrated so far (27).

Many trials comparing PCD and manual compression used the earliest versions of such devices, a learning curve for the interventionist using such devices can be assumed and bleeding has not been further characterized in some studies. Major complications such as infection, hemorrhage, and vessel occlusion have been uncommon, ranging from 0.5% to 1.9% similar to those seen with manual compression (24–26). PCDs appear to be effective in terms of reducing time to hemostasis and allow early ambulation. Whether this translates into a clinically relevant benefit such as reduced hospital stay remains to be seen (Table 5).

INTERVENTIONAL STRATEGIES—TIPS AND TRICKS

Access material recommended to be routinely available in a catheter laboratory should include sheaths sized F4 to F9 (11 cm and 25 cm), sheaths with removable hemostatic valve for catheter aspiration F6, F8, F9 (Argon®, Maxim, Medical), long sheaths F5 to F10 (45 cm, 90 cm, optional 65 cm, and 100 cm; straight and shaped) for crossover and brachial approach as well as for renal and carotid interventions.

Access site complications can be prevented by a perfect puncture technique, use of different puncture sites for staged procedures, and nurse staff training for early recognition as well as patient education (e.g., coughing, heavy lifting).

The site of femoral puncture is localized manually, in the region of maximal arterial pulsatility at the level of the inguinal ligament, appreciated, whenever possible, by palpating it along the line drawn between the anterior superior iliac spine and the pubic tubercle [Fig. 4(A) and 4(B)]. Difficult femoral access in heavily calcified, stiff femoral arteries or in obese patients can be guided by fluoroscopy, centering the direction of puncture slightly medial to the center of the femoral head. Crossover access can be troublesome in patients with heavy calcifications at the aortic bifurcation. In these cases, access should be supported by stiff wires and armed crossover sheaths. Under rare circumstances, anchoring of an inflated balloon can be helpful to advance a sheath (Fig. 5). The antegrade femoral approach can be performed, thereby minimizing risk of major complications if stringent patient triage and careful technique are employed. In case of puncture of the deep femoral artery a road map using a small-sized dilator can guide safe direct puncture of the SFA.

The retrograde puncture of the popliteal artery is usually performed under fluoroscopic guidance (calcification) or with the assistance of duplex ultrasound due to the missing postocclusive popliteal pulse [Fig. 6(A) and 6(B)]. The posterior tibial artery can be accessed next to the medial malleolus and the anterior tibial on the dorsum of the foot. Most interventionists snare the wire after lesion passage from the femoral access site and the procedure is continued

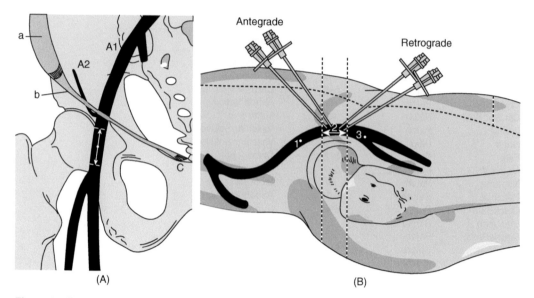

Figure 5 Femoral access route for peripheral arterial interventions below a line drawn between the anterior superior iliac spine and the pubic tubercle (inguinal ligament). **(A)** a, anterior superior iliac spine; b, inguinal ligament; c, pubic tubercle; A1, external iliac artery; A2, inferior epigastric artery. **(B)** 1, exteral iliac artery; 2, common femoral artery; 3, femoral bifurcation.

in a standard fashion from the original femoral access site to prevent larger sized access and vessel trauma distally (Fig. 7). Puncture size should be small using, for example, a 21-G micropuncture set. Usually a 0.018-inch guidewire can be advanced retrograde across the occlusion, followed by introduction of small-sized atraumatic dilator, and finally capturing of the wire with a gooseneck snare to be exteriorized at the original femoral access site.

CASE I
A 64-year-old diabetic female was referred from an outside hospital for treatment of severe recurrent claudication of the right calf. During the last six months prior to admission, the patient had undergone balloon dilatation of the SFA and popliteal artery twice [Fig. 8(A) and 8(B)], with the anterior tibial artery as the only run-off vessel [Fig. 8(C)].

What Made This Case "Complex"?
This case was considered to be complex because of severe calcifications and due to diffuse neointimal hyperplasia, resulting in a comparatively small diameter of the entire femoropopliteal

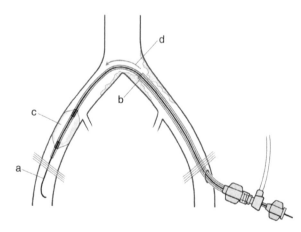

Figure 6 Complex crossover access. Balloon inflation at the level of the contra-lateral external iliac artery helps to advance an armed larger-sized sheath non-obstructive, excentric calcified plaques at the level of the aortic bifurcation. a, stiff wire; b, armed sheath; c, inflated balloon; d, crossover advancement.

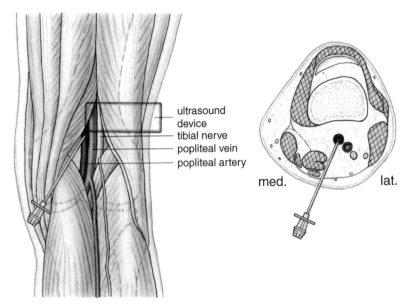

Figure 7 Transpopliteal puncture technique. (A) With the patient prone, the popliteal fossa is examined with grayscale ultrasound, and the popliteal artery (A) and vein (V) are identified on a transverse image. The two vessels can be easily differentiated based on their typical course and the degree of compressibility, thus the use of color duplex Doppler is not necessary. Note that the popliteal vein is posterior to the artery, increasing the risk of arteriovenous fistula if the puncture is performed in this position. (B) When the ultrasound probe is moved medially, the popliteal vessels can generally be visualized side by side, which helps avoid the popliteal vein. Note that the vessels are now superimposed by the semi-membranous muscle (SM) that forms the medial border of the popliteal fossa. (C) When the ultrasound probe is moved several centimeters caudally and tilted cranially, the semi-membranous muscle can be avoided because it tapers distally. The popliteal artery can now be safely punctured with a needle. Compression of the popliteal vein over the artery should be avoided to decrease risk of puncture of the vein and induction of an arteriovenous fistula (12).

arterial segment. Moreover, fibrosis of the puncture site in the groin following repeated arterial punctures rendered this case potentially challenging.

What Was the Clinical Indication for Treatment of This Patient?
Desired improvement of quality of life limited by severe calf claudication.

What Were the Potential Hazards of Treating This Patient and Anatomy?
Arterial rupture or flow-limiting dissection due to diffuse neointimal hyperplasia resulting in a comparatively small diameter of the entire femoral and popliteal arterial segments.

Which Interventional Strategies Were Considered?
- Re-intervention (redo plain balloon angioplasty and subsequent oral off-label use of rapamycin aimed at suppression of neointimal hyperplasia)
- Antegrade femoral approach allowing the use of a small sheath (4-F)
- Road mapping by injection of contrast media through the needle for advancement of a 0.035″ guidewire
- Introduction of 4-F sheath over the 0.035″ guidewire
- Percutaneous transluminal angioplasty (PTA) with low-profile balloon catheter using a 0.018″ guidewire
- Manual compression of the puncture site

Which Interventional Tools Were Used to Manage This Case?
- Antegrade puncture of the right common femoral artery resulted in a long dissection of the proximal superficial femoral artery (SFA) despite mild hand injection of contrast medium for road map (Fig. 9).

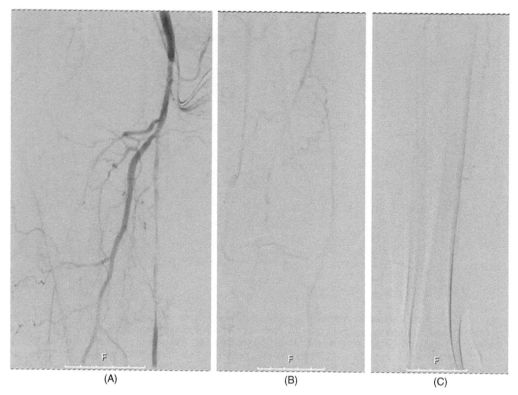

(A)   (B)   (C)

Figure 8 Baseline angiography showing severe neointimal hyperplasia of the femoropopliteal arteries and single vessel runoff via the anterior tibial artery.

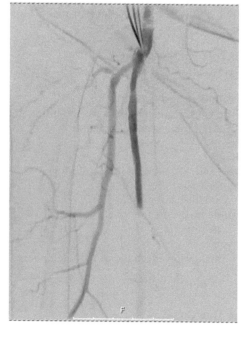

Figure 9 Long-segment dissection of the very frail superficial femoral artery after manual contrast injection.

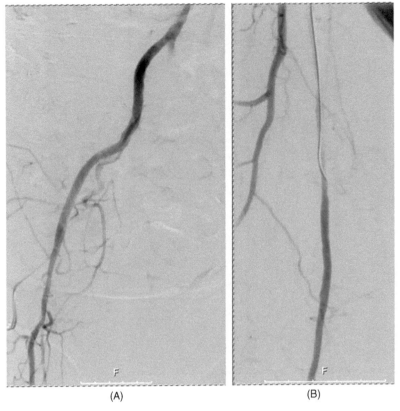

(A)   (B)

Figure 10 Crossover-access via the left common femoral artery (A) and catheterization of the true lumen of the right superficial femoral artery (B).

- Frustraneous attempt to catheterize the true lumen by advancement of a hydrophilic 0.035″ Terumo guidewire through the puncture needle using road-map technique.
- Therefore crossover access after retrograde puncture of the left common femoral artery and subsequently difficult but successful catheterization of the true lumen of the right SFA [Fig. 10(A) and 10(B)] using a 4 F single-curved supportive catheter along with a hydrophilic 0.035″ Terumo guidewire.
- Exchange of the hydrophilic 0.035″ Terumo guidewire by a 0.018″ guidewire
- Crossover balloon angioplasty of the entire femoropopliteal segment using a low profile 4–100 mm OTW-sv Fox balloon catheter [Figure 11(A) and 11(B)].
- The final angiogram demonstrated wide patency of the treated SFA and popliteal artery [Fig. 12(A) to 12(C)].

Summary: How Was the Case Managed, Is There Anything That Could Have Been Improved, and What Was the Immediate and Long-Term Outcome?

Iatrogenic dissection of a heavily calcified and thin SFA after antegrade femoral puncture was successfully managed using a crossover access and plain balloon angioplasty of the entire femoropopliteal segment.

On the basis of these experiences, we aim to use crossover approach in all patients presenting with heavily calcified ipsilateral common femoral artery and with proximally located femoropopliteal lesions and small arterial diameters.

List of Equipment Used in This Case

- Puncture needle (ANGIOKARD Medizintechnik GmbH, D-2947 Friedeburg, Germany)
- 4 F sheath (Terumo Medical Corporation, Tokyo, Japan)

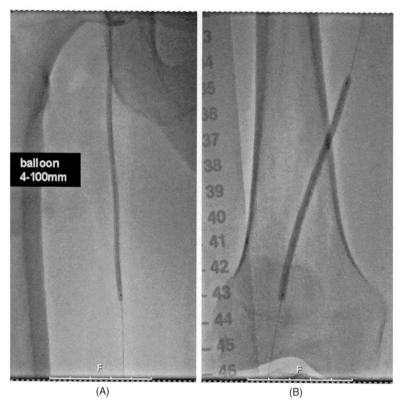

Figure 11   Crossover PTA of the entire femoropopliteal segment using a 4–100 mm balloon.

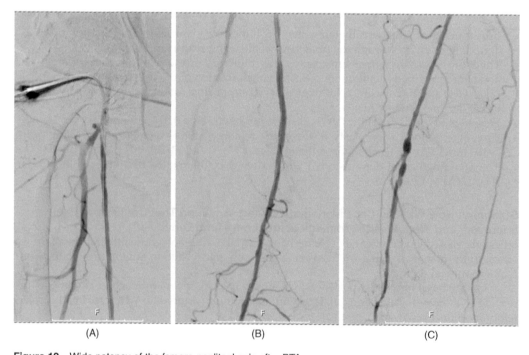

Figure 12   Wide patency of the femoro-popliteal axis after PTA.

- 0.035″ guidewire (Terumo Medical Corporation, Tokyo, Japan)
- 0.018″ guidewire (Pointer Nitinol guidewire, Angiotech, PBN Medicals, Stenlose, Denmark)
- 4 F RIM catheter (Cook Incorporated, Bloomington, IN)
- Balloon catheter 4–100 mm (svFox balloon catheter, Abbott Laboratories Vascular Enteprises Ltd. CH-8222 Beringen, Switzerland)
- Inflation device (Atrion QL2030, Atrion Medical Products, Inc. Arab. AL)

Key Learning Issues of This Specific Case

Antegrade femoral approach is associated with a considerable risk of dissection of access vessel, either by injection of contrast agent or advancement of the guidewire through the puncture needle.

In case of anterograde dissection, new access either femoral contralateral or retrograde popliteal should be used for better catheterization of the true lumen.

Chose contralateral retrograde crossover access in case of presence of ipsilateral heavily calcified access arteries and/or small caliber arteries.

CASE II

A 72-year-old male patient had undergone successful balloon angioplasty and stenting of the SFA for the treatment of severe lifestyle-limiting claudication [Fig. 13(A) to 13(C)]. Hemostasis at the arterial puncture site for which a 6-F sheath had been used was achieved using an AngioSeal® (St. Jude Medical GmbH, Eschborn, Germany) closure device. Postprocedurally, the clinical findings as well as oscillometry and measurement of ankle-brachial index revealed a

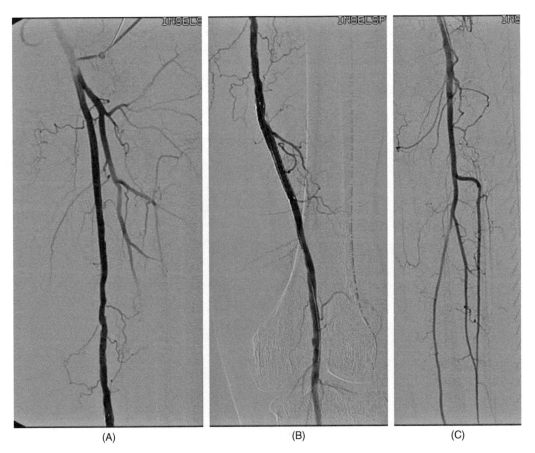

(A)   (B)   (C)

Figure 13 Angiographic result of successful balloon angioplasty and stenting of the femoropopliteal tract one day prior to readmission. The puncture site had been sealed using a closure device (AngioSeal).

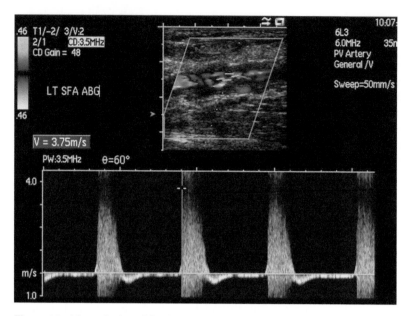

Figure 14 (*See color insert*) Duplex sonography one day postprocedurally showing a tight stenoses at the origin of the superficial femoral artery.

deterioration of lower limb perfusion at rest despite successful angiographic stenting of the SFA. Duplex sonography showed a tight stenosis with a significant increase in arterial flow velocity at the off-take of the SFA (Fig. 14). The lesion had not been visualized on the post-procedural angiogram the day before. It was suggested that the stenosis was caused by the dislocated anchor of the AngioSeal® closure device [Fig. 15(A)].

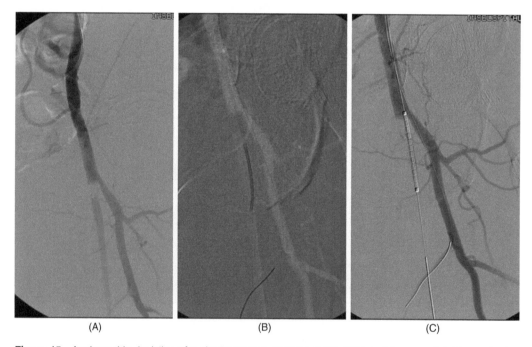

(A)   (B)   (C)

Figure 15 Angiographic depiction of a short-segment stenosis at the offtake of the superficial femoral artery most likely caused by a dislocated vascular closure device (A). Primary stenting using a Nitinol stent (B and C).

What Made This Case "Complex"?

Endovascular management of complications associated with the use of arterial closure devices has rarely been described. Bailout in the present case was considered complex due to the fact that the anchor of the closure device was located in close proximity to the orifice of the deep femoral artery.

What Was the Clinical Indication for Treatment of This Patient?

The remaining part of the closure device led to a severe stenosis at the beginning of the SFA resulting in a relevant impairment of arterial flow of the left leg.

What Were the Potential Hazards of Treating This Patient and Anatomy?

Endovascular treatment of the stenotic lesion of the arterial puncture site caused by the dislocated anchor of the closure device could have resulted in distal embolization potentially leading to further deterioration of limb ischemia.

Which Interventional Strategies Were Considered?

Surgical retrieval of the maldeployed closure device was considered. After interdisciplinary discussion, however, treating physicians agreed on an endovascular treatment attempt.

Which Interventional Tools Were Used to Manage This Case?

To secure inflow into the SFA and to prevent embolization of the anchor of the closure device, primary stenting with a self-expanded Nitinol stent in the distal common femoral, and the proximal SFA across the orifice of the deep femoral artery was performed [Figs. 15(B) and 15(C) and 16(A)]. Placement of this stent in that location led to a substantial narrowing of the deep femoral artery [Fig. 16(A)] that was managed by balloon angioplasty of the deep femoral artery through the stent struts [Fig. 16(B)], resulting in a decrease in the grade of the residual stenosis [Fig. 16(C)].

Summary: How Was the Case Managed, Is There Anything That Could Have Been Improved, and What Was the Immediate and Long-Term Outcome?

A dislocated anchor that had led to a subtotal occlusion of the proximal superficial artery was successfully treated by placement of a Nitinol stent across that device.

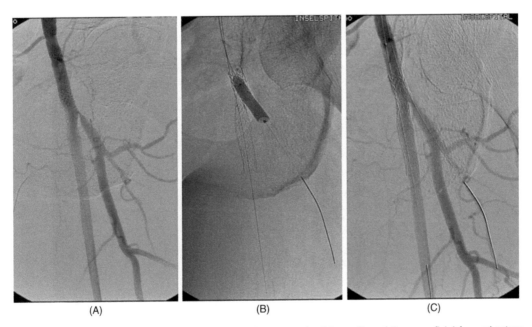

(A)   (B)   (C)

Figure 16 Placement of the Nitinol stent resulted in a stenosis of the orifice of the superficial femoral artery (A). Balloon angioplasty of the deep femoral artery through the stent (B). Final angiogram showing significant decrease of the stenosis of the deep femoral artery (C).

List of Equipment Used in This Case

- Puncture needle (ANGIOKARD Medizintechnik GmbH, D-2947 Friedeburg, Germany)
- 6-F 45-cm crossover sheath (Destination, Terumo Medical Corporation, Tokyo, Japan)
- 0.035″ guidewire (Terumo Medical Corporation, Tokyo, Japan)
- 0.018″ guidewire (Pointer Nitinol guidewire, Angiotech, PBN Medicals, Stenlose, Denmark)
- 0.014″ guidewire (Galeo Hydro Biotronik GmbH, Berlin, Germany)
- Nitinol stent 8–30 mm (X-pert, Abbott Laboratories Vascular Enteprises Ltd. CH-8222 Beringen, Switzerland)
- Balloon catheter 6–20 mm (svFox balloon catheter, Abbott Laboratories Vascular Enteprises Ltd. CH-8222 Beringen, Switzerland)
- Balloon catheter 5–20 mm (Viatrac, Guidant, USA)
- Inflation device (Atrion QL2030, Atrion Medical Products, Inc. Arab. AL)

Key Learning Issues of This Specific Case

Use of closure devices containing an intraluminal anchor can result in an obstruction of the puncture site due to the dislocated anchor. Successful endovascular treatment can be achieved by stent placement across the anchor. Balloon angioplasty of a stent-covered collateral vessel, such as the deep femoral artery, can be performed if modern Nitinol stents are used.

CASE III

A 70-year-old female presented with severe lifestyle-limiting claudication of the right lower limb. Ten years prior to admission, she had undergone kissing balloon angioplasty with stent placement of both common iliac arteries.

Present ischemic symptoms were attributed to a high-grade in-stent restenosis of the right common iliac artery [Fig. 17(A)] as well as to a significant de-novo stenosis of the right SFA [Fig. 17(B) and 17(C)].

After retrograde puncture of the left common femoral artery, a short 6-F sheath was introduced. The stenosis in the right SFA was dilated successfully using a 5–20 mm balloon.

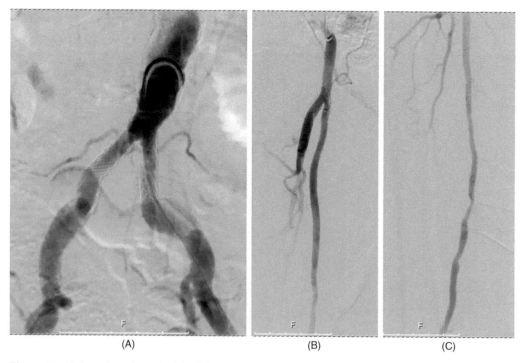

(A)   (B)   (C)

Figure 17 High-grade restenosis of the right common iliac artery (A). Widely patent proximal superficial femoral artery (B). Significant short-segment de novo stenosis in the middle superficial femoral artery (C).

Subsequently, the iliac stenosis was dilated using a 9–20 mm balloon which ruptured at nominal pressure in an oblique fashion. As a consequence, the catheter could not be retrieved.

What Made This Case "Complex"?

The oblique rupture of the balloon led to an umbrella-like configuration of the balloon so that it could not be pulled back through the crossover access.

What Were the Potential Hazards of Treating This Patient and Anatomy?

A forced pull-back of the ruptured balloon could have resulted in a severe damage or rupture of the common femoral artery.

Which Interventional Strategies Were Considered?

Besides an endovascular management of the present case, surgical extraction of the ruptured balloon would have been the only solution.

Which Interventional Tools were used to Manage this Case?

After retrograde puncture of the right common femoral artery the 0.035″ wire was retrieved using a snare (Fig. 18). A 45-cm 8-F sheath was introduced over the same wire and advanced over the aortic bifurcation in the distal segment of the left external iliac artery [Fig. 19(A)]. The same snare was advanced through the 8-F sheath to the ruptured part of the balloon [Fig. 19(B)], which was then retracted into the sheath after the shaft of the balloon catheter had been dissected using a blade. The sheath along with the ruptured part of the balloon could then be removed (Fig. 20). Figure 21 demonstrates the removed part of the balloon with the dissected catheter shaft (lower right corner), the snare, as well as the 8-F over the 0.035″ guidewire. The final angiograms showed patent femoral, popliteal, and tibial arteries on both sides without evidence of dissection and/or distal embolization (Fig. 22). The puncture sites on both sites were successfully closed with the STARCLOSE device.

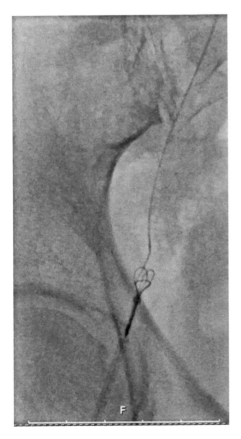

Figure 18   Retrieval of the 0.035 wire using a snare.

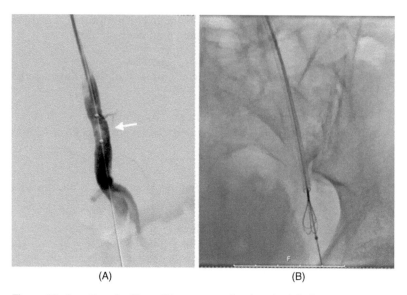

(A)   (B)

Figure 19 Insertion of a 45-cm-8F cross-over sheath to the left distal external iliac artery (A) and snaring of the ruptured balloon (B).

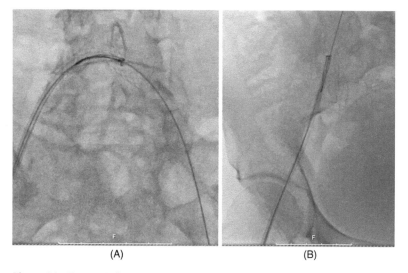

(A)   (B)

Figure 20 Removal of sheath and captured balloon (A and B).

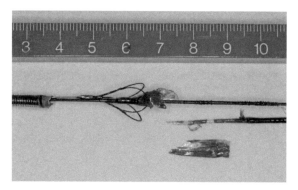

Figure 21 Photographic depiction of removed balloon and dissected catheter shaft.

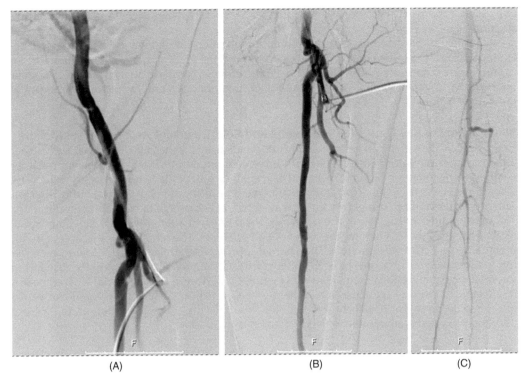

(A) (B) (C)

Figure 22 Final angiogram showing absence of peripheral embolization (A,B,C).

Final angiography showed widely patent iliac and femoropopliteal arteries without evidence of extravazation or distal embolization (Fig. 22). The arterial access site in the groin was compressed manually, whereas a PCD was used to obtain hemostasis in the left groin.

Summary: How Was the Case Managed, Is There Anything That Could Have Been Improved, and What Was The Immediate And Long-Term Outcome?

Oblique rupture of a PTA balloon in the right common iliac artery that could not be removed over the crossover access of the left groin because of an umbrella-like configuration was managed by extraction through the ipsilateral right side groin using an ENSnare system.

List of Equipment Used in This Case

- Puncture needle (ANGIOKARD Medizintechnik GmbH, D-2947 Friedeburg, Germany)
- 6-F, 10-cm sheath (Terumo Medical Corporation, Tokyo, Japan)
- 0.035″ guidewire (Terumo Medical Corporation, Tokyo, Japan)
- 4-F RIM catheter (Cook Incorporated, Bloomington, IN)
- 0.018″ guidewire (Pointer Nitinol guidewire, Angiotech, PBN Medicals, Stenlose, Denmark)
- Balloon catheter 5–20 mm (Fox Plus balloon catheter, Abbott Laboratories Vascular Enterprises Ltd. CH-8222 Beringen, Switzerland)
- Balloon catheter 9–20 mm (Fox Plus balloon catheter, Abbott Laboratories Vascular Enterprises Ltd. CH-8222 Beringen, Switzerland)
- Inflation device (Atrion QL2030, Atrion Medical Products, Inc. Arab. AL)
- ENSnare System 9–15 mm (Angiotech, Medical Device Technologies, INC. Gainesville, FL)
- 8-F, 45-cm sheath (Arrow International, Inc., Reading, PA)

Key Learning Issues of This Specific Case

Treatment of in-stent restenosis and postdilatation of a stented segment can be associated with the risk of balloon rupture due to friction between the balloon and stent struts. This risk seems to be high, especially in crossover approach for cases with in-stent stenosis after iliac kissing stenting.

During troubleshooting of interventional complications all endovascular means should be attempted prior to conversion to open surgery. Of note, the present case highlights that balloon rupture with consecutive difficulties in balloon retrieval can be managed by endovascular intervention. Awareness of adequate troubleshooting strategies and availability of dedicated tools are warranted.

Summary of the Key Issues for Successful and Safe Treatment Access/Vessel Closure
Heavy calcification at the access site and brittle small-sized arteries makes arterial access troublesome and complication prone. The most convenient access route for peripheral arterial interventions is the retrograde femoral access. The ipsilateral antegrade femoral access is advocated when there is extensive atherosclerotic involvement of infragenicular vessels, but it is technically more demanding, fraught by an increased risk of access site failure, and complications. The transpopliteal retrograde approach is a safe and efficient alternative after failed antegrade recanalization of the SFA and for the use of re-entry devices. The retrograde tibial access should be limited to experienced operators. The brachial approach is the most valuable low-risk alternative in order to avoid groin puncture in patients with absent pulse or recent surgery. Risk factors for vascular complications are patient-, procedure-, and drug related. Arterial PCD appear to be effective in terms of reducing time to hemostasis and allow early ambulation. Relative risk of access site complications such as hematoma, local bleeding, and formation of an AVF or a pseudoaneurysm is comparable to that of manual compression.

REFERENCES
1. Faglia E, Dalla Paola L, Clerici G, et al. Peripheral angioplasty as the first-choice revascularization procedure in diabetic patients with critical limb ischemia: Prospective study of 993 consecutive patients hospitalized and followed between 1999 and 2003. Eur J Vasc Endovasc Surg 2005; 29:620–627.
2. Nice C, Timmons G, Bartholemew P, et al. Retrograde vs. antegrade puncture for infra-inguinal angioplasty. Cardiovasc Intervent Radiol 2003; 26:370–374.
3. Beyer-Enke SA, Adamus R, Loose R, et al. Indication and outcome effectiveness of transpopliteal angioplasty. Aktuelle Radiol 1997; 7:297–300.
4. Feiring AJ, Wesolowski AA. Antegrade popliteal artery approach for the treatment of critical limb ischemia in patients with occluded superficial femoral arteries. Catheter Cardiovasc Interv 2007; 69:665–670.
5. Botti CFJ, Ansel GM, Silver MJ, et al. Percutaneous retrograde tibial access in limb salvage. J Endovasc Ther 2003; 10:614–618.
6. Heenan SD, Grubnic S, Buckenham TM, et al. Transbrachial arteriography: indications and complications. Clin Radiol 1996; 51:205–209.
7. Lincoff AM, Teheng JE, Califf RM, et al. Standard versus low dose weight-adjusted heparin in patients treated with the platelet glycoprotein IIb/IIIa receptor antibody fragment abciximab (c7E3 Fab) during percutaneous coronary revascularization. Am J Cardiol 1997; 79:286–291.
8. Dörffler-Melly J, Mahler F, Do DD, et al. Adjunctive abciximab improves patency and functional outcome in patients undergoing endovascular treatment of femoropopliteal occlusions. Radiology 2005; 237:1103–1109.
9. Farouque HM, Tremmel JA, Raissi SF, et al. Risk factors for the development of retroperitoneal hematoma after percutaneous coronary intervention in the era of glycoprotein IIb/IIIa inhibitors and vascular closure devices. J Am Coll Cardiol 2005; 45:363–368.
10. Kawamura A, Piemonte TC, Nesto RW, et al. Retroperitoneal hemorrhage from inferior epigastric artery: Value of femoral angiography for detection and management. Catheter Cardiovasc Interv 2006; 68:267–270.
11. Noory E, Rastan A, Sixt S, et al. Arterial puncture closure using a clip device after transpopliteal retrograde approach for recanalization of the superficial femoral artery. J Endovasc Ther 2008; 15:310–314.
12. Yilmaz S, Sindel T, Luleci E. Ultrasound-guided retrograde popliteal artery catheterization: experience in 174 consecutive patients. J Endovasc Ther 2005; 12:714–722.
13. Lupattelli T, Clerissi J, Clerici G, et al. The efficacy and safety of closure of brachial access using the AngioSeal closure device: Experience with 161 interventions in diabetic patients with critical limb ischemia. J Vasc Surg 2008; 47:782–788.

14. Abando A, Hood D, Weaver F, et al. The use of the Angioseal device for femoral artery closure. J Vasc Surg 2004; 40:287–290.
15. Koreny M, Riedmuller E, Nikfardjam M, et al. Arterial puncture closing devices compared with standard manual compression after cardiac catheterization: systematic review and meta-analysis. JAMA 2004; 291:350–357.
16. Eggebrecht H, von Birgelen C, Naber C, et al. Impact of gender of femoral access complications secondary to application of a collagen-based vascular closure device. J Invasive Cardiol 2004; 16:247–250.
17. Kahn ZN, Kumar M, Hollander G, et al. Safety and efficacy of the Perclose suture-mediated closure device after diagnostic and interventional catheterizations in a large consecutive population. Catheter Cardiovasc Interv 2002; 55:8–13.
18. Boston US, Panneton JM, Hofer JM, et al. Infectious and ischemic complications from percutaneous closure devices used after vascular access. Ann Vasc Surg 2003; 17:66–71.
19. Carere RG, Webb JG, Miyagishima R, et al. Groin complications associated with collagen plug closure of femoral arterial puncture sites in anticoagulated patients. Cathet Cardiovasc Diagn 1998; 43:124–129.
20. Eidt JF, Habibipour S, Saucedo JF, et al. Surgical complications from hemostatic puncture closure devices. Am J Surg 1999; 178:511–516.
21. Hoffer EK, Bloch RD. Percutaneous arterial closure devices. J Vasc Interv Radiol 2003; 14:865–885.
22. Ferreira AC, Eton D, de Marchena E. Late clinical presentation of femoral artery occlusion after deployment of the Angioseal closure device. J Invasive Cardiol 2002; 14:689–691.
23. Katsouras CS, Michalis LK, Leontaridis I, et al. Treatment of acute lower limb ischemia following use of the Duett sealing device: report of three cases and review of the literature. Cardiovasc Intervent Radiol 2004; 27:268–270.
24. Cremonesi A, Castriota F, Tarantino F, et al. Femoral arterial hemostasis using the Angio-Seal system after coronary and vascular percutaneous angioplasty and stenting. J Invas Cardiol 1998; 10:464–469.
25. Shammas NW, Rajendran VR, Alldredge SG, et al. Randomized comparison of Vasoseal and Angioseal closure devices in patients undergoing coronary angiography and angioplasty. Catheter Cardiovasc Interv 2002; 55:421–425.
26. Michalis LK, Rees MR, Patsouras D, et al. A prospective randomized trial comparing the safety and efficacy of three commercially available closure devices (Angio-Seal, Vaso-Seal and Duett). Cardiovasc Intervent Radiol 2002; 25:423–429.
27. Van den Berg JC. A close look at closure devices. J Cardiovasc Surg 2006; 47:285–295.

5 | Intracranial Interventions

Céline Rahman
Department of Neurology, Columbia University College of Physicians and Surgeons, New York, New York, U.S.A.

Johanna T. Fifi
Department of Radiology, St. Luke's-Roosevelt Hospital, New York, New York, U.S.A.

Philip M. Meyers
Departments of Radiology and Neurological Surgery, Columbia University, College of Physicians and Surgeons, Neurological Institute of New York, New York, New York, U.S.A.

PART 1: INTRODUCTION

Stroke exacts a great socioeconomic toll worldwide. It is the most common life-threatening neurological disease, the number one cause of adult disability, and the third leading cause of death in Europe, the Americas, and Asia. More than 780,000 people have a stroke annually in the United States alone, costing an estimated $65.5 billion in treatment and lost productivity (1,2). Intracranial atherosclerosis is a common cause of stroke, accounting for ~8% to 10% (3) to up to 29% (4) of cases of all ischemic events, and is particularly prevalent in persons of Asian (Japanese, Chinese, Korean), African, and Hispanic descent. Type 1 diabetes mellitus, cigarette smoking, and hypertension are risk factors associated with intracranial atherosclerosis (4–6).

Over the last two decades, the development of intra-arterial therapies for ischemic stroke has focused on acute recanalization therapies. More recently, angioplasty and stenting of intracranial stenosis for secondary stroke prevention in patients with intracranial stenosis has been studied. Though medical management has been the mainstay of treatment for both acute and secondary stroke management, endovascular methods are increasingly being used to prevent and treat ischemic stroke acutely and in patients who have failed medical therapy. While it is now possible in many cases to use endovascular methods such as intracranial thrombolysis, thrombectomy, angioplasty, or stenting to improve blood flow to cerebral tissue, identification of appropriate candidates remains a challenge.

WHAT MAKES A LESION "COMPLEX" IN INTRACRANIAL INTERVENTIONS?

Intracranial atherosclerotic disease is complex and endovascular treatment remains challenging due to anatomic and biomechanical differences between delicate cerebral arteries and muscular systemic arteries, specifically coronary arteries. The anatomical and structural peculiarities of cerebral arteries may in part explain the higher complication rates for intracranial revascularization procedures using techniques primarily developed for coronary applications. As such, some key anatomic features of cerebral vessels should be underscored, including the relatively small caliber and wall thickness of intracranial vessels, the lack of surrounding support of intracranial vessels, tortuous access to the intracranial circulation, the more distal location of the disease, relatively poor collateral routes, the variable configuration of intracranial atherosclerotic disease, as well as the suitability of available devices (7).

The wall composition of cerebral arteries contributes to the complexity of endovascular interventions. Cerebral arteries lack an external elastic membrane, and the boundary between media and adventitia is the outermost layer of the muscle cells (8,9). There is a dominance of the tunica media in intracranial arteries and a relative paucity of tunica adventitia. For this reason, cerebral arteries are prone to vasospasm, a potentially catastrophic complication if persistent. Furthermore, deficiency of the tunica adventitia predisposes cerebral arteries to rupture at much lower forces than coronary arteries. This has significant bearing on the revascularization procedures resulting in dilatation of cerebral arteries, where the arterial wall must be forcibly stretched. The wall composition also renders cerebral arteries stiffer in circumferential and longitudinal dimensions than other arteries, predisposing to failure with rupture at lower stretching forces (10–12).

Cerebral arteries are suspended in cerebrospinal fluid with little support from the surrounding perivascular tissue, the pia arachnoid. Furthermore, cerebral arteries are tethered to the brain by branching arteries measuring <250 μm, many of which are below the resolution of modern angiographic equipment. These fine branches can easily rupture with endovascular manipulation, leading to a catastrophic subarachnoid hemorrhage. Despite their overall small size, perforator arteries, arising from the major intracranial arteries at the base of the brain, supply functionally eloquent brain structures and occlusion of one of these perforators can lead to a functionally debilitating stroke. Therefore, a detailed anatomical knowledge of vascular and brain anatomy is mandatory in order to safely perform these procedures.

Finally, cerebral arteries are very tortuous. Compared with coronary arteries, they are located more distally in the vascular tree during transfemoral catheterization for endovascular revascularization. These anatomical features make precise and careful endovascular navigation through delicate cerebral vessels significantly more challenging.

CLINICAL INDICATIONS FOR TREATMENT OF COMPLEX LESIONS IN INTRACRANIAL INTERVENTIONS

Indications for Acute Stroke
After acute stroke onset, the core ischemic zone is surrounded by the penumbra, a region of hypoperfused brain tissue at high risk of infarction. The goal of endovascular intervention in acute stroke is to salvage the ischemic penumbra via reperfusion, thereby minimizing stroke burden and maximizing the patient's long-term recovery. Various procedures are already available for use and more are currently under investigation.

The PROACT II study, a randomized control trial, evaluated the use of intra-arterial thrombolysis with pro-urokinase, allowing for a six-hour window for stroke intervention (13). In addition, the Emergency Management of Stroke (EMS) Bridging Trial, a double blind, randomized placebo-controlled trial looked into the feasibility of combined intravenous thrombolysis followed by intra-arterial thrombolysis (14). In this trial, intravenous (IV) and local intra-arterial (IA) recombinant tissue plasminogen activator (rtPA) therapy was given in succession in patients with acute stroke who presented within a three-hour window. Bridging IA rtPA with the IV formulation appeared to provide better recanalization, although it was not associated with improved clinical outcomes in the EMS trial.

In addition, endovascular thrombectomy with the FDA-approved MERCI Retrieval System has been studied and shown to be both safe and feasible up to eight hours after stroke onset (15). The MERCI™ device is a flexible, tapered nitinol wire with a helical tip consisting of five loops of decreasing diameter, which is lodged into the clot akin to a corkscrew to allow for clot removal. Recently, the Penumbra device also received FDA approval for use in acute stroke. Penumbra is a suction microcatheter for clot aspiration (16). The FDA has approved both devices for acute recanalization of occluded cerebral vessels. Similarly, little data is available regarding the ability of the Penumbra device to improve clinical outcomes.

Basilar artery thrombosis is a special case of a devastating, potentially fatal, neurovascular insult in which acute endovascular recanalization may result in remarkable reduction in morbidity and mortality. Centers have reported successful outcomes in carefully selected cases with intervention up to 20 hours after stroke onset (17).

In the future, radiographic techniques to assess brain viability such as CT with CT perfusion and MR with MR perfusion may be used to better identify patients with salvageable ischemic penumbra. In fact, trials addressing this issue are currently ongoing. Such studies may further help with appropriate selection of patients for interventional procedures.

Indications for Elective Stenting
Patients are usually referred for elective intracranial angioplasty if they have failed "maximal medical therapy." Failure of medical therapy is a poorly defined term but connotes some persistent or recurrent ischemic neurological events, often transient ischemic attacks (TIAs) or recurrent ischemic stroke while on therapeutic doses of aspirin (≥ 81 mg/day), ticlopidine

(500 mg/day), clopidogrel (75 mg/day), warfarin [International Normalized Ratio (INR) $\geq$ 2.0], or IV heparin (prolongation of partial thromboplastin time > 1.2 $\times$ baseline value) (18–21)

The vascular evaluation of stroke patients often includes transcranial Doppler and carotid duplex ultrasonography, computerized tomography, angiography and/or magnetic resonance imaging (MRI) with magnetic resonance angiography (MRA). Intracranial stenoses in the large arteries accessible to angioplasty and stenting are usually apparent with these modalities. In individual patients, verification of the noninvasive studies with conventional cerebral angiography may be necessary prior to treatment.

The alternative to an interventional procedure is medical management of stroke, which is aimed at preventing stroke recurrence but, with the exception of IV rTPA, it does not generally address the initial presenting stroke. The current standard of medical management includes administration of IV rtPA activator (rtPA: 0.9 mg/kg body weight) if symptoms are identified within three hours of onset based upon the Neurological Disorders and Stroke rtPA Stroke Study (22,23). Several studies suggest that there may be a wider window for safe administration of IV rtPA; a pooled analysis of six randomized placebo-controlled trials showed that intravenous thrombolysis initiated within 4.5 hours of stroke onset resulted in better three-month outcomes compared with placebo (24). The safety and efficacy of IV rtPA, even in centers with little previous experience with this therapy, was also demonstrated in the European Safe Implementation of Thrombolysis in Stroke-Monitoring Study, which was required in Europe to assess the safety profile of rtPA in routine clinical practice, and the study found rtPA to be safe and effective (Wahlgren et al., 25). Still, estimates suggest that only 1% to 2% of ischemic stroke patients are in fact treated with intravenous thrombolysis in the U.S. The most common reason is delayed recognition of symptoms and patient presentation beyond the three-hour window. Large-scale public health initiatives have been undertaken to improve stroke awareness in an effort to get stroke victims to hospitals earlier. Stroke Center designation is a method to improve in-hospital policies and procedure to rapidly triage stroke victims for treatment. For patients beyond the three-hour time horizon for intravenous thrombolysis, modern neuroimaging such as MR diffusion and perfusion may help in the selection of those who may benefit from reperfusion therapies, and trials are ongoing to clarify these issues.

Medical management also includes initiation of HMG-CoA inhibitors suggested by the Pravastatin Therapy and the Risk of Stroke and SPARCL trials (26–28), and antiplatelet therapy, either with aspirin or aspirin combined with extended-release dipyridamole as suggested by numerous trials, including Chinese Aspirin Stroke Trial (CAST) (29), American Aspirin Trial (AAT) (30), Swedish ASA low dose trial (SALT) (31), the UK-TIA (United Kingdom transient ishemic attack)(32), and the ESPS 2 (European Stroke Prevention Study 2) (18) that demonstrated the efficacy of the aspirin-extended dipyridamole combination in secondary stroke prevention. In the case of intracranial atherosclerosis, the WASID trial showed that treatment with aspirin was preferable to warfarin (19,33). The CAPRIE trial showed a modest benefit of clopidogrel over aspirin in the secondary prevention of ischemic stroke (34). Angiotensin-converting enzyme inhibitors may also be used (35).

Particular attention must be paid to the differences in treating cerebrovascular infarction and myocardial infarction. Combination therapy with aspirin and clopidogrel is a commonly used regimen for cardiac patients. By contrast, dual antiplatelet therapy is not commonly used in the medical management of stroke, and has in fact been shown to be harmful in the MATCH trial (36). For acute myocardial infarction, glycoprotein IIb/IIIa inhibitors have been found useful, but they may also be quite harmful in stroke patients, as evidenced by the Abestt-II trial (Adams et al., 37), and is currently contraindicated. Largely based on coronary stent trials, dual antiplatelet regimens are still used after intracranial stenting.

HAZARDS AND COMPLICATIONS

Complications of intracranial stenting include embolic stroke, reperfusion injury, subarachnoid hemorrhage, and death. According to a recent study on the Wingspan stent, in cases with 70% to 90% intracranial stenosis, the frequency of any stroke, intracerebral hemorrhage, or death within 30 days (or ipsilateral stroke beyond 30 days) was 14.0% at 6 months, and the frequency of $\geq$50% restenosis on follow-up angiography was 25% (38). Another recent study investigated the durability of endovascular therapy for symptomatic intracranial atherosclerosis by studying 53 patients with a total of 69 intracranial lesions greater than 70% stenosis that were either angioplastied or stented. In this study, the 30-day death/stroke rate was 10.1% with one death, and within a median follow-up of 24 months, the TIA or stroke rate reached 5.8%. Restenosis rate at one year was 15.9% and was symptomatic in 18.2%. The restenosis rate was 50% for angioplasty and 7.5% for stenting (39). In a multicenter registry reporting 78 patients undergoing endovascular revascularization of intracranial stenosis, the major complication rate was 6.1% (40). High rates of early in-stent restenosis nearing 30% have raised questions about the viability of this therapy (41). An NIH-funded trial to address these and other issues is scheduled to begin in 2008.

Current data suggest a procedural mortality and morbidity in the range of 4% to 5% for intracranial angioplasty and stenting (42–63). Although one-year stroke rates differ a little from the medically treated population in patients having greater than 50% stenosis, more substantial improvements may be found in patients having greater than 70% stenosis.

INTERVENTIONAL STRATEGIES

Primary evaluation including neurological examination and noninvasive imaging is required. Generally, catheter angiography is not the primary diagnostic procedure for this condition, and it has been largely supplanted by cross-sectional imaging with CT and MRI. Conventional cerebral angiography may become necessary to assess the patient's vasculature as well as target stenotic lesions, when a revascularization procedure is contemplated. Then, the appropriate approach and devices are chosen in advance to facilitate the reperfusion procedure. A brief summary of procedure management follows.

PROCEDURE MANAGEMENT

Premedication

Combination therapy using aspirin with other antiplatelet agents has been shown in the coronary literature to help prevent early restenosis (64). The benefits of combination therapy have been extrapolated to the revascularization of cerebrovascular disease. Antiplatelet agents, typically clopidogrel or ticlopidine in addition to aspirin, are routinely administered one to three days before the procedure, if stent placement is anticipated. Some operators may administer an IV antiplatelet agent, such as abciximab before stent deployment if antiplatelet premedication is not used. However, there is both randomized trial data and anecdotal evidence that intravenous IIb/IIIa inhibitors may increase the risk of hemorrhagic complications in the ischemic brain.

Oral nimodipine may provide a neuroprotective effect, yet the benefits of this calcium channel blocking agent have been extrapolated from the subarachnoid hemorrhage literature. Intra-arterial injection of isosorbide dinitrate or calcium channel blockers such as verapamil via the guide catheter may help limit catheter-induced vasospasm. Preoperative administration of 10 mg IV dexamethasone and antibiotics have also been proposed, although the benefits remain unknown. Intraprocedural use of heparin as an IV bolus is common in neurovascular procedures, although there is little agreement on the loading dose or rate of infusion or the level of anticoagulation needed when high-level platelet inhibition is also present.

Anesthesia

Cerebral revascularization procedures have been performed successfully under both general and local anesthesia. Basilar artery lesions should be treated under general anesthesia because occlusion of the artery during balloon inflation can result in loss of consciousness and apnea. Patient immobilization facilitates visualization of severe stenoses in delicate cerebral arteries, possibly improving procedure safety.

Most intracranial procedures are often done under general anesthesia with use of paralytics to maximize safety and reduce procedure time. Complete cerebral angiography is important to determine the optimal working projection, assess collateral blood supply to the territory at risk, identify tandem lesions, characterize the length and geometry of the stenotic area, and guide further therapy if the revascularization procedure fails.

Care must be taken to limit the use of contrast during the procedure. The injured brain can be less tolerant of iodinated contrast than the uninjured brain. Nonionic, iso-osmolar contrast

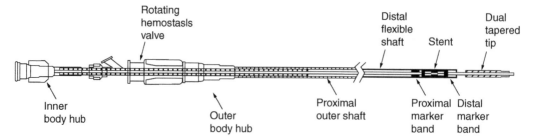

Figure 1   The Wingspan Stent System http://www.fda.gov/cdrh/MDA/DOCS/h050001.gif.

dosage should be limited as much as possible, despite good renal function with a maximum dose of 6 mg/kg.

Postprocedure Management

Ideally, the patient is extubated postprocedure, allowing for clinical assessment prior to transfer to intensive care unit with neurological specialists. However, for unstable patients, particularly those with blood pressure management concerns, extubation in the intensive care setting is prudent. The problems encountered by the neurologically injured patient are different from those seen in a standard medical–surgical ICU and warrant special attention.

Strict blood pressure control is mandatory in patients considered at risk for hyperperfusion injury. After revascularization and catheter removal, systolic and mean arterial blood pressure may need to be reduced by 25% to 30% to prevent hyperperfusion hemorrhage, which may complicate up to 5% of technically successful procedures (65), resulting in possible seizures, brain edema, hemorrhage, and even death. Cerebral perfusion imaging remains under development; however, many CT and MRI systems now offer perfusion imaging software to assess for this potentially fatal condition. Transcranial Doppler may provide surrogate information when compared with pretreatment measurements (65).

Acute or subacute stent thrombosis may result from platelet aggregation on stent struts and damaged intima. As such, clopidogrel or ticlopidine are used for up to 12 weeks postprocedure or longer. It must be stressed that these agents should be used judiciously, because both the MATCH and CHARISMA trials showed that the dangers of dual antiplatelet therapy in a stroke population outweighed their benefits.

INTERVENTIONAL TOOLS

The MERCI Retrieval System and the Penumbra device are available for acute stroke intervention while the Gateway™ balloon-Wingspan™ stent system, coronary angioplasty balloon catheters, and balloon-mounted stents are available for stroke prevention (Figs. 1–4). Angioplasty and stenting in acute stroke is experimental and not the standard of care.

SUMMARY OF OUTCOMES

Recent studies quote a high technical success rate of angioplasty and stent deployment of 96.7% to 98.8% (38–40). When compared with medical management alone (as determined in the WASID trial), no significant difference in the stroke risk at one year with treatment using a Wingspan stent was observed for the 50% to 99% stenosis group. In the 70% to 99% stenosis

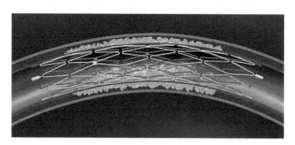

Figure 2   The Wingspan stent in place http://www.clevelandclinic.org/clevelandclinicmagazine/articles/stent.jpg.

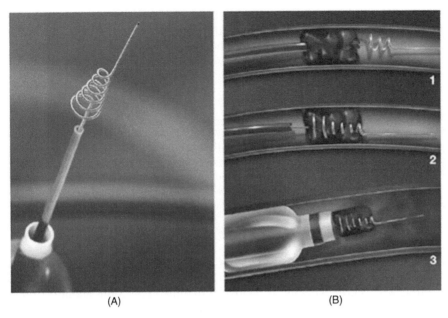

Figure 3 The MERCI Clot Retrieval System (A) The MERCI Device. (B) The MERCI Device in action http://www.nature.com/ncpneuro/journal/v3/n1/images/ncpneuro0372-f1.jpg.

group, there was a trend towards decreased risk of stroke in the stent-treated group, suggesting that the Wingspan stent may well represent a significant improvement over medical therapy in patients having a great degree of stenosis (i.e., 70%–99%).

EQUIPMENT CHECKLIST

There are numerous devices used to treat intracranial stenosis. Historically, many neurointerventionists have used devices designed for coronary revascularization on an "off-label" basis.

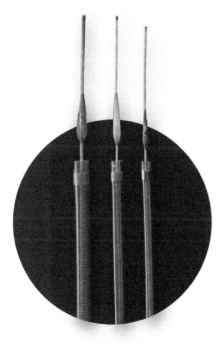

Figure 4 The Penumbra Device http://www.medgadget.com/archives/img/penumbra_system_new.jpg.

More recently, devices specific to the delicate cerebral circulation have reached the U.S. market or are under development. Currently, the only FDA-approved devices include the Gateway balloon and the Wingspan stent (Boston Scientific, Fremont, CA), the MERCI device (Concentric Medical, Inc, Mountain View, CA), and the Penumbra device (Penumbra, Inc., Alameda, CA).

PART 2: CASE PRESENTATIONS

Case 1: Intra-arterial Thrombolysis
A 62-year-old woman with multiple cardiovascular risk factors presented with quadriplegia, followed by loss of consciousness. After neurological assessment and head CT to exclude intracranial hemorrhage, she was brought directly to the interventional suite for angiography and emergent intervention. Given the short time between stroke onset and intervention, the clot is likely to be a soft, red one amenable to thrombolysis with an intra-arterial tissue plasminogen agent. However, it is hard to know in advance if the clot is a plasminogen-poor thromboembolus from the heart.

What Made the Case "Complex"?
The procedure is complex because vertebrobasilar occlusion is a life-threatening condition with a high risk of permanent morbidity and death. Patients suffer from autonomic instability due to brainstem dysfunction. Delays in diagnosis often lead to difficult decisions about treatment and risk of resultant hemorrhage. Brainstem and cerebellar infarction may require emergent neurosurgical decompression to prevent herniation syndromes and irreversible damage. Technically, the vertebrobasilar system, which supplies the brainstem, is tortuous, impeding access via transfemoral catheterization.

What was the Clinical Indication for Treatment of this Patient?
The acute life-threatening nature of basilar occlusion warrants emergent intervention in this patient. The risk of poor outcome and death following acute basilar artery occlusion is high and may exceed 80% (66).

What were the Potential Hazards of Treating this Patient and Anatomy?
The basilar system supplies the brainstem. Manipulation of this vessel system entails the risk of embolic complication as well as potential vessel rupture. Damage to the brainstem could lead to cranial neuropathies, respiratory compromise, locked-in syndrome, and potentially brain death.

Which Interventional Strategies were Considered?
Potential therapies for this lesion include intra-arterial thrombolysis and mechanical clot retrieval with the MERCI or penumbra devices.

Which Interventional Tools were used to Manage this Case?
Initially, a cerebral angiogram was performed to assess for obstructive vessel lesions. Intra-arterial thrombolysis using tissue plasminogen activator was used to dissolve the clot.

Summary
Cerebral arteriography via transfemoral approach demonstrated a distal occlusion of the basilar artery [Fig. 5 (A) and 5(B)] with absence of the bilateral posterior cerebral arteries. On high-magnification angiography, the filling defect resulting from the occlusive thromboembolism was evident [Fig. 5(B)]. A microcatheter was guided to the site of the occlusion. Microcatheter arteriography in the lateral projection further delineated the site of occlusion prior to thrombolysis with the plasminogen activator, urokinase [Fig. 5(C)]. Following lysis of the occlusive thrombus, complete restoration of flow in the vertebrobasilar system was present [Fig. 5(D)].

List of Equipment
- Prowler-14 microcatheter (Cordis Neurovascular, Miami Lakes, FL)
- Transcend EX guidewire (Boston Scientific, Fremont, CA)
- Recombinant tissue plasminogen activator (Activase, Genetec, San Francisco, CA)

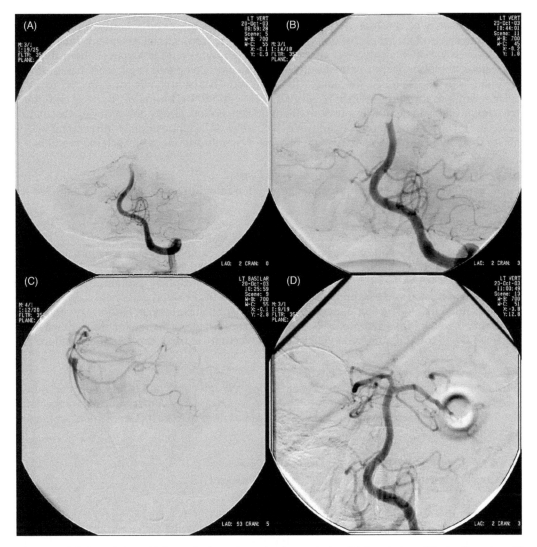

Figure 5 (A) Frontal view of left vertebral arteriography demonstrates distal occlusion of the basilar artery. (B) High-magnification angiography showing the filling defect. (C) Microcatheter arteriography in the lateral projection further delineates the site of occlusion. (D) Following intra-arterial thrombolysis with urokinases, flow in the vertebrobasilar system has been completely restored.

Key Learning Issues
A soft clot causing neurological deficits in an acute stroke patient can be successfully lysed with intra-arterial urokinase, without need for further vessel and catheter manipulation. However, mechanical thrombectomy may avoid potential hemorrhagic complications associated with thrombolytic agents.

Case 2: MERCI Retrieval System
A 75-year-old, right-handed woman with new-onset atrial fibrillation developed sudden right hemiplegia, neglect, and global aphasia during transesophageal echocardiography for evaluation for elective cardioversion. After neurological assessment and head CT showing no hemorrhage, he was brought to the interventional suite.

What Made the Case "Complex"?
Acute middle cerebral artery occlusion s associated with a high risk of major morbidity, even death. The time horizon for emergency revascularization is very brief. In general, intravenous

thrombolysis may be considered for acute ischemic strokes under three hours duration. However, large cerebral artery occlusions respond poorly to intravenous treatment. Intra-arterial thrombolysis in patients with large cerebral artery occlusions with less than six-hour duration has demonstrated improved patient outcomes at 90 days compared to placebo; however, this technique remains unproven. Mechanical thrombectomy has been shown to be effective to revascularize large cerebral arteries in 54% (MERCI device) and 80% (Penumbra), but trial end-points have not been evaluated for improved patient outcomes. Technically, the tortuous vasculature made the intervention complex. In addition, the vessel wall composition of intracranial vessels makes them more susceptible to rupture than the systemic arteries, with such intervention.

What was the Clinical Indication for Treatment of this Patient?
Emergent thrombectomy was undertaken due to the morbidity of sustaining a completed left holo-MCA stroke.

What were the Potential Hazards of Treating this Patient and Anatomy?
Given the patient's age and obvious potential for thromboembolic events, care had to be taken not to cause further embolic brain damage. As manifested by the patient's symptoms, an acute ischemic stroke involving the dominant cerebral hemisphere profoundly affected her language (expression and comprehension) and mobility (right-sided paralysis). Complications of intervention include further damage to her dominant hemisphere, potentially causing more morbidity than her initial symptoms. Reperfusion hemorrhage or malignant brain edema in the infracted tissue could require emergency hemicraniectomy to prevent cerebral herniation.

Which Interventional Strategies were Considered?
Intra-arterial thrombolysis is usually beneficial for soft clots only and is relatively contraindicated in patients with recent surgeries and those on anticoagulants. A mechanical thrombectomy device, such as the MERCI or Penumbra device, can be used to extract clots, without worsening a bleeding diathesis.

Which Interventional Tools were used to Manage this Case?
The Concentric MERCI device was used to extract the clot.

Summary
Left carotid arteriography showed intracranial occlusion of the left internal carotid artery [Fig. 6(A)]. The MERCI device, a mechanical thrombectomy device, was deployed through a microcatheter [Fig. 6(B)] using standard transfemoral catheterization technique across the site of the occlusion in the left carotid terminus and proximal left middle cerebral artery. Specimen photograph demonstrates the retrieval device and the occluding thromboembolus in two fragments [Fig. 6(C)]. Left common carotid arteriography post thrombectomy demonstrates restoration of flow in the left internal carotid, the anterior, and the middle cerebral arteries [Fig. 6(D)].

List of Equipment used in this Case
- 9-French Balloon-tip Guiding Catheter (Concentric Medical, Mountain View, CA)
- 14X Microcatheter (Concentric Medical)
- Transcend EX guidewire (Boston Scientific, Fremont, CA)
- X4 Thrombectomy Device (Concentric Medical)
- X5 Thrombectomy Device (Concentric Medical)

Key Learning Issues
Mechanical clot extraction devices can successfully revascularize acutely obstructed vessels. These devices should be considered in patients with acute large cerebral artery occlusions, contraindications to intra-arterial thrombolysis, or in those presenting for treatment between 3 and 8 hours post ictus.

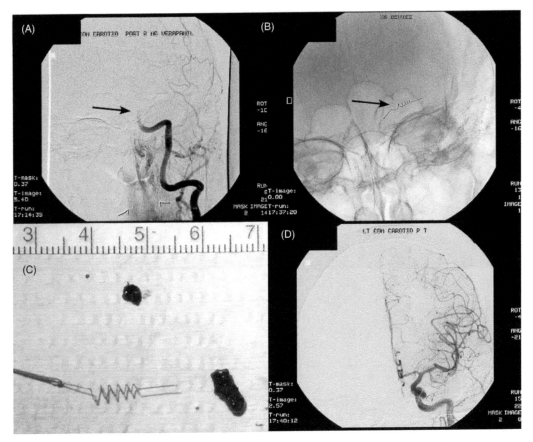

Figure 6 (A) Left carotid arteriography with opacification of the left external carotid artery branches but intracranial occlusion of the left internal carotid artery (*arrow*). (B) A mechanical thrombectomy device was deployed across the site of the occlusion in the left carotid terminus and proximal left middle cerebral artery (*arrow*). (C) Specimen photograph demonstrates the retrieval device and the occluding thromboembolus in two fragments. (D) Left common carotid arteriography post thrombectomy demonstrates restoration of flow in the left internal carotid, the anterior, and middle cerebral arteries.

Case 3: Wingspan Stent

A 68-year-old, right-handed woman presented with stereotyped episodic attacks consisting of speech arrest occurring over several weeks. She underwent a complete neurological work-up. MRA of brain revealed a critical left M1 stenosis [Fig. 7(A)], and diffusion-weighted imaging sequence showed an acute left frontal stroke [Fig. 7(B)]. She was started on antiplatelet agents and statins, but continued to suffer speech arrest TIAs. Her history was significant for ischemic cardiomyopathy with ejection fraction of 42% with diastolic dysfunction, 75-pack year tobacco history, dyslipidemia, poorly controlled hypertension, and daily alcohol use. Her examination was notable for some right/left confusion. Transcranial Doppler studies with CO_2 reactivity showed reduced cerebrovascular reserve in the left hemisphere and a risk factor for recurrent stroke (67). Because of continued symptoms despite maximal medical therapy, treatment with angioplasty and stenting of the symptomatic lesion was planned.

What made the Case "Complex"?

Intracranial revascularization using angioplasty and stenting remains an experimental therapy. On the basis of experiments performed on a small series of patients treated in Europe, Boston Scientific received provisional approval for their Gateway balloon catheter and Wingspan stent to treat symptomatic intracranial atherosclerosis with >70% stenosis refractory to medical therapy. The device has an investigational exemption and must be used with investigational review

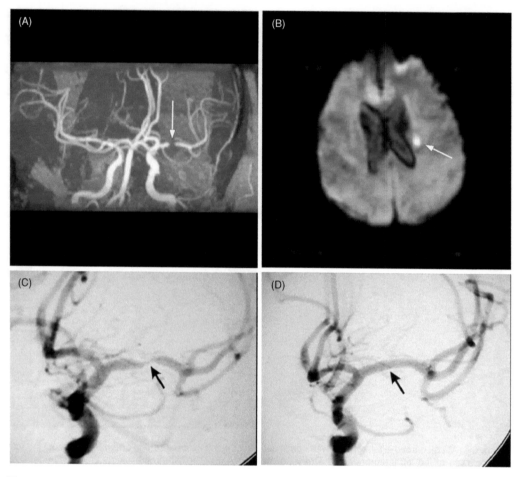

Figure 7   (A) MRA of brain shows a critical left M1 stenosis (*arrow*). (B) DWI sequence shows acute left frontal stroke (*arrow*). (C) Left internal carotid angiography demonstrates critical left M1 stenosis (*arrow*). (D) Restoration of the M1 luminal diameter after angioplasty and stenting with the Gateway balloon and Wingspan stent.

board approval. Because data on the Wingspan device remain limited, the U.S. Centers for Medicare and Medicaid Services (CMS) do not reimburse its usage. It is not yet clear that the natural history risk of intracranial atherosclerotic disease exceeds the procedural risk. Table 1 compares stroke risk at one year between medical therapy alone and stenting with the Wingspan stent.

Table 1   Comparison of Medical Management of Intracranial stenosis with Self-expanding Stents (Wingspan Stent System). Wingspan Humanitarian Device Exemption Study and WASID Study for Treatment of Intracranial Atherosclerosis

Design	Self-expanding stent (Wingspan)	Medical therapy (Aspirin versus warfarin)
Stroke risk at 1 year for:		
50%–99% baseline stenosis	9.3% (3%–22%) (4.5% procedural) $N = 45$	11% (9%–14%) $N = 569$
70%–99% baseline stenosis	10.3% (2%–27%) (4.5% procedural) $N = 29$	19% (13%–24%) $N = 206$

Table 2 Published Case Series of Intracranial Angioplasty

References (Angioplasty)	Number	Complications (%)
Higashida, RT (43)	8	38
Clark, WM (44)	22	12
Terada, T (45)	12	33
Takis, C (46)	10	40
Mori, T (47)	35	9
Callahan, AS III (48)	15	13
Marks, MP (49)	23	9
Connors, JJ III (50)	70	Variable
Nahser, HC (51)	20	5
Alazzazz, A (52)	16	13
Marks, MP (62)	37	8.3
TOTAL	259	

What was the Clinical Indication for Treatment of this Patient?

Elective stenting was undertaken in this case because the patient had failed medical therapy with antithrombotic medications, and a severe intracranial stenosis in the distribution of stroke was identified.

What were the Potential Hazards of Treating this Patient and Anatomy?

Given this patient's history of recurrent stroke and intracranial atherosclerosis, manipulation of her vessels has the potential of causing more embolic damage, particularly by perforator branch or target vessel occlusion, which may lead to a larger area of stroke and more severe disability. This would result in a permanent deficit in her dominant hemisphere in contrast to her reversible, though markedly symptomatic, ischemia during her TIAs. Vessel rupture could result in immediate death.

Which Interventional Strategies were Considered?

Angioplasty alone or angioplasty with stent placement were considered. Table 2 shows published complication rates for angioplasty alone and Table 3 shows those for combined angioplasty and stenting. A stent may provide improved short-term patency than angioplasty alone. This remains a topic of debate in the neurointerventional literature.

Which Interventional Tools were used to Manage this Case?

The Wingspan stent, specially designed for the intracranial vasculature, was chosen to keep the vessel walls open after balloon angioplasty. No residual stenosis was present following stent-supported angioplasty.

Summary

Cerebral angiography demonstrated critical left M1 stenosis [Fig. 7(C)]. A Gateway balloon and Wingspan stent were utilized to restore the M1 luminal diameter [Fig. 7(D)]. The patient recovered well and remains asymptomatic at three years clinical follow-up.

Table 3 Published Case Series of Treatment of Intracranial Atherosclerosis with Angioplasty and Balloon-mounted Stents

References	Number	Complications (%)
Mori, T (53)	12	0
Gomez, CR (54)	12	0
Levy, EI (55)	11	36
Lylyk, P (56)	34	6
De Rochemont, Rdu M (57)	18	6
Jiang, WJ (58)	40	8
Suh, DC (59)	35	11
Jiang, WJ (63)	213	7.98

List of Equipment used in this Case
- 6-French Envoy Guiding Catheter (Cordis Neurovascular, Miami Lakes, FL)
- Prowler-14 microcatheter (Cordis Neurovascular)
- Synchro-2 guidewire (Boston Scientific, Fremont, CA)
- 1.5 × 9-mm Gateway balloon catheter (Boston Scientific, Fremont, CA)
- 2.5 × 9-mm Wingspan stent (Boston Scientific, Fremont, CA)

Key Learning Issues of this Specific Case
Intracranial stenting is indicated in patients who have failed maximal medical therapy for secondary stroke prevention and can successfully revascularize severely stenotic vessels to prevent artery-to-artery embolism and improve cerebral perfusion.

PART 3: SUMMARY OF THE KEY ISSUES FOR SUCCESSFUL AND SAFE TREATMENT OF COMPLEX LESIONS IN THIS VESSEL AREA
The goal of all the described intracranial interventions is the reduction in the morbidity and mortality of ischemic strokes. Challenges to these goals include choosing the appropriate timing and type of intervention as well as identifying the appropriate candidates for the procedures. Significant advances have been made in the treatment of cerebrovascular disease, particularly through the advent of more specialized intracranial endovascular devices. However, the roles of these devices and interventions remain to be proven.

REFERENCES
1. Rosamond W, Flegal K, Furie et al. Heart disease and stroke statistics 2008 update: a report from the American Heart Association Statistics Committee and Stroke Statistics Subcommittee. Circulation 2008; 117:e25–e146.
2. Taylor TN, Torner JC, Holmes J, et al. Lifetime cost of stroke in the United States. Stroke 1996; 27:1459–1466.
3. Sacco RL Kargman DE, Gu Q, et al. Race-ethnicity and determinants of intracranial atherosclerotic cerebral infarction. The Northern Manhattan Stroke Study. Stroke 1995; 26:14–20.
4. Rundek T, Chen X. Increased early stroke recurrence among patients with extracranial and intracranial atherosclerosis: Northern Manhattan Stroke Study. Neurology 1998; 50:A75.
5. Caplan LR, Hier DB. Race, sex and occlusive cerebrovascular disease: a review. Stroke 1986; 17; 648–655.
6. Ingall TJ, Horner D, Baker HL Jr, et al. Predictors of intracranial carotid artery atherosclerosis. Duration of cigarette smoking and hypertension are more powerful than serum lipid levels. Arch Neurol 1991; 48:687–691.
7. Hurst R. Interventional Neuroradiology in Intracranial Lesions. Medlink 2007. www.medlink.com.
8. Stehbens W. Pathology of Cerebral Blood Vessels. St. Louis, MO: Mosby, 1972.
9. Ross MH, Romrell LJ, Kaye GI. Histology: a text and Atlas. Baltimore, MD: Williams & Wilkins, 1995.
10. Busby DE, Burton AC. The effect of age on the elasticity of the major brain arteries. Can J Physiol Pharmacol 1965; 43:185–202.
11. Hayashi K, Nagasawa S, Naruo Y, et al. Mechanical properties of human cerebral arteries. Biorheology 1980; 17:211–218.
12. Monson KL Goldsmith W, Barbaro NM, et al. Axial mechanical properties of fresh human cerebral blood vessels. J Biomech Eng 2003; 125:288–294.
13. Furlan A, Higashida R, Wechsler L, et al. Intraarterial prourokinase for acute ischemic stroke. The PROACT II study: a randomized controlled trial. Prolyse in Acute Cerebral Thromboembolism. JAMA 1999; 282(21):2003–2011.
14. Lewandowski CA, Frankel M, Tomsick TA, et al. Combined intravenous and intraarterial r-tpa versus intraarterial therapy of acute ischemic stroke: emergency management of stroke (EMS) bridging trial. Stroke 1999; 30:2598–2605.
15. Gobin PY, Starkman S, Duckwiler GR, et al. MERCI 1. Stroke 2004; 35:2848–2854.
16. US Food and Drug Administration. Summary for the Penumbra Device. US Food and Drug Administration, 2006. www.fda.gov/cdrh/pdf5/K053491.pdf. Accessed February 12, 2006.
17. Yu W, Foster-Barber A, Malek R, et al. Endovascular embolectomy of acute basilar artery occlusion. Neurology 2003; 61:1421–1423.
18. Diener HC, Cunha L, Forbes C, et al. European stroke prevention study 2. Dipyridamole and acetyl-salicylic acid in the secondary prevention of stroke. J Neurol Sci 1996; 143:1–13.

19. Chimowitz MI, Lynn MJ, Howlett-Smith H, et al. Comparison of warfarin and aspirin for symptomatic intracranial arterial stenosis. N Engl J Med 2005; 352:1305–1316.
20. Thijs VN. Symptomatic intracranial atherosclerosis: outcome of patients who fail antithrombotic therapy. Neurology 2000; 55:490–497.
21. Mohr JP, Thompson JL, Lazar RM, et al. A comparison of warfarin and aspirin for the prevention of recurrent ischemic stroke. N Engl J Med 2001; 345:1444–1451.
22. The National Institute of Neurological Disorders and Stroke rt-PA Stroke Study Group. Tissue plasminogen activator for acute ischemic stroke. N Engl J Med 1995; 333:1581–1587.
23. Kwiatkowski TG, Libman R, Frankel M, et al. Effects of tissue plasminogen activator for acute ischemic stroke at one year. National institute of neurological disorders and stroke recombinant tissue plasminogen activator stroke study group. N Engl J Med 1999; 340:1781–1787.
24. Schellinger PD, Hacke W. An update on thrombolytic therapy for acute stroke. Curr Opin Neurol 2004; 17:69–77.
25. Wahlgren N, Dávalos A, Ford GA, et al. SITS-MOST investigators. Thrombolysis with alteplase for acute ischaemic stroke in the safe implementation of thrombolysis in stroke-monitoring study (SITS-MOST): an observational study. Lancet 2007; 369:275–282.
26. White HD, Simes RJ, Anderson NE, et al. Pravastatin therapy and the risk of stroke. N Engl J Med 2000; 343:317–326.
27. Amarenco P, Callahan A III, Goldstein LB, et al. Stroke prevention by aggressive reduction in cholesterol levels (SPARCL) investigators. N Engl J Med 2006; 355:549–559.
28. Heart Protection Study Collaborative Group. MRC/BHF heart protection study of cholesterol lowering with simvastatin in 20,536 high-risk individuals: a randomised placebo-controlled trial. Lancet 2002; 360:7–22.
29. CAST (Chinese Acute Stroke Trial) Collaborative Group. CAST: randomised placebo-controlled trial of early aspirin use in 20,000 patients with acute ischaemic stroke. Lancet 1997; 349:1641.
30. Fields WS, Frankowski RF, Hardy RJ. Controlled trial of aspirin in cerebral ischemia. Stroke 1977; 8:301.
31. The SALT Collaborative Group. Swedish aspirin low-dose trial (SALT) of 75 mg aspirin as secondary prophylaxis after cerebrovascular ischaemic events. Lancet 1991; 338:1345.
32. Farrell B, Richards S, Warlow C. The United Kingdom transient ischaemic attack (UK-TIA) aspirin trial: final results. J Neurol Neurosurg Psychiatry 1991; 54:1044.
33. Chimowitz MI, Kokkinos J, Strong J, et al. The warfarin-aspirin symptomatic intracranial disease study. Neurology 1995; 45:1488–1493.
34. CAPRIE Steering Committee. A randomised, blinded, trial of clopidogrel versus aspirin in patients at risk of ischaemic events (CAPRIE). Lancet 1996; 348:1329–1339.
35. The Heart Outcomes Prevention Evaluation Study Investigators. Effects of an angiotensin-converting-enzyme inhibitor, ramipril, on cardiovascular events in high-risk patients. N Engl J Med 2000; 342:145–153.
36. Diener HC, Bogousslavsky J, Brass LM, et al. Aspirin and clopidogrel compared with clopidogrel alone after recent ischaemic stroke or transient ischaemic attack in high-risk patients (MATCH): randomised, double-blind, placebo-controlled trial. Lancet 2004; 364:331–337.
37. Adams HP Jr, Effron M, Torner J, et al. Emergency administration of abciximab for treatment of patients with acute ischemic stroke: results of an international phase III trial: Abciximab in Emergency Treatment of Stroke Trial (AbESTT-II). Stroke 2008; 39(1):87–99.
38. Zaidat OO, Klucznik R, Alexander MJ, et al. The NIH registry on use of the Wingspan stent for symptomatic 70–99% intracranial arterial stenosis. Neurology 2008; 70(17):1518–1524.
39. Mazighi M, Abou-Chebl A. Durability of endovascular therapy for symptomatic intracranial atherosclerosis. Stroke 2008; 39(6):1766–1769.
40. Fiorella D, Levy E, Turk AS, et al. US multicenter experience with the wingspan stent system for the treatment of intracranial atheromatous disease: periprocedural results. Stroke 2007; 38:881–887.
41. Levy EI, Turk AS, Albuquerque FC, et al. Wingspan in-stent restenosis and thrombosis: incidence, clinical presentation, and management. Neurosurgery 2007; 61:644–650.
42. Eckard DA, Zarnow DM, McPherson CM, et al. Intracranial internal carotid artery angioplasty: technique with clinical and radiographic results and follow-up. AJR Am J Roentgenol 1999; 172:703–707.
43. Higashida RT, Tsai FY, Halback VV, et al. Transluminal angioplasty for atherosclerotic disease of the vertebral and basilar arteries. J Neurosurg 1993; 78:268–272.
44. Clark WM, Nesbit G, O'Neill OR, et al. Safety and efficacy of percutaneous transluminal angiolasty for intracranial atherosclerotic stenosis. Stroke 1995; 26:1200–1204.
45. Terada T, Higashida RT, Halbach VV, et al. Transluminal angioplasty for atherosclerotic disease of the distal vertebral and basilar arteries. J Neurol Neurosurg Psychiatry 1996; 60:377–381.

46. Takis C, Pessin MS, Jacobs DH, et al. Intracranial angioplasty: experience and complications. Am J Neuroradiol 1997; 18:1661–1668.
47. Mori T, Kazita K, Mori K. Percutaneous transluminal cerebral angioplasty: serial angiographic follow-up after successful dilatation. Neuroradiology 1997; 39:111–116.
48. Callahan AS III. Balloon angioplasty of intracranial arteries for stroke prevention. J Neuroimaging 1997; 7:323–325.
49. Marks MP, Norbash AM, Steinberg GK, et al. Outcome of angioplasty for atherosclerotic intracranial stenosis. Stroke 1999; 30:1065–1069.
50. Connors JJ III. Percutaneous transluminal angioplasty for intracranial atherosclerotic lesions: evolution of technique and short-term results. J Neurosurg 1999; 91:415–423.
51. Nahser HC, Henkes H, Weber W, et al. Intracranial vertebrobasilar stenosis: angioplasty and follow-up. Am J Neuroradiol 2000; 21:1293–1301.
52. Alazzazz A, Aletich VA, Debrun GM, et al. Intracranial percutaneous transluminal angioplasty for arteriosclerotic stenosis. Arch Neurol 2000; 51:1625–1630.
53. Mori T, Chokyu K, Mima T, et al. Short-term arteriographic and clinical outcome after cerebral angioplasty and stenting for intracranial vertebrobasilar and carotid atherosclerotic occlusive disease. Am J Neuroradiol 2000; 21:249–254.
54. Gomez CR, Misra VK, Liu MW, et al. Elective stenting of symptomatic basilar artery stenosis. Stroke 2000; 31:95–99.
55. Levy EI, Horowitz MB, Koebbe CJ, et al. Transluminal stent-assisted angioplasty of the intracranial vertebrobasilar system for medically refractory posterior circulation ischemia: early results. Neurosurgery 2001; 48:1215–1221.
56. Lylyk P, Ceratto R, Ferrario A, et al. Angioplasty and stent placement in intracranial atherosclerotic stenoses and dissections. Am J Neuroradiol 2002; 23:430–436.
57. De Rochemont Rdu M, Buchkremer M, Sitzer M, et al. Recurrent symptomatic high-grade intracranial stenoses: safety and efficacy of undersized stents – initial experience. Radiology 2004; 231:45–49.
58. Jiang WJ, Wang YJ, Du B, et al. Stenting of symptomatic M1 stenosis of middle cerebral artery: an initial experience of 40 patients. Stroke 2004; 40:6.
59. Suh DC, Kim SJ, Lee DH, et al. Outcome of endovascular treatment in symptomatic intracranial vascular stenosis. Korean J Radiol 2005; 6:1–7.
60. Mori T, Kazita K, Mori K. Follow-up study after percutaneous transluminal cerebral angioplasty. Eur Radiol 1998; 8:403–408.
61. Song JK. Intracranial angioplasty and thrombolysis. Neurosurg Clin N Am 2000; 11:49–65.
62. Marks M. Intracranial angioplasty without stenting for symptomatic atherosclerotic stenosis: long-term follow-up. AJNR Am J Neuroradiol 2005; 26:525–530.
63. Jiang W. Comparison of elective stenting of severe vs moderate intracranial atherosclerotic stenosis. Neurology 2007; 68:420–426.
64. Berger P. Clopidogrel after coronary stenting. Curr Interv Cardiol Rep 1999; 1:263–269.
65. Meyers PM, Higashida R, Phatouros, et al. Cerebral hyperperfusion syndrome after percutaneous transluminal stenting of the craniocervical arteries. Neurosurgery 2000; 47:335–343.
66. Schonewille WJ, et al. Outcome in patients with basilar artery occlusion treated conventionally. J Neurol Neurosurg Psychiatry 2005; 76(9):1238–1241.
67. Marshall R. Monitoring of cerebral vasodilatory capacity with transcranial Doppler carbon dioxide inhalation in patients with severe carotid artery disease. Stroke 2003; 34:945–949.

6 | Complex Cases in Vascular Interventions—Carotid Arteries

Klaus Mathias

Department of Radiology, Klinikum Dortmund, Academic Teaching Hospital of the University of Muenster, Dortmund, Germany

PART 1: INTRODUCTION AND ACTUAL EVIDENCE

Several randomized trials comparing surgery with medical therapy have shown that prophylactic carotid endarterectomy (CEA) reduces the incidence of stroke in properly selected patients with high-grade symptomatic and asymptomatic carotid artery stenosis (1,2). Carotid angioplasty has a history of 30 years and can be considered an alternative treatment option after a period of technical development and growing clinical experience (3,4). Recent trials and numerous registries have shown a similar outcome of CEA and carotid artery stenting (CAS) concerning morbidity, mortality, and long-term results (5,6). Presently, it is not evident what for patients would have more benefit, whether from one or the other treatment modality. But the huge amount of CAS data, delivers some information about subgroups of patients who have an increased risk of endovascular therapy. Old age, anatomical variations, additional pathologic findings besides the carotid artery stenosis, may influence the choice of treatment. Some special cases will be presented and the technical peculiarities will be described.

CAS is a particularly complex intervention, and although skills acquired in other vascular territories are helpful, specific training is necessary to achieve personal competence and good results. Although it is difficult to set exact thresholds for competence in CAS due to the relative paucity of data, several reports in the literature give a hint that the learning curve extends much longer than some might be inclined to think (7). In evaluating the applications of stent operators who wanted to participate in the CREST trial, it was found that 94 operators who had performed fewer than 15 CAS procedures in NASCET-equivalent cases had a stroke and a death rate of 7.1%, as compared to 3.7% of the 9 operators who had performed 15 or more procedures (8). However, probably the learning curve for CAS extends even far beyond the first 15 cases, because an analysis of the learning curve for the use of distal protection devices in the "global carotid artery stent registry" (7,9) revealed that the incidence of procedure-related complications was clearly lower in institutions where several hundred procedures had been performed as compared to centres with less experience.

This is in line with data from Pro-CAS, the prospective registry of CAS organized by the German Societies of Angiology and Radiology. A multivariate analysis of 5341 interventions that had been documented in Pro-CAS between 1 July 1999 and 30 June 2005, was carried out in search of predictors of peri-interventional complications. It was found that neurological complications and/or death occurred 1.77 times more often (95% confidence interval 1.11 to 2.81) in the first 50 interventions of an institution as compared to later, when experience with 150 or more interventions had been accumulated (7,10).

TECHNIQUE OF CAS

Over the years, carotid angioplasty and stenting went through several steps of technical improvement. The first interventions were performed in an "over-the-wire-technique" without sheath or guiding catheter. Presently, we use three different techniques for the access to the lesion:

anchoring technique	aortic arch type I and II
telescoping technique	aortic arch type I and II
guiding catheter technique	aortic arch type I to III

The *anchoring technique* uses the external carotid artery (ECA) for placement of a stiff guidewire, which serves for the positioning of the sheath in the common carotid artery (CCA). First the CCA is probed with a diagnostic catheter with a vertebral, sidewinder, head hunter, Vitek, or right Judkins tip configuration. The guidewire—preferably a Terumo J-wire—is navigated into the ECA and the diagnostic catheter follows the wire in this artery. The guidewire is exchanged for a stiffer wire like the Amplatz stiff guidewire, the diagnostic catheter is removed, and the sheath is advanced over the wire in the CCA.

The *telescoping technique* saves some steps in comparison to the anchoring technique. The sheath is introduced into the femoral artery and placed in the descending thoracic aorta. The guidewire and mandrin are pulled out. The sheath is connected with a permanent saline flushing. A Vitek catheter with a stiff Terumo wire is inserted in the sheath. The curve of the catheter tip is formed in the descending thoracic aorta. The catheter is then gently pushed forward until it enters the orifice of the left common carotid or innominate artery. An angiogram shows the carotid bifurcation and the stenosis. The guidewire is now navigated into the ECA, the catheter is pushed into the artery, and afterwards the sheath is advanced into the CCA. The diagnostic catheter and guidewire are pulled out.

The *guiding catheter technique* is the third method to place a "working channel" in the CCA. Some interventionists routinely use a guiding catheter, often combined with a short 8-French sheath. The puncture holes in the femoral artery are larger with guiding catheters than with a 6-French sheath.

We prefer a guiding catheter with a sidewinder (1 or 2 configuration) in patients with a type III aortic arch. The shape of the guiding catheter is formed in the iliac arteries in a crossover maneuver. The catheter is then pushed up into the aortic arch and hooked in the CCA. This technique avoids the shaping of the tip of the catheter in the aortic arch, the left subclavian artery, or at the aortic valve. The risk of embolization in the cerebral circulation is prevented (Fig. 1).

Cerebral protection is used routinely with different embolic protection devices.

Filter protection	
Fixed basket	
Symmetrical	Accunet, Emboshield Pro
Asymmetrical	Filterwire EZ
Bare wire	
Symmetrical	Emboshield Pro
Asymmetrical	Spider
Balloon protection	
Proximal	Mo.Ma, NPS
Distal	Percusurge

Filters are used in more than 80% of the cases, but have their limits in tortuous internal carotid arteries (ICAs), in which they cannot be placed properly and may induce spasm. The lesion is crossed unprotected, which can release embolic particles. *Balloon protection* is technically more demanding and causes transient ischemic reactions in patients with exhausted neurovascular reserve capacity. With the reversed flow system, thrombolysis and thromboaspiration are made possible in acute carotid artery occlusions.

The debate is still on about the ideal *stent*. At the level of the carotid bifurcation only self-expandable stents should be used. These stents must meet several requirements like radial force, conformability, flexibility, visibility, and scaffolding. In symptomatic patients a small mesh size of the stent has been shown to have a lower complication rate compared to large free cell areas, which can be explained by the fact that less plaque material protrudes through the stent meshes. On the other hand, stents with small meshes are less flexible, straighten the carotid artery, and remodel the bifurcation. In asymptomatic carotid artery stenosis the mesh size seems to be unimportant. A hybrid stent (Cristallo™; Invatec) was developed with closed cells in its

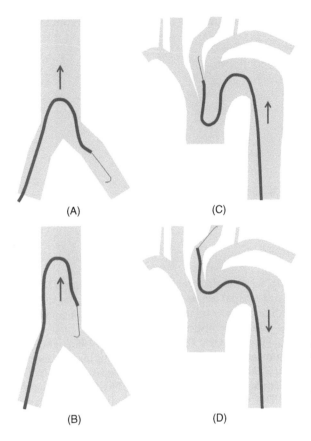

(A)

(C)

(B)

(D)

Figure 1 Guiding catheter technique for CCA access. (A) The tip of the SIM-2 or SIM-3 guiding catheter is formed in a crossover maneuvre in the contralateral iliac artery. (B) The catheter is gently pushed forward through the aorta into the aortic arch. (C) The guiding catheter is moved forward until it hooks in the CCA. (D) The guiding catheter is carefully pulled to insert its tip in the CCA as deep as possible.

middle part and open cells at its ends. More than three-quarters of the stents are placed across the bifurcation. Drug-eluting stents are not necessary in the treatment of bifurcational disease because the recurrence rate is low at 3% to 7%, and the re-intervention rate is below 3% of all CAS.

INDICATIONS
The indications for CAS are derived from the experiences of vascular surgery and the randomized trials on CEA and CAS (1,2,5,6). *Symptomatic* older men with a recent event and a stenosis of more than 70% according to the NASCET method have the highest benefit. The numbers needed to treat to prevent an ipsilateral stroke are between three and four patients when the complication rate stays below 5%.

Asymptomatic patients should have a degree of stenosis exceeding 80%. Rapid progression of the degree of stenosis, an incomplete Circle of Willis, a contralateral carotid occlusion, and an insufficient neurovascular reserve capacity are strong arguments for removal of the stenosis in these patients. CAS will prevent one stroke out of 17 at risk when the complication rate is below 3%.

The risk of CAS is lower than that of CEA in patients with an occluded contralateral carotid artery, and in patients with recurrent stenosis after endarterectomy (1). On the other hand the risk of CAS increases in patients older than 80 years due to generalized atherosclerosis, elongation of the vessels, and diminished biological reserve. Also severe calcifications of the stenosis and kinks of the CCA or ICA may be reasons to abstain from an endovascular procedure and to prefer CEA. The table that follows lists medical findings that are in favor of CAS in comparison to CEA.

Tandem stenoses
Bifurcation at the C2 level
Recurrent stenosis after CEA or CAS
Radical neck dissection
Radiotherapy
Inflammation or tumor of the neck
Paresis of the contralateral laryngeal nerve
Tracheostomy
Bechterew's disease
Severe obesity (weight limits of angiographic tables 160–200 kg)

PART 2: UNUSUAL CASES

CASE 1: CAS after CEA

CEA has a recurrence rate between 5% and 10% in the first year after the procedure (11). Re-operations have an increased risk of stroke and cranial nerve injury, which amounts to up to 10%. Patients have a better outcome with CAS because cranial nerve injuries do not occur and strokes are rare when the recurrent stenosis is due to myointimal proliferation.

The 71-year-old woman suffered from a symptomatic stenosis of the right ICA and was treated by CEA. Nine months later, a recurrent stenosis was detected by duplex ultrasound with a systolic peak flow velocity in the ICA of 322 cm/sec and only 44 cm/sec in the CCA. The finding of a recurrent ICA stenosis was confirmed by CT angiography (CTA), which revealed additionally a stenosis of the CCA (Fig. 2). The diagnostic results were discussed with the patient. The risk of the disease with an annual stroke rate of about 1% to 3% and the chances of endovascular treatment were explained. The patient desired removal of the stenoses despite the fact that she was asymptomatic.

CAS was performed with a femoral access in local anaesthesia. An aortic arch angiogram revealed a type III arch with a deeply seated origin of the innominate artery, a 3 cm long stenosis of the proximal CCA, an 80% carotid stenosis at the bifurcation, and no opacification of the ECA. The lesion was approached by a telescoping technique using a 90-cm long, 6-French Cook shuttle sheath, a 5-French Vitek catheter, and a 0.035″ stiff Terumo guidewire. An anchor technique was not considered because the ECA seemed to be occluded. It was decided to treat first the bifurcational recurrent stenosis and then the CCA stenosis under cerebral protection with a filter system (Acculink; Abbott). The innominate artery was probed with a Vitek catheter, and the guidewire was navigated into the CCA and advanced close to the bifurcation. In that manner enough support was given to place the sheath at the orifice of the CCA. After crossing of both lesions with the delivery sheath of the filter and deployment of the filter a 3 × 40-mm balloon catheter was introduced and the distal lesion predilated. The idea was to facilitate the crossing of the stenosis with the stent catheter; pushing the stent catheter against a tight stenosis may otherwise displace the sheath. After predilatation, a self-expandable nitinol stent (Acculink 10 × 40 mm; Abbott) was placed, and an in-stent dilatation with a balloon catheter (8 × 40 mm) was performed. The stenosis could be completely removed, but the flow was still slow with the sheath in the orifice of the CCA. A second stent (Acculink 10 × 40 mm) was then deployed in the CCA without predilatation ending proximally at the origin of the artery. The balloon of 8 × 40 mm was used again. Control angiograms demonstrated a good result of CCA and ICA stenting, a normal opacification of the ECA due to a normalized perfusion pressure, and a filling of the middle cerebral artery (MCA), but not of the anterior cerebral artery territory.

The Acculink stents were chosen because of their large cell size and high flexibility. The arterial segment covered by a stent becomes mechanically stiffer. Two stents in a neck artery, which follows every head movement, will increase the mechanical stress between them. The mechanical stress may induce a myointimal proliferation or, with a short gap between the two stents, even aneurysm formation. Using stents with good conformability and sufficient distance

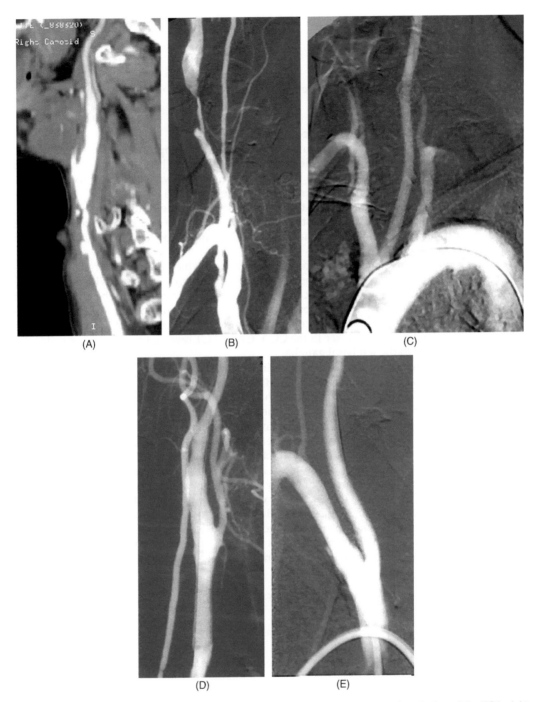

Figure 2 71-year-old woman with recurrent stenosis of the right CCA artery and occlusion of the ECA eight months after CEA. (A) CT-angiography reveals a distal CCA stenosis. (B) Additional stenosis of the proximal CCA. (C) Elongated aorta: type III aortic arch. (D) Removal of the distal CCA stenosis. (E) Removal of proximal CCA stenosis.

between the stents, CAS may have a good long-term prognosis. Follow-up examinations have shown no recurrence up to 18 months.

What is special about this case?

– recurrent stenosis after CEA
– combined proximal and distal CCA stenosis
– selection of stent

CASE 2: CAS—Vascular Surgery Impossible

A 74-year-old patient was referred to our department with a symptomatic stenosis of the left ICA and an occlusion of the right ICA. He observed a weakness of his left side, which persisted for half an hour and disappeared within four hours completely, five weeks prior to admission. Normally, such a combination of bilateral carotid artery disease should be treated by CAS because vascular surgery has a higher stroke rate as shown in the NASCET trial with 14.7%, and the SPACE trial with 13% (1,5). The stroke rate of carotid artery stenting in a patient with an occluded contralateral carotid artery is not increased in comparison to unilateral stenosis with endovascular treatment.

But our patient presented an additional problem and which ruled out surgery as a treatment option. He suffered for several decades from severe Bechterew's disease with a completely frozen neck (Fig. 3). There was no surgical access to the carotid artery with the chin in a fixed position close to the sternum. He had coronary artery disease with an older anteroseptal myocardial infarction. Duplex ultrasound detected a peak systolic flow velocity of 344 cm/sec in the ICA stenosis and a flow of 53 cm/sec in the CCA. Cranial CT revealed moderate brain atrophy and a lacunar infarct in the left basal ganglia.

CAS was performed with a SIM-2 guiding catheter (Cordis), a FilterWire EZ (Boston Scientific), and a Precise stent (Cordis). The guiding catheter was chosen for smooth atraumatic probing of the left CCA in a type III aortic arch and an innominate artery of the bovine type. The SIM-2 tip was formed in a crossover maneuver in the iliac artery. The guiding catheter was then connected with the saline line for permanent flushing, was gently pushed up into the aorta, and hooked in the innominate artery. A Terumo wire was then placed in the left CCA and the guiding catheter pulled back to let the catheter tip glide in the left CCA. The FilterWire EZ was then navigated through the stenosis, a 6 × 20-mm Precise stent was deployed in the ICA, and an in-stent dilatation was carried out with a 5 × 20-mm balloon catheter.. We placed the stent only into the ICA, because the lesion was very short and was located 1.5 cm distal to the normally wide bifurcation. After angiographic documentation of the treatment result we closed the puncture site with 8-French Angioseal (St. Jude). The patient received 5000 IU of heparin and 1 mg atropine during the intervention. He was under aspirin and clopidogrel before, during, and after the procedure. Clopidogrel was prescribed for eight weeks after CAS.

The special features of the case were:

– the positioning of the C-arm with 50% caudocranial tilting
– the type III aortic arch
– the bovine type origin of the left CCA
– stenting of only the ICA

In more than 80% of CAS the stent is placed across the bifurcation.

CASE 3: CAS in Tandem Stenosis

A 74-year-old man suffered an acute stroke (modified Rankin Scale 3) and was referred to us for treatment of his symptomatic left ICA stenosis. MRI showed two fresh separate smaller infarctions in the MCA territory, and color-coded Duplex ultrasound confirmed the diagnosis of a severe ICA stenosis with a peak systolic flow velocity of 488 cm/sec. A medication with 100 mg aspirin and 75 mg clopidogrel was started, and CAS planned three days later. Selective carotid angiography confirmed the ICA stenosis at the level of the bifurcation, but revealed an additional stenosis in the petrous part of the distal ICA (Fig. 4).

The intervention was planned with a shuttle sheath (Cook), cerebral protection with FilterWire EZ (Boston Scientific), predilatation with a balloon diameter of 3 mm, a Carotid

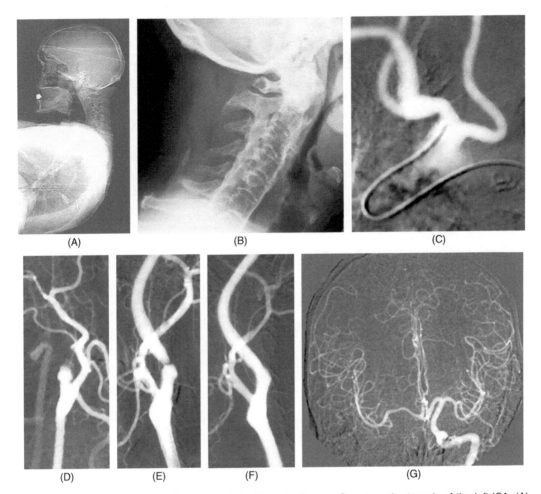

Figure 3 74-year-old man with far advanced Bechterew's disease. Symptomatic stenosis of the left ICA. (A) Head in vertical position with the patient on the angiographic table. (B) Frozen cervical neck, nor surgical window for CEA. (C) Occluded right ICA. (D) Type III aortic arch and bovine trunk; the SIM-2 guiding catheter is in place. (E) Short 88% left ICA stenosis. (F) Stent placement and in-stent angioplasty with good result. (G) Left ICA supplies ACA and MCA of both hemispheres.

Wallstent (Boston Scientific) for the bifurcational stenosis, and a Herculink stent (Abbott) of the distal ICA stenosis. The sheath was brought in position with the aid of a Vitek diagnostic catheter and a stiff Terumo J wire. The filter was placed below the distal ICA stenosis to protect the cerebral circulation during treatment of the bifurcational stenosis. After removal of that stenosis and retrieval of the filter, a 0.014″ guidewire was used (Choice PT, Boston Scientific) for probing of the distal ICA stenosis. The stent was placed without predilatation and cerebral protection. Control angiography showed a normal width of the ICA at both treatment sites. The puncture site was closed with 6-French Angioseal (St. Jude). The blood pressure was monitored, and the systolic pressure was kept below 120 mm Hg to prevent a hyperperfusion syndrome.

What is special about this case?

– CAS in acute stroke
– blood pressure monitoring
– selection of stent
– second stenosis of the distal ICA
– partial cerebral protection

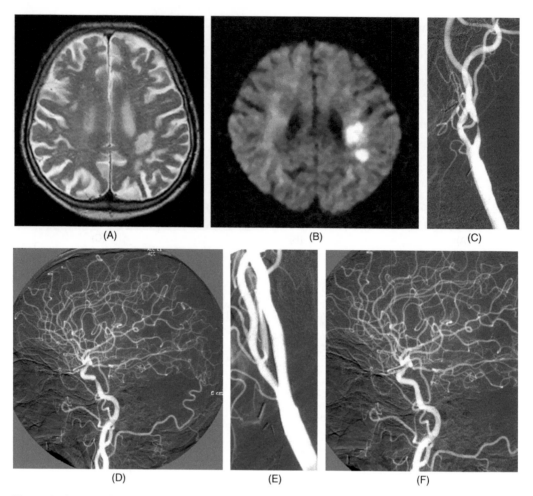

Figure 4 Acute stroke in a 74-year-old man. (A and B) Acute infarction of the left MCA territory in the T2- and Diffusion Weighted MR scans. (C) Short 90% stenosis of the left ICA. (D) Additional stenosis of the petrous part of the ICA. (E) ICA stenosis treated with stent placement and angioplasty with slight residual stenosis of less than 20%. (F) Distal ICA stenosis removed by balloon-expandable stent.

The risk from a second stroke after an acute cerebral ischemic event is highest in the first few weeks and decreases within six months to a risk level of an asymptomatic stenosis. Early treatment is therefore desirable, but larger strokes may endanger patients with cerebral hemorrhage. A degree of stenosis of about 90%, as in this case, reduces the pressure of the cerebral circulation of the affected side. Cerebrovascular autoregulation will open cerebral arteries and arterioles as much as possible. With removal of the stenosis, a sudden increase in pressure and flow occurs and leads to hyperperfusion. The patient may develop head ache, brain edema, and in the worst case cerebral bleeding. The risk of cerebral hemorrhage is growing considerably with the combination of hyperperfusion, double platelet function inhibition, and infarction necrosis. In such cases we keep the blood pressure as low as reasonably possible with systolic pressures between 90 and 120 mm Hg. The blood pressure is not only measured during the stay in the angiographic unit, but pressure monitoring continues for the next few hours in the ward. We could keep the incidence of cerebral hemorrhage in more than 4000 CAS in the range of 1% to 2%.

In symptomatic patients the fibrous cap of the plaque is eroded and thrombus forms on the plaque surface. This soft material will protrude through the wide stent meshes and may embolize in the cerebral circulation. Narrow meshes reduce the risk of plaque and thrombus

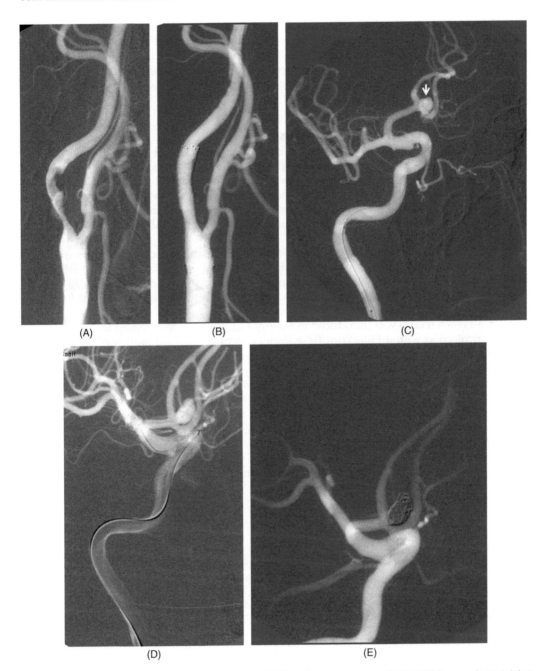

(A)   (B)   (C)

(D)   (E)

Figure 5 Irregular symptomatic stenosis of the right ICA in a 63-year-old man. (A) 75% ICA stenosis containing thrombus. (B) Removal of the stenosis under cerebral protection with stenting and angioplasty. (C) The cerebral angiogram reveals an aneurysm of the anterior communicating artery 5 × 5 × 10 mm. (D) A microcatheter is introduced and its tip is navigated into the aneurysmal sack. (E) Complete exclusion of the aneurysm after coiling.

prolapse. The Wallstent has the smallest cell size of all carotid stents has with about 1-mm² free cell area. This fact determined our choice of stent in that case.

It is well known from the surgical literature that patients benefit from endarterectomy of a bifurcational stenosis despite an additional distal ICA stenosis. CAS is more advantageous in such cases of tandem stenoses because both lesions can be treated in one session with complete normalization of blood flow.

We routinely use cerebral protection devices. In this case we had a filter device in place performing CAS at the bifurcation. We thought that this tight lesion may be the cause for the stroke. The embolic risk of placing a balloon-expandable stent in the distal ICA seemed much lower, and the procedure was performed without cerebral protection. It can be discussed whether proximal balloon protection (Mo.Ma, Invatec; NPS, Gore) would have increased the safety of the intervention.

CASE 4: CAS and Cerebral Artery Aneurysm

The incidence of cerebral artery aneurysms is about 50 to 60 out of 100,000 people (12). The risk of aneurysmal rupture peaks in the sixth decade. That is the same age group in which carotid artery stenosis is encountered most frequently. The incidental finding of cerebral artery aneurysms and carotid artery stenosis must be expected from time to time. The question arises how to treat patients with a tight ICA stenosis when the cerebral aneurysm is located at the affected side, and how the risk of subarachnoidal hemorrhage is influenced by removal of a pressure-reducing ICA stenosis.

A 63-year-old man was referred for CAS after a right hemispheric transient ischemic attack three weeks ago. An irregular ulcerated ICA stenosis was found by CTA and DSA. Additionally, an aneurysm of the anterior communicating artery was detected. We determined the size of the aneurysm as $5 \times 5 \times 10$ mm. It was decided to treat both lesions in one session to prevent subarachnoidal hemorrhage (Fig. 5).

A 6-French sheath was introduced in the right CCA with a telescoping technique. Under cerebral protection with a FilterWire EZ a Protégé stent ($7–10 \times 40$ mm) was placed and an in-stent dilation was performed with a balloon 5-mm in diameter. The control angiogram demonstrated a good stenting result.

Immediately afterwards a microcatheter was guided via the sheath in the aneurysmal sack. Seven GDC coils (Boston Scientific) with decreasing diameter and length were placed in the aneurysmal sack until the aneurysm was completely excluded from the blood stream.

What is special about this case?

– combination of a high-degree ICA stenosis with an ipsilateral cerebral artery aneurysm
– treatment of both lesions in one session
– prevention of subarachnoidal hemorrhage

REFERENCES

1. North American Symptomatic Carotid Endarterectomy Trial Collaborators (NASCET). Beneficial effect of carotid endarterectomy in symptomatic patients with high-grade carotid stenosis. N Engl J Med 1991; 325:445–453.
2. European Carotid Surgery Trialists' Collaborative Group. Randomised trial of endarterectomy for recently symptomatic carotid stenosis: final results of the MRC European Carotid Surgery Trial (ECST). Lancet 1998; 351:1379–1387.
3. Mathias K. Ein neuartiges Katheter-System zur perkutanen transluminalen Angioplastie von Karotisstenosen. Fortschr Med 1977; 95:1007–1009.
4. Mathias K, Mittermayer Ch, Ensinger H, et al. Perkutane Katheterdilatation von Karotisstenosen. Fortschr Röntgenstr 1980; 133:258–261.
5. Ringleb PA, Allenberg J. Bruckmann H, et al. 30 day results from the SPACE trial of stent-protected angioplasty versus carotid endarterectomy in symptomatic patients: a randomised non-inferiority trial. Lancet 2006; 368:1239–1247.
6. Mas JL, Chatellier G, Beyssen B, et al. Endarterectomy versus stenting in patients with symptomatic severe carotid stenosis. N Engl J Med. 2006; 355:1660–1671.
7. Theiss W, Hermanek P, Mathias K, et al. Predictors of death and stroke after carotid angioplasty and stenting. A subgroup analysis of the Pro-CAS data. Stroke 2008; 39:2325–2330.
8. Al-Mubarak N, Roubin GS, Hobson RW, et al. Credentialing of Stent Operators for the Carotid Revascularization Endarterectomy vs. Stenting Trial (CREST). Stroke 2000; 31:292.
9. Wholey MH. Al-Mubarek N, Wholey MH. Updated review of the global carotid artery stent registry. Catheter Cardiovasc Interv 2003; 60:259–266.

10. Mudra H, Buchele W, Mathias K, et al. Interventional treatment of extracranial carotid stenoses: current status, requirements and indications. Vasa 2006; 35:125–131.
11. Rugonfalvi-Kiss S, Dosa E, Madsen HO, et al. High rate of early restenosis after carotid eversion endarterectomy in homozygous carriers of the normal mannose-binding lectin genotype. Stroke 2005; 36:944–948.
12. Taylor AD, Byrne JV. Cerebral arterial aneurysm formation and rupture in 20767 elderly patients: hypertension and other risk factors. J Neurosurg 1995; 83:812–819.

7 | Subclavian Interventions

Edward B. Diethrich

Arizona Heart Institute and Arizona Heart Hospital, Phoenix, Arizona, U.S.A.

PART 1: INTRODUCTION

What Makes a Lesion "Complex" in Subclavian Interventions?

While most interventional procedures in the subclavian region are fairly straightforward, there are conditions that increase the complexity of intervention. Flush occlusions of the subclavian artery, usually occurring on the left side, can make passage of a wire difficult, particularly from the retrograde femoral approach. The retrograde brachial approach is more satisfactory in this setting, since a wire and guiding catheter can be placed to assist in penetration of the plaque. Nonetheless, the wire may still deviate, producing a dissection or procedural failure. The relationship of the vessel orifice and the occlusion or stenosis can create the potential for vertebral artery compromise. Aortic arch configurations are variable and, in some cases, it can be difficult to manipulate the wire and catheter. Any or all of these types of complications (as well as others) can add to the complexity of subclavian intervention.

Although carotid–subclavian bypass and transposition of the carotid artery to the subclavian for revascularization of the upper extremity and correction of subclavian steal syndrome were areas of particular interest in earlier days (1–3), endovascular treatment of these conditions is the norm today. The left subclavian artery is most frequently diseased, and intervention may involve antegrade and retrograde access. Right subclavian artery intervention is often the most difficult because fluoroscopic visualization is harder to achieve, and there is a tendency for stenoses to develop in the very short segment between the origin and take-off of the right vertebral artery. The subclavian artery is a thin-walled vessel and is susceptible to closed trauma and operative injury, even during conventional procedures. Although perforation is rare, the tortuosity in subclavian arteries may contribute to the potential for wire injury when there is an attempt to maneuver through the lesion or manipulation occurs inadvertently at the level of the branches.

Clinical Indications for Treatment of Complex Lesions in Subclavian Interventions

Subclavian stenting is frequently used for treatment of stenotic and occlusive disease; pathologic lesions of the subclavian arteries may be the result of Takayasu's arteritis, Behcet's disease, fibromuscular dysplasia, radiation-induced stenosis, true aneurysms, mycotic aneurysms, post-traumatic pseudoaneurysms, arteriovenous fistulas, and spontaneous or iatrogenic dissections. Most of the procedures, however, are for the treatment of atherosclerotic stenotic or occlusive arterial lesions, producing subclavian steal or upper extremity claudication. The common clinical indications for intervention are described in Table 1. Stents, usually covered, are also used to repair traumatic injuries following motor vehicle accidents and such; however, intervention can be extremely challenging, and endovascular procedures to treat these injuries should be performed only by those who are able to convert quickly to an open procedure. Subclavian stenting has also been used to salvage left internal mammary artery (LIMA) grafts, and to treat vertebrobasilar ischemia, which results from severe atherosclerosis or dissection of the vertebral or subclavian artery. For atherosclerotic lesions, the results of balloon angioplasty alone are not as satisfactory as those of stenting. Therefore, our preference is to use stents routinely under these conditions. In general, the results of these procedures have been highly successful; complications such as stent deformation, fracture, and infection yielding aneurysm formation, have been reported very infrequently.

Hazards and Complications

Although lesions in the subclavian arteries tend to be firm, concentric, localized, and relatively smooth, potential complications of treatment still include dissection, perforation, disruption,

Table 1 Indications for Endovascular Treatment of Subclavian Disease

Subclavian steal syndrome
Transient ischemic attack (TIA)
Stroke
Amaurosis fugax
Arm claudication
Upper limb ischemia
Vertebrobasilar ischemia
Angina in patients with LIMA graft
Leg claudication in patients with axillofemoral grafts
Anticipation of coronary artery bypass (+ need for a patent IMA)
Pulsatile tinnitus
Aneurysm
Trauma
Rupture

thrombosis, and embolization (Table 2); the rates of these complications are extremely variable. Calcific atherosclerotic plaques affecting either the subclavian arteries are prone to dissection, which is probably the most common complication related to angioplasty, and a potential cause of extensive damage and procedural failure. In occlusive lesions, creation of false channels can also complicate the procedure and even cause it to be unsuccessful. When contrast migration is indicative of dissection outside the central channel, the operator must determine if the procedure should be abandoned. In our experience, coaxial passage of the wire is more difficult when a false channel has been created but most lesions can be crossed safely. Though entering *under* (subintimally) a plaque in high-grade lesions and re-entering into the true lumen may be a successful strategy, it is not always possible, especially in an occluded subclavian artery. While it is tempting to proceed in a subintimal plane, balloon angioplasty and stenting here may result in perforation of the vessel or even a dissection across the aortic arch.

The nearly universal use of the LIMA as a conduit for bypassing coronary artery obstructions may lead to complications in subclavian endovascular procedures. When there is an obstructed lesion at the origin of the left subclavian artery (the side usually preferred with the left internal mammary bypass), flow is limited and can result in graft failure. Stent deployment at the origin of the left subclavian can ensure uncompromised flow to the LIMA prior to coronary revascularization. Given that restenosis is unlikely, long-term success can be anticipated. In some patients, angina may resolve initially after a LIMA bypass to the left anterior descending artery; later, however, progressive occlusive disease may develop in the left subclavian

Table 2 Potential Complications of Subclavian Endovascular Intervention

Thrombosis
Bleeding
AV fistula
Peripheral nerve injury
Peripheral atheroembolism
Peripheral atheroembolism: to limbs, visceral, cerebral
Subintimal dissection
Perforation
Dissection
Pseudoaneurysm
Plaque rupture
Vertebral artery compromise
Obstruction of left subclavian artery origin limits LIMA bypass flow → graft failure
Stent blocks artery orifice
Restenosis (rare)
Persistence of symptoms

artery and cause a recurrence of symptoms. Stenting under these circumstances restores normal coronary flow through the internal mammary artery.

A complication that can occur relates to the origin of the internal mammary artery and positioning of the stent in the left subclavian artery. Atherosclerotic plaque may be present near the internal mammary artery orifice, and an improperly positioned stent can actually compromise the vessel. Proper sizing and positioning of the device using adequate imaging techniques are required to eliminate this complication. Another potential and similar complication of subclavian stenting is related to the position of obstructing plaque and the vertebral artery origin. Frequently, there are several millimeters of artery free of significant disease, and a stent can be safely deployed. If vertebral artery compromise is a potential problem, a second, protective wire can be inserted in the vertebral artery. This permits access for ballooning if the subclavian stent impinges upon the vertebral artery during the procedure. We have occasionally seen cases in which a stent blocked an artery orifice, and it was necessary to thread a wire through the stent and dilate it to restore flow to the branched vessel. Overall, restenosis is relatively rare and can be effectively treated using additional endovascular intervention. Small-size stent diameters, more than one stent implantation, and a difference in upper limb systolic blood pressures after intervention are independent predictors of restenosis (4).

Interventional Strategies

Subclavian lesions frequently affect the left side more often than the right because of the intrathoracic segment and are generally limited to the proximal segment. Overall, endovascular manipulation of the subclavian is relatively safe. Disease in the subclavian is most commonly found at the arch origins, and there often remains a 1 to 2 cm stump of subclavian artery from the aortic lumen. Normally, subclavian lesions are concentric, although the proximal aortic stump may present some asymmetry secondary to flow disturbances caused by plaque formation, particularly at the 90-degree origin of the left subclavian artery.

The best way to access the target lesion is still controversial, and the risks and benefits of different approaches (femoral, brachial) have to be assessed on a case-by-case basis. Our preference, especially in a tight or occluded lesion, is the percutaneous brachial approach through a 5- to 6-F sheath because proximity to the site of the lesion allows better "pushability" and directing of the device. In general, the closer the puncture site is to the area of therapy, the easier it is to maneuver and access the area of interest.

Noninvasive assessment with duplex imaging of the arch, vertebral, and extracranial arteries is important, and computed tomography (CT) examination of the brain is often performed as well. Duplex imaging of the arch vessels is sometimes technically difficult because of the intrathoracic location of left subclavian artery origin. Nevertheless, it can reveal hemodynamic patterns of subclavian steal. Using several imaging modalities, including angiography and magnetic resonance angiography, help ensure adequate procedural planning and often assist the clinician in identifying patients who may be at high risk for a perioperative cerebrovascular accident during a stenting procedure.

Although angiography is still the main imaging method during endovascular procedures, the ostial location of most subclavian artery lesions may be difficult to visualize using standard arch views because of superimposed images of the subclavian artery origin over the aorta. Additional oblique views are of utmost importance for accurate diagnosis. The newer 64-slice CT angiography is extremely useful for high-quality resolution of occlusive lesions, and we have also found that intravascular ultrasound (IVUS) is particularly helpful in assessing lesions and determining accurate stent placement at the level of the arch vessel origin. IVUS produces high-resolution, real-time images and reassembled three-dimensional reconstructions that provide longitudinal or volume views. Longitudinal views are assembled rapidly by specialized computer software and are available to the clinician in the operating room, facilitating rapid clinical decisions following a catheter pull-through and permitting exact positioning of the intravascular stent.

Oral antiplatelet therapy is optimal for these procedures. Some teams prefer to use Plavix before the operation; however, there are no data to support this treatment. We have routinely used antiplatelet therapy for 30 days following stent deployment.

Local anesthesia with mild sedation allows the assessment of neurological episodes, but there are disadvantages to using local anesthesia, because patient movement during the procedure can be problematic when "road mapping" is being used for stent deployment or to guide balloon angioplasty.

The most common and, usually, easiest-to-correct lesions are those occurring at the origin of the left subclavian artery. Plaque formation in this location often extends a few millimeters into the aortic arch itself, a trait that is characteristic of all the arch vessel lesions. Although subclavian lesions are often calcific in nature, most are easily crossed, ballooned, and stented. Lesions in the second part of the subclavian artery, however, should be evaluated very carefully to ensure that stent placement will not interfere with patency of the vertebral artery or the internal mammary artery. In chronic disease, the subclavian artery is frequently occluded at its origin, a condition referred to as a flush occlusion. This presentation is often difficult to treat, particularly with the retrograde femoral approach, since the true lumen of the subclavian artery may be hard to locate. Therefore, our general preference is to use a percutaneous left brachial artery approach. After entry and 6-F sheath placement, a 0.035-inch Glidewire (Cook, Bloomington, IN) is passed forward to engage the lesion. Because the artery is often tortuous at this point, an angled guide catheter is directed to the lesion and positioned in a coaxial position. In many cases, substituting the former for a straight wire allows the catheter to be gently advanced with the wire probing through the plaque into the aortic arch. Balloon angioplasty and stent deployment follow; sizing and selection of a device depend on the nature of the lesion. In highly calcified lesions, a balloon-expandable stent may be preferable, but more often a self-expanding model is deployed. If it is difficult to cross the occlusion, a smaller wire may be selected and a combined approach with a catheter and wire from the femoral artery may be used. In lesions that are nonocclusive, either brachial or femoral techniques are acceptable.

Right subclavian artery intervention is usually more difficult than left subclavian because fluoroscopic visualization is obscured, and there is a tendency for stenoses to develop in the very short segment between the right subclavian origin and the take-off of the right vertebral artery. When treating the right subclavian, even simply crossing the lesion with a wire risks embolization to the common carotid artery, which is in close proximity. If a lesion appears highly calcific or difficult to cross due to high-grade occlusion, a temporary occlusion of the common carotid artery may be performed using a dual brachiofemoral approach in a kissing balloon fashion to access the target vessel from the brachial artery. In addition, aspiration of any debris before deflation of the occluding balloon may be accomplished using a long femoral sheath placed at the ostium of the common carotid artery. The sizes of the carotid protection devices, such as filters, limit their use in the subclavian arteries. Double-balloon techniques may be useful when there is concern of vertebral artery compromise (via occlusion or dissection) secondary to subclavian manipulation.

Interventional Tools (Table 3)
Ordinarily, the subclavian artery is selectively catheterized with a 5-F diagnostic catheter, and the lesion is crossed with a 0.035 wire to support either the sheath or guide as the delivery system. Self-expanding nitinol stents or balloon-expandable stainless steel stents may be used. For lesions involving the ostium, expandable stents can be deployed with more precision because self-expanding stents often exhibit some proximal movement during deployment. Nevertheless, we have used self-expanding stents for areas that are potentially compressible since balloon-mounted stents are subject to crush injury.

Summary of Outcomes
Endovascular surgery has become a multispecialty domain with rapid growth in the number of cases performed and pathologies addressed. Technical success is as high (5–18) as 100% in some cases, and midterm patency rates of over 90% have been reported (10). Subclavian stenting is frequently used for treatment of stenotic (8,9) and occlusive (10–12) disease. In addition, stents have also been used to repair traumatic arterial injuries (13,14). Vertebrobasilar ischemia, which results from severe atherosclerosis or dissection of the vertebral or subclavian artery and is often unresponsive to medical intervention, has also been treated using balloon angioplasty and stenting (15). In general, the results of these procedures have been highly successful;

Table 3 List of Tools for Subclavian Intervention

Equipment for Subclavian Stenting (Brachial Approach)

- 18-gauge Cook (Cook Bloomington, IN) needle / Cook micropuncture set
- Indeflator (ACS, Santa Clara, CA)
- Guidewire: 0.035-inch × 180-cm angled Glidewire (Terumo, Somerset, NJ) or 0.035-inch, 180-cm straight Glidewire (Terumo)
- Guidewire: 0.035-inch × 180-cm Amplatz (Cook)
- Guidewire: 0.035-inch × 180-cm straight-stiff Glidewire (Terumo)
- Catheter: 5-F × 65-cm Berenstein (Boston Scientific, Natick, MA)
- Sheath: 6-F × 11-cm Cordis Brite-tip (Cordis, Miami Lakes, FL)
- Sheath: 6-F × 55-cm Cordis Brite-tip (Cordis)
- Balloons: Cordis Opta-Pro 80-cm (Cordis), or Abbott Fox PTA 75-cm (Abbott Laboratories, Abbott Park, IL)
- Balloon-expandable stent (size/type to be determined by physician)

Equipment for Subclavian Stenting (Femoral Approach)

- 18-gauge Cook needle (Cook, Bloomington, IL)
- Indeflator (ACS, Santa Clara, CA)
- Guidewire: 0.035-inch × 260-cm angled Glidewire (Terumo, Somerset, NJ)
- Guidewire: 0.035-inch × 260-cm Amplatz (Cook)
- Catheter: 5-F × 100-cm Bentson 2 (Cook), or 5 F × 100-cm Headhunter (Terumo)
- Sheath: 7-F × 11-cm Cordis Brite-tip (Cordis, Miami Lakes, FL)
- Sheath: 7-F × 90-cm Cook Flexor Shuttle (Cook)
- Balloons: Cordis Opta-Pro 110-cm (Cordis), or Abbott Fox PTA 135-cm (Abbott Laboratories, Abbott Park, IL)
- Balloon-expandable stent (size/type to be determined by physician)

complications, such as stent deformation (16), fracture (17), and infection yielding aneurysm formation (18) are rare.

Equipment Checklist
Equipment for Subclavian Stenting (Brachial Approach)

- 18-gauge Cook (Cook Bloomington, IN) needle / Cook micropuncture set
- Indeflator (ACS, Santa Clara, CA)
- Guidewire: 0.035-inch × 180-cm angled Glidewire (Terumo, Somerset, NJ) **or** 0.035-inch, 180-cm straight Glidewire (Terumo)
- Guidewire: 0.035-inch × 180-cm Amplatz (Cook)
- Guidewire: 0.035-inch × 180-cm straight-stiff Glidewire (Terumo)
- Catheter: 5-F × 65-cm Berenstein (Boston Scientific, Natick, MA)
- Sheath: 6-F × 11-cm Cordis Brite-tip (Cordis, Miami Lakes, FL)
- Sheath: 6-F × 55-cm Cordis Brite-tip (Cordis)
- Balloons: Cordis Opta-Pro 80-cm (Cordis), or Abbott Fox PTA 75-cm (Abbott Laboratories, Abbott Park, IL)
- Balloon-expandable stent (size/type to be determined by physician)

Equipment for Subclavian Stenting (Femoral Approach)

- 18-gauge Cook needle (Cook, Bloomington, IL)
- Indeflator (ACS, Santa Clara, CA)
- Guidewire: 0.035-inch × 260-cm angled Glidewire (Terumo, Somerset, NJ)
- Guidewire: 0.035-inch × 260-cm Amplatz (Cook)
- Catheter: 5-F × 100-cm Bentson 2 (Cook), or 5-F × 100-cm Headhunter (Terumo)
- Sheath: 7-F × 11-cm Cordis Brite-tip (Cordis, Miami Lakes, FL)
- Sheath: 7-F × 90-cm Cook Flexor Shuttle (Cook)
- Balloons: Cordis Opta-Pro 110-cm (Cordis), or Abbott Fox PTA 135-cm (Abbott Laboratories, Abbott Park, IL)
- Balloon-expandable stent (size/type to be determined by physician)

PART 2: COMPLEX CASES

Case #1: Long Total Occlusion of the Left Subclavian Artery

An 80-year-old female presented with dizziness and headaches when using her left arm for extended periods. She was evaluated with duplex ultrasound of the left arm and carotids, revealing total occlusion of her left subclavian artery and reversal of flow in her left vertebral artery.

Procedure:
Access to the left brachial artery was obtained in a retrograde fashion, with an 18-gauge Cook needle and a 0.035-inch × 180-cm angled Glidewire using Seldinger technique. A 6-F × 1-cm sheath was then placed in the artery, and 5000 units of heparin were given intravenously; the activated clotting time was maintained at 200 to 250 for the remainder of the case. A retrograde hand-injected arteriogram was performed, showing a long-segment total occlusion of the prevertebral left subclavian artery, with a large, patent left vertebral artery in close proximity. To obtain better working leverage, the short sheath was exchanged for a 6-F × 55-cm Cordis sheath. A repeat arteriogram was performed. Once again, the regular 0.035-inch × 180-cm angled Glidewire was advanced through the sheath and attempts were made to cross the lesion. These were unsuccessful, so a 5-F × 90-cm Berenstein catheter was advanced over the wire to obtain even greater working leverage. Multiple attempts at subintimal dissection were made using the regular-angled 0.035-inch × 180-cm Glidewire. Eventually, a tight loop was formed but re-entry was not established. To obtain greater leverage, the Berenstein catheter was exchanged for a 5-F LIMA catheter. New attempts to cross the lesion with the regular angled 0.035-inch × 180-cm Glidewire failed, so it was exchanged for a straight stiff 0.035-inch × 180-cm Glidewire. Using the combination of the long sheath, LIMA catheter, and straight-stiff Glidewire, we were able to cross the lesion subintimally and re-enter the true lumen at the ostium of the subclavian artery. After crossing the lesion, confirmation of re-entry into the true lumen was obtained by back bleeding through the catheter and injection of a puff of contrast. The wire and catheter were then advanced into the descending thoracic aorta. To gain support for the planned intervention, the wire was exchanged for an Amplatz 0.035-inch × 180-cm wire. The lesion was then predilated with a 5-mm × 7-cm semi-compliant Fox balloon. An angiogram was done to mark the landing zone. A Bridge Assurant 8-mm × 30-mm balloon-expandable stent was then deployed, with care not to cover the vertebral artery (Figs. 1 and 2). A second stent was required to obtain sufficient overhang into the aorta. Pressure gradients after balloon angioplasty were 60 mm Hg, but this resolved with stenting. A completion angiogram was then obtained, demonstrating completely patent subclavian, vertebral, and mammary arteries. The sheath was then removed under pressure in the recovery room.

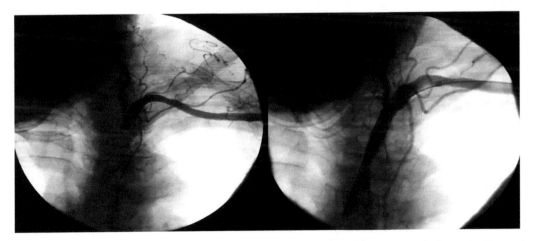

Figure 1 Angiogram showing occlusion of the left subclavian artery and post-stent deployment with good arterial flow.

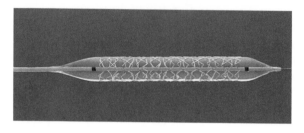

Figure 2 Photo of Bridge Assurant stent, 8 mm × 30 mm.

What Made the Case Complex?

The hazards involved in treating this patient were primarily anatomical. The lesion was complex—a long total occlusion of the left subclavian artery, requiring stent extension near the vertebral vessel. Great precision in landing the stent was required to prevent coverage of this vessel. Further, the risk of failure in treating a long subclavian artery occlusion has historically been high.

What was the Clinical Indication?

On the basis of the patient's symptoms and the noninvasive tests, a diagnosis of subclavian steal syndrome was made.

What were the Potential Hazards of Treating this Patient and Anatomy?

The hazards involved in treating this patient were primarily anatomical as described earlier.

Which Interventional Strategies were Considered?

We chose a brachial approach on the basis of our extensive experience with such complex lesions. A femoral approach was not appropriate due to the inherent lack of catheter and wire support it affords. Once the lesion has been crossed using a retrograde brachial approach, placement of a stiff guidewire (such as the Amplatz wire used in this case) provides sufficient support for most interventions. However, in treating long, highly calcified lesions, we sometimes employ a brachiofemoral wire when additional support is needed.

Which Interventional Tools were used to Manage this Case?

(See list of equipment used in this case)

Summary: How was the Case Managed, is There Anything That Could Have Been Improved, and What was the Immediate and Long-Term Outcome?

In treating proximal branch vessels arising from the aorta, we almost always employ balloon-expandable stents; it is our belief that their greater radial force is of benefit. In this particular case, we could have judged better by selecting the length of the initial stent, and therefore avoided the need for a second stent. The patient is currently 12 months out from her intervention and is doing well. No recurrent symptoms have been noted.

List of Equipment used in this Case

18-gauge Cook needle (Cook, Bloomington, IN)
6-F × 11-cm Cordis sheath (Cordis, Miami Lakes, FL)
6-F × 55-cm Cordis sheath (Cordis)
0.035-inch × 180-cm regular angled Glidewire (Terumo, Somerset, NJ)
0.035-inch × 180-cm straight stiff Glidewire (Terumo)
0.035-inch × 180-cm Amplatz wire (Cook)
5-F × 90-cm Berenstein catheter (Boston Scientific, Natick, MA)
5-F × 90-cm IMA catheter (Cordis)
7-mm × 4-cm Fox balloon (Abbott Labs, Abbott Park, IL)
(2) 8-mm × 30-mm Bridge Assurant balloon-expandable stents (Medtronic, Santa Rosa, CA)

Key Learning Issues of this Specific Case
As mentioned earlier, in this particular case, we could have judged better by selecting the length of the initial stent, and therefore avoided the need for a second stent.

Case # 2: Heavily Calcified High-Grade Stenosis of the Left Subclavian Artery With Total Occlusion of the Innominate Artery and High-Grade Stenosis of the Left Common Carotid

A 72-year-old male who presents with coronary artery bypass grafting with three vein grafts in the remote past.

Procedure:
After addressing the right common carotid lesion from a femoral approach using an I-Cast covered stent, we proceeded with intervention on the subclavian lesion. Access to the left brachial artery was obtained in a retrograde fashion with an 18-gauge Cook needle and a 0.035-inch × 180-cm angled Glidewire using Seldinger technique. A 6-F × 11-cm sheath was then placed in the artery. The Glidewire was then advanced across the lesion with ease. The short sheath was exchanged for a 7-F × 55-cm Cordis sheath, which was advanced into the postvertebral left subclavian artery. A hand-injected retrograde arteriogram was then obtained, demonstrating a short-segment, highly calcified ostial lesion of >90% stenosis, with a large and patent vertebral artery. With the dilator re-inserted into the sheath, it was advanced across the lesion into the aorta. A puff of contrast was then used to confirm placement in the aorta. A pull-back arteriogram was then obtained to mark the landing zones. The sheath was re-advanced into the aorta, using the dilator. Because of the lesion's heavy calcification and the risk of embolizing into the patient's only vertebral artery, we chose to proceed with primary stenting using a covered, balloon-expandable stent. A 7-mm × 22-mm I-Cast stent was selected. The stent was advanced over the wire into the sheath, which had been advanced distal to the lesion. The sheath was pulled back to uncover the stent and prepare it for deployment. A predeployment angiogram was obtained through the sheath to confirm correct positioning. The stent-graft was slowly deployed, allowing the balloon to form an hourglass shape. After deployment, the stent's proximal overhang was flared by advancing the balloon partially into the aorta and inflating it. The wire and balloon were removed and a completion arteriogram was obtained, showing excellent results (Figs. 3 and 4). A Boomerang device was then used to close the artery (Fig. 5).

What made the Case Complex?
Because of innominate artery occlusion, severe coronary disease, and highly calcific carotid and subclavian lesions, the patient is considered a complex case. In addition, the subclavian lesion in this case was considered complex, because of the lesion's high degree of calcification and

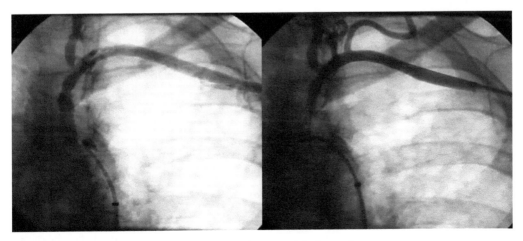

Figure 3   Angiogram showing 90% ostial lesion and post-stent deployment.

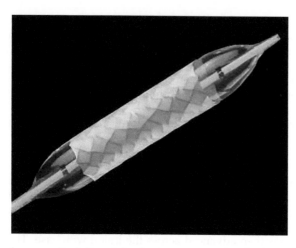

Figure 4   Photo of I-Cast stent, 7 mm × 20 mm (note covering of stent).

because the left vertebral artery appeared to be the only patent vessel connecting to the patient's posterior cerebral circulation.

What was the Clinical Indication for Treatment of this Patient?
He had a recent cardiac event that lead to repeat catheterization, revealing coronary disease not amenable to revascularization, total occlusion of the innominate artery, and high-grade stenosis (> 90%) of both the left common carotid and left subclavian arteries.

What were the Potential Hazards of Treating this Patient and Anatomy?
Stenting was considered important in this case, as balloon angioplasty would not have been a viable long-term treatment in this very calcified lesion. Embolization appears to be a true risk in highly calcified lesions and, given the importance of this patient's left vertebral artery, we believed steps should be taken to minimize this risk. Therefore, we chose to proceed with primary stenting in the hope this would minimize the potential for free fragmentation of debris.

Which Interventional Strategies were Considered?
In similar cases, one option might have been the use of a protection device such as the Emboshield (Abbbott Labs, Abbott Park, IL) but, in this case, the vertebral artery was smaller than the device was designed for.

Which Interventional Tools were used to Manage this Case?
We selected a covered stent (I-Cast, Atrium Medical, Hudson, NH), believing this would further reduce the possibility of embolization.

Summary: How was the case Managed, is There Anything that Could Have Been Improved, and What was the Immediate and Long-Term Outcome?
The stent-graft was slowly deployed, allowing the balloon to form an hourglass shape. After deployment, the stent's proximal overhang was flared by advancing the balloon partially into

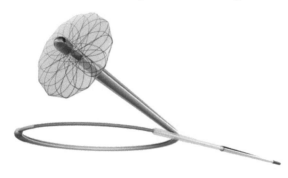

Figure 5 Photograph of the Boomerang Device for arterial closure.

the aorta and inflating it. The wire and balloon were removed, and a completion arteriogram was obtained, showing excellent results (Figs. 3 and 4). A Boomerang device was then used to close the artery. The patient is now six months out from his procedure and doing well.

List of Equipment used in this Case
18-gauge Cook needle (Cook, Bloomington, IL)
6-F × 11-cm Cordis sheath (Cordis, Miami Lakes, FL)
7-F × 55-cm Cordis sheath (Cordis)
0.035-inch × 180-cm regular angled Glidewire (Terumo, Somerset, NJ)
7-mm × 22-mm I-Cast stent graft (Atrium Medical, Hudson, NH)
5/6 Boomerang closure device (Cardiva, Mountain View, CA)

Key Learning Issues of this Specific Case
The vertebral artery is very fragile, so risk of dissection is of great concern. Another option might have been abandoning endovascular therapy altogether and proceeding with carotid–subclavian bypass after stenting the left common carotid. This was not a good option for this patient because of his severe cardiac disease and recent cardiac event.

Case #3: Difficult Left Carotid–Subclavian Bypass Stenosis
This is a 50-year-old male, who had undergone an ascending aortic graft for a Type I dissection three years ago. He then developed a large aortic arch aneurysm that was treated by a rerouting procedure, with grafts from the ascending aorta (anastomosed to the previous graft) to the innominate and left common carotid arteries. The arch aneurysm was excluded with a Gore TAG thoracic endoprosthesis (WL Gore Associates, Flagstaff, AZ). The left subclavian artery was intentionally covered with this graft. The patient did well until six weeks postprocedure, at which time he developed left upper extremity claudication necessitating a left carotid–subclavian bypass. Recurrent symptoms developed two months later, and duplex scanning showed increased velocities at the carotid anastomosis.

Procedure:
Access to the left brachial artery was obtained in a retrograde fashion with an 18-gauge Cook needle and a 0.035-inch × 180-cm angled Glidewire, using Seldinger technique. A 6-F × 11-cm sheath was then placed in the artery. Heparin was given intravenously, and the activated clotting time was kept at 200 to 250 seconds for the remainder of the case. A 4-F × 90-cm angled Glide catheter was advanced over the wire to the proximal subclavian, and a hand-injected arteriogram obtained. This revealed an occluded proximal left subclavian artery, a patent left vertebral artery, and a patent carotid–subclavian bypass. The bypass was selectively cannulated, and an arteriogram of the bypass performed. This showed significant evidence of a carotid-to-graft anastomotic stenosis, greater than 50%. The bypass was crossed with a 0.035-inch × 180-cm Glidewire. Because of the angle and severity of stenosis, a Glide catheter would not advance over the wire into the common carotid artery. A Spectranetics "Quick-cross" catheter was placed over the wire into the common carotid and rerouting bypass graft. The wire was removed, and pull-back gradients obtained across the carotid–subclavian bypass, demonstrating a 40 mm Hg systolic gradient with significant dampening of the waveform. The bypass was re-crossed with a 0.035-inch × 180-cm regular angled Glidewire, advanced to the proximal rerouting bypass and into the ascending aorta. The Spectranetics catheter was used to exchange this for a 0.035-inch × 450-cm angled stiff Glidewire. Fortunately, the Glidewire tracked easily into the thoracic endograft and down to the aorta into the left iliac artery. Left femoral access was obtained using an 18-gauge Cook needle with a 0.035-inch × 260-cm regular angled Glidewire and a 9-F × 11-cm Cordis sheath placed in a retrograde fashion. The 450-cm Glidewire was snared and pulled out of the left femoral sheath, establishing a left-brachial-to-left-femoral wire.

After establishing the left-brachial-to-left-femoral wire, tension was applied at each end by grasping the wire with hemostats and pulling. The left brachial sheath was exchanged for a 7-F × 11-cm Cordis sheath, and a Multi-track 7-F monorail angiocatheter was advanced over the brachial aspect of the wire into the left carotid–subclavian bypass. A power injector angiogram was obtained showing the stenosis. Next, a balloon angioplasty was performed using first a

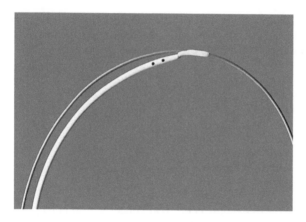

Figure 6 Spectranetics Multi-track angiographic catheter.

4-mm × 2-cm, then a 6-mm × 2-cm OptiPro balloon. The Multi-track (Spectranetics) catheter (Fig. 6) was used for a postangioplasty arteriogram, which showed significant rebound of the lesion. Due to the rebound, a 6-mm × 17-mm Express LD stent was deployed, leaving a 2-mm overhang into the common carotid artery (Figs. 7 and 8). The Multi-track catheter was again used to obtain a completion angiogram, which now showed resolution of the stenosis. Gradients were re-evaluated, showing improved waveform and resolution of pressure differences. The brachial and femoral sheaths were removed in the recovery room.

What Made the Case Complex?
The complexity of this case is reflected in the inability to use traditional techniques, to evaluate and treat the lesion because of the lack of "pushability" of the catheters in relation to the lesion.

What was the Clinical Indication for Treatment of this Patient?
This patient had undergone an ascending aortic graft for a Type I dissection three years ago. He then developed a large aortic arch aneurysm that was treated by a rerouting procedure, with grafts from the ascending aorta (anastomosed to the previous graft) to the innominate and left common carotid arteries. He developed left upper extremity claudication necessitating a left carotid–subclavian bypass. Recurrent symptoms developed two months later, and duplex scanning showed increased velocities at the carotid anastomosis.

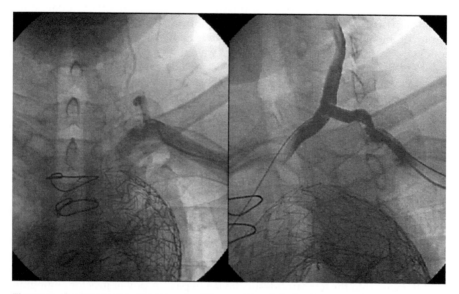

Figure 7 Angiogram showing stenosis of the carotid–subclavian bypass and post-stent deployment.

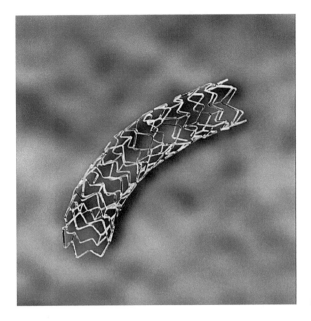

Figure 8 Photo of Express LD stent (6 × 17 mm) used to correct subclavian bypass stenosis.

What were the Potential Hazards of Treating this Patient and Anatomy?

Because of the angulation and stenosis of the bypass, we were unable to pass even a simple catheter over a wire into the common carotid. This was initially overcome using the Spectranetics "quick-cross" catheter, with its very low-profile tapered tip. This is one of our workhorse catheters for difficult lesions and total occlusions. Next, we were faced with a defined problem that we could not treat because no balloon/stent would cross the lesion from the brachial approach.

Which Interventional Strategies were Considered?

One option that we considered was the placement of a very stiff wire, such as an Amplatz wire, across the lesion for support. The downside of such an approach is the potential for injury or dissection of the left common carotid artery. Ultimately, we chose to obtain femoral access and establish a brachial-to-femoral wire for the added support needed, with less risk of injury to the carotid artery.

Which Interventional Tools Were Used to Manage this Case?

Given the nature of the patient's previous rerouting, the intervention was challenging. The maneuver would not have been possible without the extended-length (450-cm) Glidewire.

Summary: How was the Case Managed, is There Anything that Could Have Been Improved, and What was the Immediate and Long-Term Outcome?

After establishing the brachial-to-femoral wire, the final challenge was how to perform angiograms while maintaining the wire in place. This problem was easily overcome using the Multi-track angiocatheter, which has a monorail design, allowing power-injection imaging while maintaining the wire. The patient is now two months postprocedure and is free of symptoms.

List of Equipment used in this Case

(2) 18-gauge Cook needle (Cook, Bloomington, IN)
6-F × 11-cm Cordis sheath (Cordis, Miami Lakes, FL
7-F × 11-cm Cordis sheath (Cordis)
9-F × 11-cm Cordis sheath (Cordis)
0.035-inch × 180-cm regular angled Glidewire (Terumo, Somerset, NJ)
0.035-inch × 260-cm regular Glidewire (Terumo)

0.035-inch × 450-cm angled stiff Glidewire (Terumo)
Spectranetics "Quick-cross" catheter (Spectranetics, Colorado Springs, CO)
7-F Multi-track angiographic catheter (NuMed, Hopkinton, NY)
4-mm × 2-cm OptiPro Balloon (Cordis, Miami Lakes, FL)
6-mm × 2-cm OptiPro Balloon (Cordis)
6-mm × 17-mm Express LD Stent (Boston Scientific, Natick, MA)

Key Learning Issues of this Specific Case

This was a patient with significant disease and at risk from prior intervention. Because of angulation and stenosis of the bypass, we were unable to pass even a simple catheter over a wire into the common carotid. It is important to consider all options in such a case and to have a variety of tools at hand. Considerable experience with these tools and an experienced team is a must in these situations.

SUMMARY OF KEY ISSUES FOR SAFE, SUCCESSFUL TREATMENT OF SUBCLAVIAN LESIONS

Endovascular therapy of the subclavian arteries has been in wide use for a number of years and has proven safe and effective. Complications associated with endovascular therapy are often preventable, and the use of appropriate technique is one of the most important ways to limit complications. Preoperative imaging is extremely important in determining the indication and optimal approach for subclavian intervention. Although angiography remains the gold standard, CT and magnetic resonance angiography offer additional diagnostic value, as does IVUS imaging. IVUS may be particularly useful in vessel diameter determination so that overdilatation and arterial injury can be prevented. It is also helpful in accurate stent placement at the origins of the subclavian or aortic arch. Gentle manipulation of endovascular equipment is very important in reducing the risk of embolization and other complications. While restenosis does not represent a considerable problem in the subclavian arteries, it may present as a complication later. As such, ongoing clinical follow-up and imaging is mandatory in those who have undergone endovascular intervention.

REFERENCES

1. Diethrich EB, Garrett HE, Ameriso J, et al. Occlusive disease of the common carotid and subclavian arteries treated by carotid-subclavian bypass. Analysis of 125 cases. Am J Surg 1967; 114:800–808.
2. DeBakey ME, Diethrich EB, Garrett HE, et al. Surgical treatment of cerebrovascular disease. Postgrad Med 1967; 42:218–230.
3. Diethrich EB, Koopot R. Simplified operative procedure for proximal subclavian arterial lesions: direct subclavian anastomosis. Am J Surg 1981; 142:416–421.
4. Przewlocki T, Kablak-Ziembicka A, Pieniazek P, et al. Determinants of immediate and long-term results of subclavian and innominate artery angioplasty. Catheter Cardiovasc Interv 2006; 67(4):519–526.
5. Motarjeme A. Percutaneous transluminal angioplasty of supra-aortic vessels. J Endovasc Surg 1996; 3(2):171–181.
6. Martinez R, Rodriguez JA, Torruella L, et al. Stenting for occlusion of the subclavian arteries: Technical aspects and follow-up results. Tex Heart Inst J 1997; 24:23–27.
7. Mathias KD, Luth I, Haarmann P. Percutaneous transluminal angioplasty of proximal subclavian artery occlusions. Cardiovasc Intervent Radiol 1993; 16(4):214–218.
8. Nomura M, Kida S, Yamashima T, et al. Percutaneous transluminal angioplasty and stent placement for subclavian and brachiocephalic artery stenosis in aortitis syndrome. Cardiovasc Intervent Radiol 1999; 22:427–432.
9. Maskovic J, Jankovic S, Lusic I, et al. Subclavian artery stenosis caused by non-specific arteritis (Takayasu disease): treatment with Palmaz stent. Eur J Radiol 1999; 31:193–196.
10. Rodriguez-Lopez J, Werner A, Martinez R, et al. Stenting for atherosclerotic occlusive disease of the subclavian artery. Ann Vasc Surg 1999; 13:254–260.
11. Al-Mubarak N, Liu MW, Dean LS, et al. Immediate and late outcomes of subclavian artery stenting. Catheter Cardiovasc Interv 1999; 46:169–172.
12. Korner M, Baumgartner I, Do DD, et al. PTA of the subclavian and innominate arteries: long-term results. Vasa 1999; 28:117–122.

13. d'Othee BJ, Rousseau H, Otal P, et al. Noncovered stent placement in a blunt traumatic injury of the subclavian artery. Cardiovasc Intervent Radiol 1999; 22:424–427.
14. Bruninx G, Wery D, Dubois E, et al. Emergency endovascular treatment of an acute traumatic rupture of the thoracic aorta complicated by a distal low-flow syndrome. Cardiovasc Intervent Radiol 1999; 22:515–518.
15. Malek AM, Higashida RT, Phatouros CC, et al. Treatment of posterior circulation ischemia with extracranial percutaneous balloon angioplasty and stent placement. Stroke 1999; 30:2073–2085.
16. Sitsen ME, Ho GH, Blankensteijn JD. Deformation of self-expanding stent-grafts complicating endovascular peripheral aneurysm repair. J Endovasc Surg 1999; 6:288–292.
17. Phipp LH, Scott DJ, Kessel D, et al. Subclavian stents and stent-grafts: cause for concern? J Endovasc Surg 1999; 6:223–226.
18. Malek AM, Higashida RT, Reilly LM, et al. Subclavian arteritis and pseudoaneurysm formation secondary to stent infection. Cardiovasc Intervent Radiol 2000; 23:57–60.

8 | Vertebral Interventions

J. Stephen Jenkins

Interventional Cardiology Research, Ochsner Heart and Vascular Institute, New Orleans, Louisiana, U.S.A.

COMPLEX VERTEBRAL INTERVENTIONS

The complexity of vertebral artery intervention is determined by the anatomical location of the lesion being treated (1). The anatomic course of the vertebral artery is divided into four segments (V1–V4) (Fig. 1). The complexity of ostial vertebral artery angioplasty presents a challenge as does angioplasty in the ostial location of any vessel. Precise stent placement covering the ostium without protruding excessively into the parent artery can always be a challenge. One to two millimeters of stent hanging into the parent artery is necessary to prevent missing ostial disease (2).

The V1 segment originates at subclavian artery and extends to the transverse foramina of either the fifth or sixth cervical vertebrae. This segment can be treated percutaneously with relative ease provided it is not tortuous or redundant, as it tends to be in the more elderly patient. Percutaneous angioplasty is relatively simple in straight V1 segment arteries (3).

The V2 segment courses through the bony canal of the transverse foramina from C2 to C6. This is the easiest vertebral segment to treat percutaneously due to favorable anatomic features such as its short distance from the subclavian artery and its straight course.

The V3 segment continues as the artery exits the transverse foramina at C2 and ends as the vessel penetrates the dura mater and becomes an intracranial vessel. The complexity of angioplasty in the V3 segment increases as this segment is extremely tortuous to allow mobility of the alanto-axial and the alanto-occipital joint. Care should be taken to avoid balloon expandable stents in this flexible joint region. Short self-expanding stents and avoiding extreme tortuousity increase success in this segment.

The V4 segment courses along the inferior portion of the pons until joining the contralateral vertebral artery to form the basilar artery. The anterior spinal communicator arteries originate from the V4 segments bilaterally and join in the midline to supply the anterior two-thirds of the spinal cord. For this reason, angioplasty in the V4 segment should be approached with extreme caution, as occlusion of the anterior spinal communicators can cause major deficits.

CLINICAL INDICATIONS FOR TREATMENT OF COMPLEX LESIONS IN VERTEBRAL INTERVENTIONS

Vertebral artery revascularization is indicated when medical therapy has failed to alleviate symptoms of vertebral basilar insufficiency (VBI) (4,5). Accepted posterior circulation (vertebrobasilar) ischemic symptoms include: diplopia, dizziness, drop attacks, gait disturbance, dysphasia, and bilateral homonymous hemianopia (6). Prior to consideration for revascularization, the anatomy of the anterior and posterior circulation and the circle of Willis should be defined. A diagnostic aortic arch and four-vessel angiography including selective carotid and vertebral artery angiography is required. The anatomy is then correlated with the posterior circulation symptom complex to determine which artery requires revascularization. In the absence of proximal atherosclerotic occlusive disease, unilateral vertebral artery stenosis or occlusion is well tolerated. Revascularization therapy for symptomatic VBI should be pursued in patients with:

1. bilateral vertebral stenosis greater than 70% luminal diameter stenosis;
2. unilateral stenosis greater than 70% luminal diameter stenosis in the presence of an occluded or hypoplastic contralateral vertebral artery;
3. artery-to-artery embolism from a stenosis in the vertebral artery even in the presence of a unilateral stenosis (7,8).

Additional indications include instances where vertebral angioplasty would increase total cerebral blood flow to patients with diffuse atherosclerotic disease involving occlusions of both

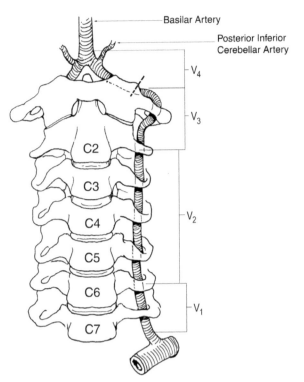

Figure 1 Vertebral artery anatomy.

carotid arteries (9). Vertebral angioplasty should not be attempted once the vessel is totally occluded. Although some percentage of total occlusions could technically be treated, the distal embolic debris would be clinically devastating due to territory supplied by V4 and basilar artery causing cerebellar, midbrain, pons, medullary or brainstem infarctions. Total occlusion of the vertebral artery is a contraindication to endovascular treatment (10).

HAZARDS AND COMPLICATIONS

Procedural complications of vertebral artery stenting include major and minor stroke, Transient Ischemic Attacks (TIA), and all other complications that accompany percutaneous procedures including death, access site bleeding, vessel rupture, and renal failure (11,12) (Table 1).

Important branches of the V4 segment include the posterior inferior cerebellar artery (PICA) and the anterior spinal artery. The anterior spinal artery from each V4 artery joins in the midline and supplies the anterior two-thirds of the spinal cord. It is because of these branches that angioplasty of the V4 segment is extremely risky and is rarely attempted except for acute stroke intervention or severe symptoms unresponsive to medical treatment.

INTERVENTIONAL STRATEGIES

Contrast angiography using digital subtraction techniques is the gold standard to identify vertebral basilar atherosclerotic disease. Angiographic evaluation includes an aortic arch and

Table 1

Peri-interventional complications		
	Proximal vertebral artery	**Distal vertebral artery**
TIA	1–2%	1%
Major stroke	1–2%	10%
MI	0	0
Death	<1%	3%

four-vessel study with selective angiography of bilateral carotid and vertebral arteries including intracranial imaging. The intracranial distribution of the anterior and posterior circulation and the circle of Willis should also be defined in several views making certain to identify any collateral blood supply.

A 5-F Berenstein is the diagnostic catheter of choice to perform selective angiography of the vertebral artery. A 4-F, 5-F or 6-F Judkins right, internal mammary, or Vitek curved catheters are acceptable if the vertebral artery cannot be cannulated with a Berenstein catheter. A multipurpose curve is useful when procedures are performed using a brachial access. A 0.035-in. hydrophilic wire or J-wire should be used to place the diagnostic catheter in the subclavian artery distal to the vertebral artery ostium. A manifold is connected and continuous pressure monitored while engaging the vertebral artery ostium. A 0.014-in. soft guidewire or filterwire is recommended for use with a rapid exchange or monorail balloon to predilate the stenotic lesion. Embolic protection devices are not FDA approved for use in the vertebral artery; however, it should be strongly considered if there is a comfortable landing zone distal to the index lesion. The predilation balloon should be 0.5 mm less than that of the reference vessel diameter. One must be very diligent to keep the tip of the guidewire within view at all times during the procedure as guidewire perforation can cause fatal intracranial hemorrhage. This can happen with any guidewire, but is of particular concern when a hydrophilic guidewire is used. Balloon expandable coronary or peripheral stents on a 0.014-in. platform work well in the vertebral artery ostium. The proximal stent should be extended 1 to 2 mm into the subclavian artery to ensure coverage of the vertebral artery ostium. Both balloon expandable and self-expanding stents are acceptable in the V1 and V2 segments of the vertebral artery. Balloon expandable stents should be used when the stenosis is in proximity of the vertebral artery ostium (13).

INTERVENTIONAL TOOLS

	Size	Device
Guide catheters	6-Fr	Envoy
		Judkins right
		Internal mammary
		Multipurpose
Guidewires	0.014 in.	Balance Middle Weight (Abbott)
		Wisper (Abbott)
		Choice PT (Cordis)
Embolic protection	4–6 mm	Filterwire (BSC)
Stents balloon expandable	3–6 mm	Vision (Abbott)
		Liberte (BSC)
		Express Biliary SD (BSC)
		Palmaz Blue (Cordis)
Stents self-expanding	4–7 mm	Xpert (Abbott)

SUMMARY OF OUTCOMES

Symptomatic vertebral artery stenosis (VAS) has a five-year stroke risk of 30% to 35%. Mortality associated with posterior circulation (PC) strokes is high, ranging from 20% to 30% (10,14,15). Surgical revascularization is rarely performed due to high morbidity and mortality. Surgical morbidity includes recurrent laryngeal nerve palsy, Horner's syndrome, lymphocele, chylothorax, and thrombosis (Table 2). Endovascular revascularization with stents offers a potential treatment option for these patients (Table 2) (16,17).

Percutaneous angioplasty and stent placement of PC, symptomatic, vertebrobasilar atherosclerotic disease is a safe and effective approach that avoids the morbidity associated with major surgery. Balloon angioplasty alone or combined with stenting is associated with high success rates and low to moderate restenosis rates when bare metal stents are used. Most available data are limited to single-center retrospective reports. There is a scarcity of data using drug-eluting stents in PC territory and it will not be included in this review (Table 3) (2,12,18–20).

Table 2   Surgical Morbidity

Recurrent Laryngeal nerve palsy	2%
Horner's syndrome	15%
Lymphocele	4%
Chylothorax	5%
Thrombosis	1%

The only randomized data to date comparing vertebral artery stenting to medical therapy was reported by Coward in 2007 (21). The CAVATAS study (Carotid and Vertebral Artery Transluminal Angioplasty Study) included a total of 16 vertebral stenosis patients randomized equally to endovascular or medical therapy. Endovascular treatment was successful in all eight patients with two procedural TIAs giving a 25% morbidity in the percutaneous arm. At mean follow-up of 4.7 years there were no vertebral strokes in either group. The composite of myocardial infarction, stroke, and death occurred in three patients in the medical treatment arm and in four patients in the endovascular arm. The authors concluded from this study that there was no benefit from endovascular therapy and stroke was more common in the carotid territory. Although the data benefit from being randomized, the numbers are too small to draw conclusions.

In the Cochrane Review reported by Coward et al. (22), the literature was searched for English papers that reported at least three cases of vertebral artery intervention. He identified 313 cases of vertebral artery intervention, which included 173 cases of primary stent placement. In these 20 studies combined, there was a 30-day major stroke and death rate of 3.2% and a 30-day TIA and nondisabling stroke rate of 3.2%. These published case series combined suggest that endovascular treatment of the vertebral artery is safe and effective although selection bias exists. Although this data is nonrandomized, it is much stronger than the one randomized vertebral trial published to date.

EQUIPMENT CHECKLIST (TABLE 4)

Interventional Guidewires
0.014″ soft guidewire is recommended for use with a rapid exchange (RX) or monorail balloon. A filterwire should be used in all vertebral arteries with an adequate landing zone distal to the index lesion. Although there is no data to support this statement, the author feels the obligatory embolization of atherosclerotic debris with balloon angioplasty in a territory as sensitive as the PC can potentially be minimized with distal protection devices.

Interventional Guide Catheters
A 6-F or 5-F Judkins right, multipurpose or envoy guiding catheter can be used to perform the intervention. A curve similar to the diagnostic imaging catheter should be chosen.

PTA Balloons
The balloon length is determined by the lesion length and should cover the lesion completely. The balloon diameter should be at least 0.5 mm less than the reference vessel diameter.

Table 3   Studies of Vertebral Artery Stenting

References	N	Technical success rate (%)	Procedural complications	Improvement in symptoms	Mean follow-up	Late stroke	Restenosis
12	32	100	TIA (1)	31/32	10.6 mo	0/32	1/32
2	33	97	CVA (1)	27/33	16.2 mo	1/33	43%
18	50	98	None	48/50	25 mo	1/50	10%
19	58	100	CVA (3)	56/58	31.3 mo	0/58	25%
20	38	100	TIA (1)	23/26	11 mo	0/38	36%

CVA = cerebral vascular event.

Table 4 Vertebral Angioplasty Equipments list

Guidewires	0.014 soft guidewire, rapid exchange
Guides	5-F or 6-F Judkins right, multipurpose or Envoy
Balloons	3.0–5.0 × 15–20 mm, moderately compliant balloon
Stents	Balloon expandable or self-expanding stents
Embolic protection devices	Filterwire, spiderwire, accunet, angioguard, emboshield

Stents

Balloon expandable coronary or peripheral stents on a 0.014 platform work well in the ostial or V1 position. One needs to be certain that the proximal portion of the stent covers the vertebral ostium. It is not uncommon for the proximal stent to extend back into the subclavian artery by 1 to 2 mm. Both balloon expandable and self-expanding stents are acceptable in the V1, V2, and V3 position when the lesion does not involve the ostium of the vertebral artery. Stents should be avoided if possible in the V4 position unless needed for bail out indications.

Embolic Protection Devices

Embolic protection devices (mentioned above) are not FDA approved for use in the vertebral artery, however, they should be considered if there is a comfortable landing zone distal to the index lesion.

CASE PRESENTATIONS

Complex Case 1

Relevant Clinical Information

This is a 50-year-old male with a history of atherosclerotic coronary artery disease treated with percutaneous intervention, hypertension, diabetes mellitus, hypercholesterolemia, and smoking. Medications included Glyburide, Maxide, and aspirin. Meclozine was begun for symptoms of dizziness two weeks prior to presentation by his primary care physician. Physical exam and laboratory exam were unremarkable. On presentation to our institution, this patient complained of profound dizziness, drop attacks, and vertigo. He reported many near fainting spells, which were not necessarily related to position or exertion; however, one position did tend to exacerbate his symptoms. The patient worked as a diesel engine boat mechanic and reported frequently falling into the engine portion of the boats when he was bending over attempting to perform his job. Prior to the patient's referral he underwent an arch and four-vessel cerebral study that demonstrated bilateral VAS. He was referred to our institution for further management and treatment of vertebrobasilar insufficiency.

Angiographic Images—Diagnostic and Intervention
Commentary
The diagnostic images demonstrate critical narrowing of both vertebral arteries in a patient with typical symptoms of VBI. The interventional results show bilateral vertebral ostium that are widely patent with adequately expanded stents and good angiographic results. The interesting scenario that surrounds this case is the presentation of VBI in this patient and the response to revascularization, first in the left vertebral artery and then two months later the right vertebral artery, as well as in-stent restenosis occurring six months after intervention on the left vertebral artery.

This patient had recurrent episodes of dizziness, vertigo, near fainting spells, and drop attacks. On several instances, he physically hurt himself by falling and cutting his head while at work. Of note, the basilar artery was intact and the posterior cerebral arteries were normal. This would lead one to believe that revascularization of one vertebral artery would provide adequate flow to the PC relieving the VBI symptoms. However, after revascularization of the left vertebral artery, the patient reported a definite improvement but partial resolution in the severity of his symptoms. He was instructed that only one patent vertebral artery was necessary to supply adequate flow to the PC and should relieve symptoms of VBI, as long as the basilar

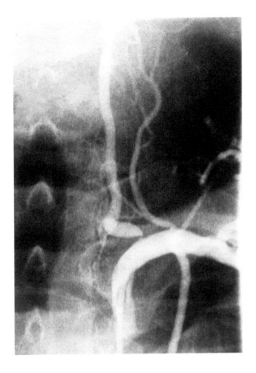

Figure 2 This image demonstrates a high-grade ostial stenosis of the left vertebral artery. Approximately 2 cm distal to the ostium the vessel makes a 90° turn cephalad. This gives an adequate window for angioplasty and stenting with a short stent.

artery and posterior cerebrals are normal. Only partial resolution of his symptoms occurred with a patent left vertebral artery and he requested on multiple occasions that intervention be performed on the other vertebral artery. After much persistence, the right vertebral artery was angioplastied and stented two months later with complete resolution of symptoms. Although it has been reported that one vertebral artery is adequate to prevent symptoms of VBI in man (23,24), this was clearly not adequate to relieve symptoms in this patient.

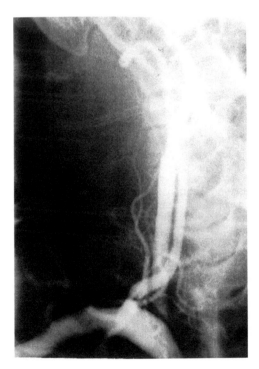

Figure 3 The final result demonstrates a well-deployed stent with a distal step down. Angioplasty was performed using 8-Fr coronary equipment. Anticoagulation with 8000 units of intravenous heparin was given to maintain an activated clotting time (ACT) > 300 seconds and a diagnostic 6-Fr JR4 catheter was used to selectively cannulate the left vertebral artery ostium. A 0.035-in guidewire was then inserted into the V2 segment of the artery and the diagnostic catheter was exchanged for an 8-Fr JR4 coronary guiding catheter. A 4 × 2 peripheral angioplasty balloon was used to perform predilation. A J&J P104 biliary stent (Cordis Corporation, Miami, FL) was then mounted on a 5 × 2 balloon and deployed in the ostium of the left vertebral artery. Note that the short stent has allowed the tortuous segment of this artery to remain unchanged.

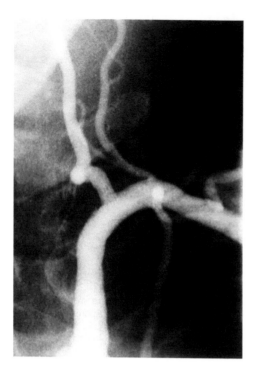

Figure 4 This image represents a 95% stenosis of the right vertebral artery ostium. Transition to the bony canal of the V2 segment is smooth, lending this vessel more favorable anatomy for percutaneous angioplasty with less risk of distal dissection.

The patient remained asymptomatic and free of VBI symptoms with two patent vertebral arteries and could once again perform his duties as a diesel boat mechanic. Four months later, he presented again with VBI symptoms that were consistent with the symptoms he experienced with one patent vertebral artery. There was definite improvement but only partial resolution in severity of the VBI symptoms when compared to his initial presentation. Repeat angiography was performed demonstrating in-stent restenosis of the left vertebral artery. Simple

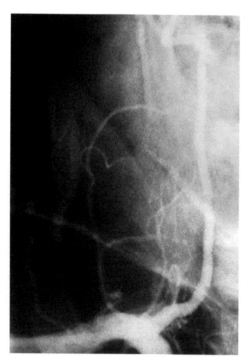

Figure 5 This image demonstrates the final angioplasty result in the ostial right vertebral artery. Anticoagulation with heparin was given to maintain an ACT > 300 seconds and a 5-Fr Van Andle catheter was used to cannulate the right vertebral artery ostium. A 0.035-in. guidewire was then advanced into the V2 segment of the artery taking care not to traumatize the V4 segment with the wire. Two important branches, the posterior inferior cerebellar artery and anterior spinal communicators, arise from this segment and care should be exercised to protect these small vessels from the guidewire. The diagnostic catheter was then exchanged for an 8-Fr multipurpose coronary guiding catheter. Predilation was performed with a 5 × 2 balloon. A J&J P104 biliary stent was mounted on the balloon and deployed in the ostium of the right vertebral artery with high-pressure inflations. The final result demonstrates a widely patent ostium with a step down seen at the distal end of the stent.

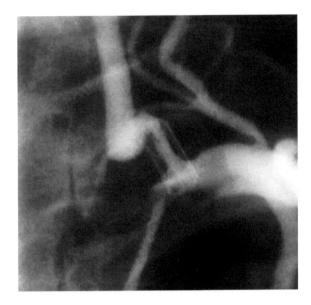

Figure 6 This image of the left vertebral artery was taken six months after stent implantation. It demonstrates a critical 90% in-stent restenosis lesion.

balloon angioplasty was performed with adequate results and the patient's symptoms once again resolved completely.

Contrary to the published literature with regards to the number of vertebral arteries necessary to relieve VBI symptoms, this patient clearly needed two patent vertebral arteries to relieve his symptoms. Whether the right vertebral was patent with an occluded left vertebral artery or vice versa, symptoms persisted that prevented this patient from performing his job.

(a) What made the case "complex"? This case is considered complex as it was necessary to treat both vertebral arteries in order to render this patient asymptomatic.
(b) What was the clinical indication for treatment of this patient? The indication to treat this patient was drop attacks and dizziness.
(c) What were the potential hazards of treating this patient and anatomy? The hazards include dissection, stroke, and TIA.
(d) Which interventional strategies were considered? A strategy that would allow the guidewire to sit in the subclavian artery without intubating the vertebral artery was necessary to successfully treat both of these ostial lesions.

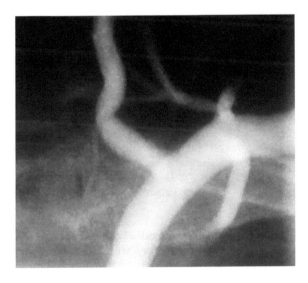

Figure 7 Left vertebral artery is shown after treatment of in-stent restenosis with a 5 × 2 balloon at 18 atm. There is approximately a 10% residual stenosis.

(e) Which interventional tools were used to manage this case? A Judkins right coronary guide and sportwire were used to image and cross these lesions. Palmaz P154 stents were mounted on a 5 × 20 balloon and deployed at 12 atm.

(f) Summary: How was the case managed, is there anything that could have been improved, what was the immediate and long-term outcome? The outcome was suboptimal with only partial improvement after treatment on only one vertebral artery. The symptoms in this patient resolved completely after stenting of both vertebral arteries.

(g) List of equipments used in this case: Plamaz P154 stent, 5 × 20 angioplasty balloon, sportwire, and Judkins right 4 guide.

(h) Key learning issues of this specific case: Two patent vertebral arteries are necessary in some patients to provide adequate PC flow.

Complex Case 2

This patient is an 83-year-old male with a history of dilated cardiomyopathy, peripheral vascular disease, and non-Hodgkin's lymphoma treated with chemotherapy 10 years prior who presented with two transient ischemic attacks in the previous month. The symptoms were described as dizziness and blurred vision that lasted between 15 to 20 minutes and resolved. Initial work-up included a computed tomography scan of the head that was normal and carotid duplex scan that demonstrated 20% to 39% stenosis bilaterally. The patient was initially treated with coumadin maintaining a therapeutic INR for two months before the identical symptoms as above returned.

Physical examination revealed a blood pressure of 154/70 mm Hg and heart rate 60 beats per minute. The patient was alert and oriented × 3. There was no carotid bruit, no neurologic findings, and the rest of the physical exam was normal.

At this point, he was referred for an arch and four-vessel angiography with intracranial imaging due to break through symptoms on coumadin with a therapeutic INR. Angiographic imaging revealed an occluded right V4 artery that ended in PICA. The left vertebral artery had a 90% stenosis in the V4 segment at the vertebral basilar junction.

This scenario of angiographic findings represents a high-risk case with potential for several complications. First, one should remember that angioplasty in the basilar artery can cause major stroke if plaque shift occurs into anterior inferior cerebellar or pontine arteries that arise from the basilar artery. Likewise, the posterior inferior cerebellar and anterior spinal communicator arteries arise from the V4 segment of the vertebral artery and can cause major stroke if balloon inflations compromise these branches. It is therefore wise to attempt plain old balloon angioplasty in these segments with an undersized balloon if an adequate angiographic result can be obtained without a flow limiting dissection. Stents should only be used for bail out with suboptimal balloon angioplasty results.

Angiographic Images
Commentary

This case represents successful percutaneous balloon angioplasty in the most risky segment of the vertebral artery. The vertebral basilar junction deserves respect due the tiny branches that arise from the V4 segment and the basilar artery. Major deficits or life-threatening cerebral vascular accidents can occur if these small branches are compromised with percutaneous angioplasty. With the use of an undersized balloon and no stent, this patient was successfully treated with no complications. Conservatism should be practiced when considering percutaneous therapy in this segment of the vertebral artery, and percutaneous therapy should not be attempted if there is resolution of symptoms with antiplatelet or anticoagulant therapy alone.

(a) What made the case "complex"? This case was complex because of the location of the stenosis in the V4 segment.

(b) What was the clinical indication for treatment of this patient? There were symptoms of dizziness and blurred vision while the patient was taking coumadin with therapeutic INR levels. Failure of medical therapy to relieve symptoms constitutes an indication for arch and four-vessel angiography to determine if percutaneous therapy is a therapeutic option.

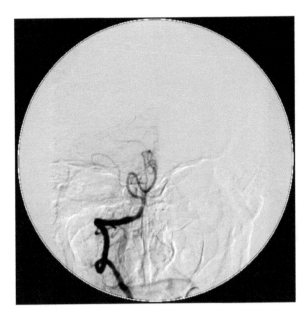

Figure 8 This image demonstrates an occluded right V4 at PICA.

(c) What were the potential hazards of treating this patient and anatomy? First, one should remember that angioplasty in the basilar artery can cause major stoke if plaque shift occurs into anterior inferior cerebellar or pontine arteries that arise from the basilar artery. Likewise, the posterior inferior cerebellar and anterior spinal communicator arteries arise from the V4 segment of the vertebral artery and can cause major stroke if balloon inflations compromise these branches.

(d) Which interventional strategies were considered? The only interventional strategy that should be considered in the basilar artery is provisional stenting. If an adequate result can be obtained with plain old balloon angioplasty then this is the best approach.

(e) Which interventional tools were used to manage this case? A guiding catheter, guidewire, and angioplasty balloon were used to manage this case.

(f) Summary: How was the case managed, is there anything that could have been improved, what was the immediate and long-term outcome? The procedure was completed

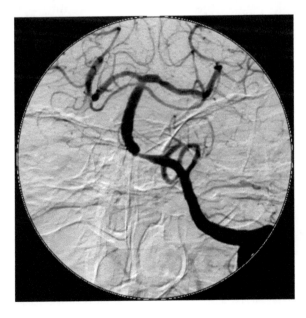

Figure 9 There is a 90% stenosis of the left vertebral artery in the V4 segment at the vertebral basilar junction.

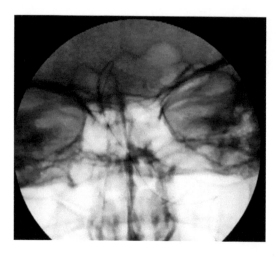

Figure 10 The reference vessel diameter in the basilar artery was 3.0 mm by quantitative analysis. A 2.5-mm balloon was chosen and plain old balloon angioplasty was attempted.

successfully with no TIA or stroke. The balloon inflations were tolerated well and at one-year follow-up the patient remained asymptomatic.

(g) List of equipments used in this case: Choice PT wire, Envoy guide, and a 2.5-mm balloon.
(h) Key learning issues of this specific case: Conservatism should be practiced in the V4 segment of the vertebral and stents should be placed only in bail out situations.

Complex Case 3

The patient is a 58-year-old Caucasian female with dyslipidemia, hypertension, and tobacco abuse referred for evaluation of symptomatic bilateral VAS. She had an extensive cardiac history including CABG 12 years prior with a left internal mammary artery (LIMA) to the left anterior descending coronary artery (LAD) and multiple coronary angioplasty procedures including brachytherapy on two occasions. Symptoms included frequent dizziness and imbalance for one year and occasional left arm and hand weakness that resulted in dropping objects on occasion. She denied left arm claudication or syncope.

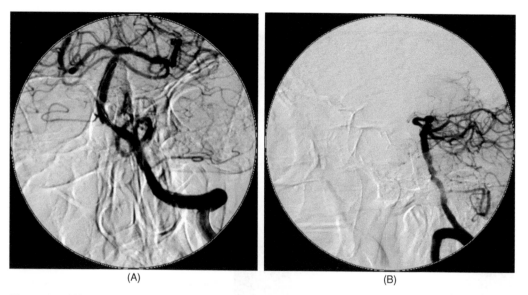

(A) (B)

Figure 11 (**A**) anterior posterior projection, (**B**) lateral projection. This image demonstrates an acceptable angiographic result with a 20% to 30% residual stenosis and no dissection that was accepted as the final result.

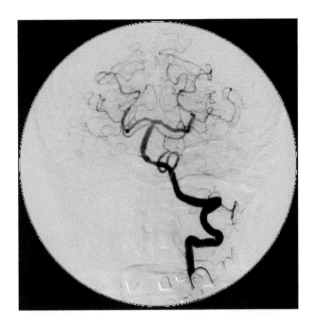

Figure 12 One-year follow-up angiography.

The physical exam was pertinent for a soft bruit over the right carotid artery and equal pulses bilaterally. The systolic blood pressure was 140/70 mm Hg bilaterally. There were no other significant physical findings. The patient was placed on dual antiplatelet therapy 18 months prior for coronary stenting with no improvement in her mentioned symptoms. She was referred for evaluation after nonselective coronary angiography of the LIMA graft demonstrated moderate left subclavian stenosis and significant left VAS.

Angiographic Images

Equipments and Strategies
A 5-Fr Bernstein diagnostic catheter was used to engage the brachieocephalic trunk and place a 0.035-guidewire into the right subclavian artery. The diagnostic catheter was exchanged for a 6-Fr Judkins right coronary guiding catheter that was withdrawn to select the ostium of the

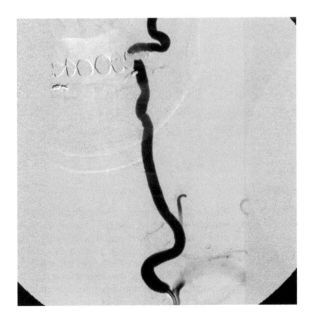

Figure 13 Ostial angiography of the left vertebral artery demonstrates an 80% stenosis with a 25-mm Hg gradient. There was a 50% stenosis of the left subclavian artery with no significant gradient.

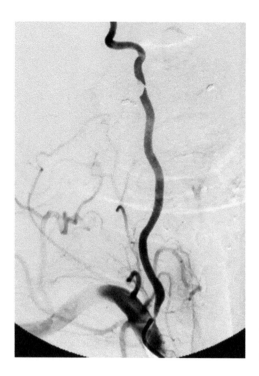

Figure 14 Critical 95% ostial stenosis of the right vertebral artery. Quantitative analysis was performed using this image, and a balloon size of 0.5 mm less than the reference vessel diameter was chosen.

right vertebral artery. A 0.014-coronary guidewire was then used to cross the ostial stenosis and a 3.0 × 20 mm balloon was inflated to 6 atm in the vertebral artery. A 4.0 × 12 mm stent was then deployed at 12 atm in the ostium of the artery. The use of a Judkins right curve in the subclavian artery allows precise positioning of the stent in ostial vertebral lesions. Gentle right or left torque on the catheter will position the stent in or out of the artery to allow precise placement when used in conjunction with contrast injections. The Judkins right curve allows visualization of the vertebral artery with the catheter sitting well into the subclavian artery so as not to interfere with the stent deployment. Regardless of the territory intervened

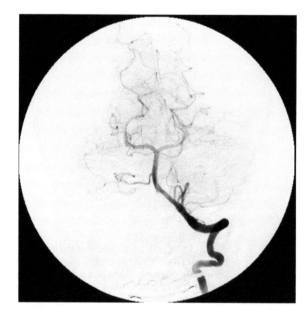

Figure 15 This image demonstrates baseline cerebral flow when injecting the left vertebral artery. Although both posterior cerebral, both anterior inferior cerebellar, and both superior cerebellar arteries are filled from this injection, there is no retrograde flow through the right V4 segment filling the right posterior inferior cerebellar artery.

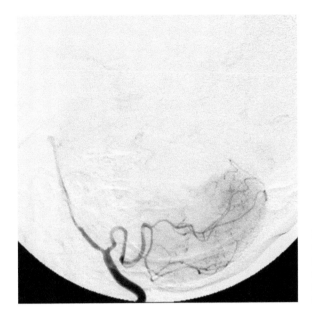

Figure 16 Intracranial imaging of the right vertebral artery demonstrates a hypoplastic, atherosclerotic V4 segment that isolates the right posterior inferior cerebellar artery. This represents the most likely ischemic territory per angiography.

upon, ostial stent positioning can always be a challenge and this is no different in the vertebral artery.

Commentary
There are several factors that make this case complex. First, one needs to determine clinically which lesion is the culprit when both subclavian arteries are moderately stenosed and both vertebral arteries have significant stenoses. A team approach is necessary with neurology evaluation to determine which lesion is the most symptomatic. In this case, the neurologist determined that the left PICA was the most likely cause of the patient's symptoms. Angiographically this seemed appropriate as there was a 5-mm Hg gradient across both subclavian stenoses and the patient had no anterior ischemia on nuclear stress imaging, and there was no claudication symptoms in either arm.

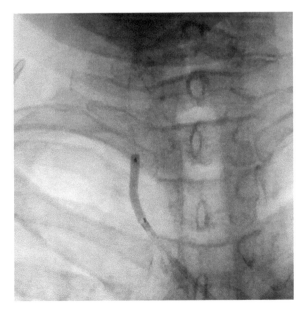

Figure 17 Balloon predilation is performed to both optimize stent positioning and to verify appropriate vessel diameter determined by quantitative analysis. Adequate predilation is also very important in facilitating stent placement in ostial lesions, as in this patient.

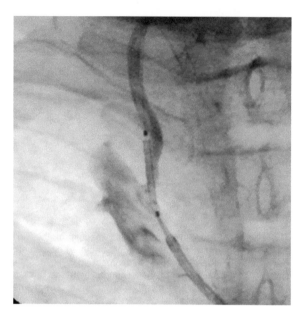

Figure 18 Contrast injections are performed to position the stent 1 to 2 mm into the subclavian artery. The vertebral artery ostium can be missed if this step is omitted.

The second complex factor in this case was the critical stenoses that were truly ostial in location. Careful stent positioning and hanging the stent 1 to 2 mm into the subclavian ostium will prevent missing the ostium and the need for an additional stent.

There was complete resolution of this patient's symptoms on neurologic exam at three months post procedure. This demonstrates that the untreated 80% stenosis of the left vertebral artery was not contributing to the patient's symptoms and that the right posterior inferior cerebellum was the ischemic territory. It is also possible that angioplasty of the left vertebral would allow enough retrograde flow through the hypoplastic V4 segment to render the patient asymptomatic. This approach was not chosen as it would be less likely to provide flow to the right PICA and because of the possibility of interfering with the LIMA graft. This patient was

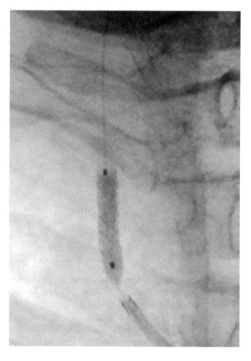

Figure 19 During deployment, the stent should be inflated slowly to prevent watermelon seeding forward or backward. This allows repositioning if necessary by placing the indeflator on neutral and making small movements with the stent delivery system.

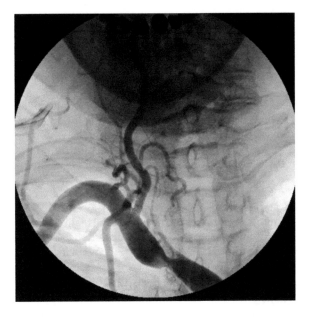

Figure 20 The final result is demonstrated with 1 to 2 mm of the stent hanging into the subclavian artery.

followed with serial duplex ultrasound exams to evaluate antegrade vertebral flow and bilateral arm blood pressure checks to monitor the bilateral subclavian stenoses.

(a) What made the case "complex"? This case was complex because both subclavian arteries and both vertebral arteries were diseased requiring a neurologic exam and a team approach to determine which lesion was the culprit. Both the anatomy and the neurologic exam were used to dictate which lesion to treat.

(b) What was the clinical indication for treatment of this patient? Symptoms included frequent dizziness and imbalance for approximately one year.

(c) What were the potential hazards of treating this patient and anatomy? The complexity of this anatomy with a diseased vertebral artery arising from a diseased subclavian that could potentially compromise both the right upper extremity and the PC. Also, the ostial location of this lesion requires special care in placing the stent to prevent missing the lesion.

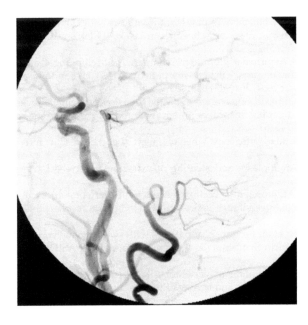

Figure 21 The final intracranial image demonstrates brisk flow in the right posterior inferior cerebellar artery and flow through the hypoplastic right V4 segment.

(d) Which interventional strategies were considered? The strategy was to treat the vertebral artery without compromising the subclavian artery. A primary stenting approach to the right vertebral artery ostium was planned.

(e) Which interventional tools were used to manage this case? A 6-Fr Judkins right guiding catheter, a 0.014 coronary guidewire, and a balloon expandable stent were used to primarily stent the vertebral artery.

(f) Summary: How was the case managed, is there anything that could have been improved, what was the immediate and long-term outcome? There was complete resolution of this patient's symptoms on neurologic exam at three months post procedure. This demonstrates that the untreated 80% stenosis of the left vertebral artery was not contributing to the patient's symptoms and that the right posterior inferior cerebellum was the ischemic territory.

(g) List of equipments used in this case: A 6-Fr Judkins right guiding catheter, a 0.014 wisper wire, and a 4.0 × 12 balloon expandable stent were used to perform this procedure.

(h) Key learning issues of this specific case: This case reinforces the need to take a team approach when performing vertebral angioplasty. Only the lesions that are symptomatic should be revascularized and the rest should be managed medically with routine surveillance.

SUMMARY OF THE KEY ISSUES FOR SUCCESSFUL AND SAFE TREATMENT OF COMPLEX VERTEBRAL ARTERY LESIONS

In summary, it is necessary to first know the anatomy of the PC by performing an arch and four-vessel diagnostic angiogram. A complete neurologic exam is also necessary to determine the symptomatic vessel that will provide the best revascularization to the PC. Proper guide selection and the use of coronary angioplasty equipment will allow safe and effective treatment of complex vertebral lesions. When anatomy allows, embolic protection devices should be used to prevent distal embolic complications. Following these rules will improve the chances of successful angioplasty in complex vertebral lesions.

REFERENCES

1. Jenkins JS, Subramanian R. Endovascular treatment for vertebrobasilar insufficiency. Curr Treat Options Cardiovasc Med 2002; 4(5):385–391.
2. Albuquerque FC, Fiorella D, Han P, et al. A reappraisal of angioplasty and stenting for the treatment of vertebral origin stenosis. Neurosurgery 2003; 53(3):607–614; discussion 14–16.
3. Nomura M, Hashimoto N, Nishi S, et al. Percutaneous transluminal angioplasty for intracranial vertebral and/or basilar artery stenosis. Clin Radiol 1999; 54(8):521–527.
4. Diener HC, Bogousslavsky J, Brass LM, et al. Management of atherothrombosis with clopidogrel in high-risk patients with recent transient ischaemic attack or ischaemic stroke (MATCH): study design and baseline data. Cerebrovasc Dis 2004; 17(2–3):253–261.
5. Diener HC, Bogousslavsky J, Brass LM, et al. Aspirin and clopidogrel compared with clopidogrel alone after recent ischaemic stroke or transient ischaemic attack in high-risk patients (MATCH): randomised, double-blind, placebo-controlled trial. Lancet 2004; 364(9431):331–337.
6. Whisnant JP, Cartlidge NE, Elveback LR. Carotid and vertebral-basilar transient ischemic attacks: effect of anticoagulants, hypertension, and cardiac disorders on survival and stroke occurrence–a population study. Ann Neurol 1978; 3(2):107–115.
7. Jenkins JS, White CJ, Ramee SR, et al. Vertebral insufficiency: when to intervene and how? Curr Interv Cardiol Rep 2000; 2(2):91–94.
8. Henry M, Polydorou A, Henry I, et al. Angioplasty and stenting of extracranial vertebral artery stenosis. Int Angiol 2005; 24(4):311–324.
9. Wehman JC, Hanel RA, Guidot CA, et al. Atherosclerotic occlusive extracranial vertebral artery disease: indications for intervention, endovascular techniques, short-term and long-term results. J Interv Cardiol 2004; 17(4):219–232.
10. Chimowitz MI, Lynn MJ, Howlett-Smith H, et al. Prognosis of patients with symptomatic vertebral or basilar artery stenosis. The Warfarin-Aspirin Symptomatic Intracranial Disease (WASID) Study Group. Stroke 1998; 29(7):1389–1392.
11. Eberhardt O, Naegele T, Raygrotzki S, et al. Stenting of vertebrobasilar arteries in symptomatic atherosclerotic disease and acute occlusion: case series and review of the literature. J Vasc Surg 2006; 43(6):1145–1154.

12. Jenkins JS, White CJ, Ramee SR, et al. Vertebral artery stenting. Catheter Cardiovasc Interv 2001; 54(1):1–5.
13. Mukherjee D, Roffi M, Kapadia SR, et al. Percutaneous intervention for symptomatic vertebral artery stenosis using coronary stents. J Invasive Cardiol 2001; 13(5):363–366.
14. Chimowitz MI, Lynn MJ, Howlett-Smith H, et al. Comparison of warfarin and aspirin for symptomatic intracranial arterial stenosis. N Engl J Med 2005; 352(13):1305–1316.
15. Fields WS, North RR, Hass WK, et al. Joint study of extracranial arterial occlusion as a cause of stroke. I. Organization of study and survey of patient population. JAMA 1968; 203(11):955–960.
16. Berguer R, Flynn LM, Kline RA, et al. Surgical reconstruction of the extracranial vertebral artery: management and outcome. J Vasc Surg 2000; 31(1, pt 1):9–18.
17. Thevenet A, Ruotolo C. Surgical repair of vertebral artery stenoses. J Cardiovasc Surg (Torino) 1984; 25(2):101–110.
18. Chastain HD II, Campbell MS, Iyer S, et al. Extracranial vertebral artery stent placement: in-hospital and follow-up results. J Neurosurg 1999; 91(4):547–552.
19. Lin YH, Juang JM, Jeng JS, et al. Symptomatic ostial vertebral artery stenosis treated with tubular coronary stents: clinical results and restenosis analysis. J Endovasc Ther 2004; 11(6):719–726.
20. Weber W, Mayer TE, Henkes H, et al. Stent-angioplasty of intracranial vertebral and basilar artery stenoses in symptomatic patients. Eur J Radiol 2005; 55(2):231–236.
21. Coward LJ, McCabe DJ, Ederle J, et al. Long-term outcome after angioplasty and stenting for symptomatic vertebral artery stenosis compared with medical treatment in the Carotid and Vertebral Artery Transluminal Angioplasty Study (CAVATAS): a randomized trial. Stroke 2007; 38(5):1526–1530.
22. Coward LJ, Featherstone RL, Brown MM. Percutaneous transluminal angioplasty and stenting for vertebral artery stenosis. Cochrane Database Syst Rev 2005 (2):CD000516.
23. Berguer R, Feldman AJ. Surgical reconstruction of the vertebral artery. Surgery 1983; 93(5):670–675.
24. Molnar RG, Naslund TC. Vertebral artery surgery. Surg Clin North Am 1998; 78(5):901–913.

9 | Thoracic Aortic Dissection and Nondissective Thoracic Aortic Disease

Martin Czerny and Michael Grimm

Department of Cardiothoracic Surgery, University of Vienna Medical School, Vienna, Austria

INTRODUCTION

Within the last decade, thoracic endovascular aortic repair (TEVAR) has been increasingly performed on patients with more advanced age as well as on thoracic aortic pathology being located within the aortic arch as supra-aortic transpositions have become an established, safe, and reproducible procedure (1–7). Indications for treatment contain dilatative as well as obliterative pathology, primarily aneurysms, being followed by a steadily increasing number of penetrating atherosclerotic ulcers (8). Furthermore, TEVAR has become the modality of choice in patients with complicated type B dissections (9,10). By a better understanding of the mechanisms of intramural hematoma (IMH), TEVAR is also applied in patients presenting with IMH of the entire thoracic aorta (11).

Atherosclerotic Thoracic Aortic Aneurysms

More than 50% of patients presenting with thoracic aortic aneurysms have to be regarded as complex, being defined by the need of an additional procedure prior to stent-graft placement in order to pave the route for a successful and durable endovascular procedure (12,13). The majority of these additional procedures are rerouting procedures primarily of the supra-aortic branches in order to gain a sufficient proximal landing zone for extensive sealing and prevention of endoleak formation. The length of the proximal landing zone has been shown to independently predict avoidance of early as well as late endoleak formation (5). The same is true for the distal landing zone; nevertheless visceral rerouting procedures are complex and invasive and it is still controversial if visceral rerouting prior to TEVAR really is less invasive than a conventional surgical approach with all safety nets available (14,15).

Penetrating Atherosclerotic Ulcers

Penetrating atherosclerotic ulcers (PAU) have been recently defined as a distinct entity of acute aortic syndromes gaining increasing importance by improved diagnostic means and by sensibilization of the scientific community to the pathology itself (16). Being the result of an advanced obliterative atherosclerotic process, PAU may also be associated with other severe manifestations of the underlying disease such as coronary artery disease as well as peripheral arterial occlusive disease. The natural history of PAU, especially when being symptomatic, is dismal (17,18). PAU may be complex due to their location, as at least one-third of them are located in the aortic arch as well as to the fact that—in contrast to aneurysms—many intercostal arteries are still patent and the risk of spinal cord injury is higher. Furthermore, vascular access may be challenging as more than 50% of patients require a retroperitoneal approach to the common iliac artery or even to the infrarenal aorta in order to be able to advance the introduction sheath of the stent graft (8).

Type B Dissections

Merely 1 out of 10 type B dissections is or turns complicated (19). Due to the results from the INSTEAD trial (yet unpublished), it is now generally accepted that uncomplicated type B dissections should be treated with a primary conservative approach. Nevertheless, complicated type B dissections are the ideal target for TEVAR as procedural morbidity and mortality are substantially less than any other approach (9,10). Complicated type B dissections define themselves by rupture or malperfusion irrespective of the affected vascular bed, that is, intercostal, visceral, renal or peripheral.

Intramural Hematoma

IMH of the aorta has been recently defined as a subtype of acute aortic wall dissection with no detectable intimal tear and consequently, lack of false lumen flow (20). Lack of presence of intimal disruption or flap has been the prerequisite for IMH diagnosis (16). With the recent advances in imaging, in particular via ECG-gating techniques, a more precise evaluation of IMH is possible. The presumed mechanism of IMH, rupture of vasa vasorum (21), however, may be doubted since in many IMH patients a small primary entry tear can be found (11). Rupture of a small atherosclerotic plaque at the free lateral wall or at the concavity of the distal aortic arch may be found as the underlying disease mechanism. Following plaque rupture, antegrade and/or retrograde progression of the pathology affects the aortic wall. If the primary lesion is located at the convexity of the aortic arch, supra-aortic branches may serve as a natural anatomical barrier against retrograde progression, thus resulting in predominant antegrade development as observed in type B dissection. However, in case of a primary lesion located at the free lateral wall or at the concavity of the distal aortic arch, the lack of a natural anatomical barrier may permit retrograde progression down to the level of the aortic root. This mechanism seems valid for both variants of acute aortic syndromes, IMH as well as dissection (11).

IMH is regarded as complex when the entire thoracic aortic up to the level of the aortic root is affected and empiric surgical replacement of the ascending aorta as well as of the concavity of the aortic arch is the mainstay of therapy if the described mechanism of plaque rupture cannot be retraced.

CLINICAL INDICATIONS

Atherosclerotic Thoracic Aortic Aneurysms

Treatment of thoracic aortic aneurysms is indicated when the risk of the yearly rate of rupture exceeds the remaining risk of treatment. It is generally accepted that the cutoff point is at a maximum diameter of 6 cm being adjusted for age, sex, and body mass index. TEVAR has become the therapy of first choice due to its clearly lower procedural morbidity and mortality.

Penetrating Atherosclerotic Ulcers

In contrast to the decision making in patients with atherosclerotic thoracic aortic aneurysms, the maximum diameter of PAU plays a minor role. Morphology and, if applicable and traceable, progression of the lesion are the cornerstones of decision making besides clinical symptoms or already sustained rupture.

Type B Dissections

TEVAR in type B dissections is indicated in contained rupture as well as in patients with any kind of malperfusion in downstream vascular beds.

Intramural Hematoma

Treatment of IMH is indicated in contained rupture as well as if the ascending aorta is affected. Malperfusion in IMH is rarely an issue.

HAZARDS AND COMPLICATIONS

Atherosclerotic Thoracic Aortic Aneurysms

As the underlying disease is atherosclerotic, manipulation especially within the aortic arch may cause embolization of debris. As a consequence, manipulation should be kept to a minimum. As a long covered segment may be necessary for total exclusion of the lesion, a high number of intercostal arteries may have to be sacrificed. Therefore, a high level of alertness for spinal cord malperfusion has to be there. Cerebrospinal fluid drainage may add as an important adjunct to prevent this dreadful complication. Overstenting of the left subclavian artery may add to spinal cord malperfusion and should be done only in emergency situations.

Penetrating Atherosclerotic Ulcers

Patients with PAU are frail and are generally in an advanced stage of their aggressive underlying disease. Furthermore, the rough intravascular surface of the lesions may cause tear of the stent-graft fabric as well as atheroembolic embolization.

Type B Dissections

It is of utmost importance to reaffirm to beside within the true lumen, as stent-graft placement in the false lumen may have dreadful consequences. Therefore, serial angiographies should be performed and the CT scans have to be studied in detail in advance in order to know about the individual functional anatomy. Furthermore, balloon dilatation after TEVAR has to be avoided, as rupture of the dissecting membrane might be the consequence. Furthermore, the so-called floating visceral sign has to be ruled out, as despite filling of the visceral bed with contrast medium, significant malperfusion may be present.

Intramural Hematoma

As in dissections, balloon dilatation should not be performed due to the risk of rupture. Furthermore, oversizing of the stent graft should not be more than 10% in order not to expose the friable aortic wall to a high amount of radial force.

IMAGING, INTERVENTIONAL STRATEGIES, AND TOOLS

Imaging

All CT examinations prior to treatment should be performed on a 64-row CT scanner. To allow pulsation-free visualization of the thoracic aorta up to the aortic root, a retrospective ECG-gating technique should be used.

In our setting, all CT angiograms are performed in the arterial phase during the intravenous administration of nonionic iodinated contrast material. A bolus triggering technique assesses the contrast medium transit time. A threshold of 150 HU (absolute) is used. One hundred and thirty milliliters of contrast agent is administered in a biphasic fashion: the first 30 mL is injected at a flow rate of 6 mL/sec followed by the second 100 mL administered at 5 mL/sec. A saline flush of 40 mL is administered to all the patients after the contrast medium injection to optimize contrast utilization. With a post-threshold delay of eight seconds, ECG-gated CT angiography of the entire aorta is performed using the following imaging parameters: a slice collimation of 64×0.625 and a pitch of 0.29 is used. The matrix size is 512×512. Images are reconstructed with a slice thickness of 1.4 and a slice increment of 1 mm as well as with a slice thickness of 3 and a slice increment of 2 mm without using the ECG-triggering ("untagged images"). Additionally, image redistribution according to the heart action is performed after scanning (retrospective ECG-triggering). Usually, images are triggered in a midphase at 55% of a RR-interval. If pulsation artifacts occur, other phases of the heart cycle are reconstructed. For every phase, two series are reconstructed (1.4/1 as well as 3/2 mm).

Interventional Strategy

Stent grafts are placed under anesthesia. Access vessel exposure is being performed surgically. A 5-French pigtail catheter is advanced via the right brachial artery into the aortic arch to reconfirm characterization of the morphology and extent of the lesions. After systemic heparinization with 80 IU/kg, arteriotomy is performed and the catheter is advanced under fluoroscopic guidance. Afterwards, a change to an ultrastiff guidewire (Backup Meier) is being performed. Stent grafts are deployed during systemic hypotension with a systolic pressure of 70 mm Hg. The more proximal the stent graft is being deployed the more liberal we do use rapid pacing via a temporary pacemaker electrode being inserted via the right subclavian vein into the right ventricle. Pacing is performed up to 180 beats per minute. With this method blood pressure control seems most effective.

Interventional Tools

Three different, commercially available stent-graft systems are used namely, the modified Valiant endovascular stent graft (Medtronic, Santa Rosa, CA), the Relay stent graft (Bolton Medical, Sunrise, FL) as well as the Gore TAG stent graft (Gore Inc. Phoenix, AZ).

Quality Control

Patients undergo a completion CT scan to verify the effectiveness of the procedure before discharge, then at one, three, and six months and annually thereafter.

SUMMARY OF OUTCOMES

Atherosclerotic Thoracic Aortic Aneurysms

Results after supra-aortic transpositions in various extents followed by endovascular stent-graft placement for the treatment of various pathology affecting the aortic arch are promising. Endoleak formation is directly related to the number of prostheses and may be reduced by longer devices (5). Each type of arch rerouting, irrespective of extent, has turned out to be effective (1–8). Therefore, extended applications of these combined treatment strategies substantially augment the therapeutic options.

Penetrating Atherosclerotic Ulcers

Endovascular stent-graft placement in patients with PAU is an effective palliation for a life-threatening sign of a severe systemic process. Hemodynamic instability at referral and a high preoperative risk score predict adverse outcome. During midterm follow-up, patients are mainly limited by sequelae of their underlying disease (8).

Type B Dissections

TEVAR has emerged as the therapy of first choice in patients sustaining complicated type B dissections. Nevertheless, these patients have to be subjected to serial follow-up CT scans as aneurysm formation requiring treatment in downstream aortic segments occurs in up to 20% of patients. Uncomplicated type B dissection should be initially managed with best medical treatment. TEVAR remains an option in these patients if a progression of the underlying disease occurs (9,10,22).

Intramural Hematoma

Plaque rupture may be identified as the cause of IMH in a previously unrecognized subgroup of patients. If at the convexity of the distal arch, supra-aortic branches prevent retrograde extension toward the ascending aorta. If at the free lateral wall or at the concavity, IMH may affect the entire thoracic aorta, due to the lack of the natural barrier of the supra-aortic branches. Endovascular stent-graft placement of this plaque-associated IMH may be more effective and less invasive than conventional surgery in order to treat the entire thoracic aortic disease (11).

EQUIPMENTS CHECKLIST

The following chart shall supply the reader with a detailed list of all medical supplies needed in TEVAR as well as with the costs of these supplies (23).

	Ordering #	Costs/unit (€)	N	Total costs (€)
Introduction sheath PTA Angio 407850 9-F 12 cm Ulti	30031427	10.67	2	21.34
Introduction sheath Angio Terumo RSB50 N 5-F 10 cm	30201542	10.40	1	10.40
FD PTCA SCH 30601 0.35″ 300 cm ger. Backup	30022227	154.38	1	154.38
Kath. Diagn. Pigtail 5-F 451503V5 65 cm 5 SL	30018107	15.04	1	15.04
Abd. Angio. t. femor 203 × 280 cm	30004841	9.21	1	9.21
Abd. BV cover 85 × 95	30014695	1.16	1	1.16
Abd. draping nsk 100 × 150 251220/4	30020443	1.44	1	1.44
Flushing set Angiofill II MDD520 H	30032630	9.51	1	9.51
Cannula arterial 099326 18G Seldinger	30012286	3.98	1	3.98
Syringe 20 mL	30001692	0.04	6	0.27
Syringe 10 mL	30001691	0.03	4	0.11
Cannula inject 20G × 1-1/2 0.90 × 40 Nr. 01	30001700	0.01	2	0.02
Scalpel No. 11 sterile	30003225	0.21	1	0.21
Gazin MK 9/7.5 16-F 13682 1 Set	113314	0.41	4	1.65

Gloves OP Derma Plus Gr. 7.5	30042051	0.26	4	1.05
Gown OP large 133 cm	30016949	2.61	4	10.44
Angiography coil San 1939	117802	2.39	2	4.78
Phys. NaCl Inffl. 200 mL	114960	0.32	1	0.32
Xenetix 300 mg/mL Inffl. 200 mL	168650	62.95	1	62.95
Fentanyl Amp. 10 mL	183313	0.54	1	0.54
Dormicum Amp. 5 mg/1 mL	110797	0.15	1	0.15
Heparin-Imm Dstfl. 5000 IE/mL 5 mL	115120	3.44	1	3.44
Rö.Film Drystar TM 1B NIF 35 × 43 1 sheath	30097999	1.49	6	8.93
Introduction sheath RCF 18.0-P-38-30-JRB Checkflo	30093713	200.79	1	200.79
Introduction sheath XLCFW 24.0-38-30 Endostent	30092185	274.51	1	274.51
FD Bentson 035″ 7/260 cm M001491031 ger.	30067544	7.93	1	7.93
Pressure tube angio 1520010 1200PSI 200	30095803	4.81	1	4.81
Syringe 200 mL for Illumena 900105	30209174	9.17	1	9.17
Stent graft	30207964	10,045.00	1	10,045.00
Cath. Ballon Reliant AB46 10–46 mm (TAA)	30117306	226.64	1	226.64
Abd. C arm multipart DBL 990716	30099509	41.23	1	41.23
				11,131.40

COMPLEX CASES

Case 1—Atherosclerotic Thoracic Aortic Aneurysm

A 79-year-old male was referred for treatment of a huge aortic arch aneurysm with a maximum diameter of 8 cm (Fig. 1). Due to his frail general status and due to his risk factors (extracardiac arteriopathy as well as COPD) a conventional surgical replacement of the aortic arch was deemed high risk. Median numeric EuroSCORE was 12 and median logistic EuroSCORE was 37.

Therefore, a combined vascular and endovascular approach was chosen. As a first step, total arch rerouting was performed. Access was gained via an upper median sternotomy and the pericardium was opened. As a next step, the supra-aortic branches were circumferentially dissected. Afterwards, 80 IU of heparin per kilogram bodyweight was applied. For total arch rerouting, a 18/9 mm Dacron prosthesis was chosen. The ascending aorta was tangentially clamped and an end-to-side anastomosis between the proximal portion of the Dacron prosthesis and the ascending aorta was performed. Afterwards the brachiocephalic trunk was clamped at its origin, the trunk was transected and an end-to-end anastomosis between the first branch

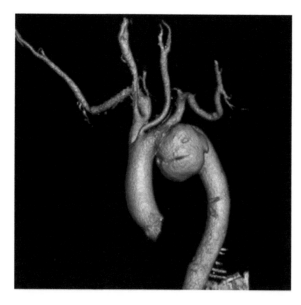

Figure 1 Aortic arch aneurysm at the time of diagnosis.

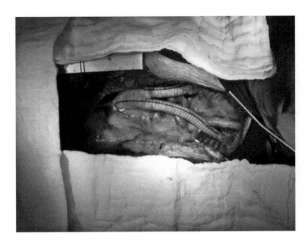

Figure 2 Final intraoperative result after total arch rerouting.

of the Dacron prosthesis and the trunk was being performed. Then, the left subclavian artery was transected and an end-to-end anastomosis between the second branch of the prosthesis and the left subclavian artery was done. Finally, the left common carotid artery was reinserted into the branch to the left subclavian. Figure 2 shows the final intraoperative result. Afterwards, the wound was closed in layers.

After a recovery period of one week, the patient underwent stent graft placement. The right common femoral artery was exposed and 80 IU of heparin per kilogram bodyweight was applied. A pigtail catheter was advanced via the right subclavian artery for serial angiography. After insertion of an ultrastiff Backup-Meier guidewire, a 42/250 mm stent graft (Bolton, Relay, Sunrise, FA) was advanced into the aortic arch. Rapid pacing was begun and after having reached functional circulatory arrest, the stent graft was deployed. Afterwards, rapid pacing was gradually reduced and normal circulation was thereby restored. All catheters and guidewires were removed, the wound was closed in layers and the patient woke up on the operating table. Recovery was uneventful. Completion CT scan showed regular supra-aortic perfusion, the stent graft in place as well as no signs of any kind of endoleak. Follow-up is regular for three years (Fig. 3).

The complexity of this case is underlined by a limiting thoracic aortic pathology in a very delicate anatomical region encomprising all brain and upper extremity supplying great vessels. By this combined concept, a durable result could be achieved and the patient was able to reassume a normal life soon after the procedure. Quality of life was preserved and the threat of aneurysmal rupture was averted with a stable and durable result.

Case 2—Penetrating Atherosclerotic Ulcers
A 64-year-old male was referred for treatment of multiple PAU of the thoracic aorta originating from the level of the left common carotid artery to below the thoracoabdominal transition (Fig. 4). The patient suffered from severe generalized atherosclerosis, was on dialysis for glomerulonephritis, and had substantial COPD. Median numeric EuroSCORE was 13 and median logistic EuroSCORE was 41. The patient was symptomatic with new onset of chest pain corresponding to the multisegmental location of the lesions.

Therefore, a combined vascular and endovascular approach was chosen. As a first step, autologous double transposition of the supra-aortic branches was performed in order to gain a sufficient proximal landing zone for stent-graft insertion. A median upper hemisternotomy access was chosen and the supra-aortic branches were circumferentially dissected (Fig. 5). Eighty IU of heparin per kilogram bodyweight was applied. The common carotid artery was transected at the level of the arch and an end-to-side anastomosis between the brachiocephalic trunk and the left common carotid artery was performed. Afterwards, the left subclavian artery was transected and an end-to-side anastomosis between the already transposed left common carotid artery and the subclavian artery was performed (Fig. 6). Then, the wound was closed in layers.

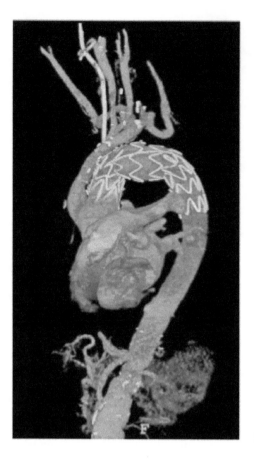

Figure 3 Completion CT scan after stent-graft placement.

After a recovery period of one week, stent-graft placement was performed. Vascular access was gained via the right common iliac artery, as the external iliac artery was very narrow due to the underlying obliterative disease. A 9 mm Dacron graft was sewn onto the native vessel in an end-to-side fashion. After heparinization, two stent grafts were deployed (Bolton, Relay, Sunrise, FA) beginning at the level of the brachiocephalic trunk down to the level of the celiac trunk. Afterwards, due to severe narrowing of the iliac bifurcation as well as of the external iliac artery, the Dacron graft was extended to the right groin as an iliaco-femoral bypass. Then, the wound was closed in layers. The patient woke up uneventfully. After two hours the patient became paraplegic. Mean arterial pressure was elevated at once and cerebrospinal fluid drainage was installed. Symptoms disappeared and further recovery was uneventful. The final complication CT scan is depicted in Figure 7.

The complexity of this case is underlined by multisegmental thoracic aortic disease, requiring extension of the proximal landing zone by rerouting as well as by symptomatic spinal cord malperfusion. In this context, it is essential to remind onto the four spinal cord supplying vascular territories, the left subclavian artery, the intercostal arteries, the lumbar arteries as well as the hypogastric arteries. Normally, sacrifice of one supplying territory does not subject these patients to a higher risk of symptomatic spinal cord malperfusion. Previous or procedure-related sacrifice of two territories, however, may highly likely result in malperfusion. Cerebrospinal fluid (CSF) drainage as well as elevation of mean arterial blood pressure are highly valuable tools in reversing this complication whereas CSF drainage acts like a fasciotomy to the spinal cord.

Case 3—Intramural Hematoma

A 72-year-old male was referred with a symptomatic IMH of the entire thoracic aorta with an accompanying pericardial effusion (Fig. 8). The general condition was weak and conventional

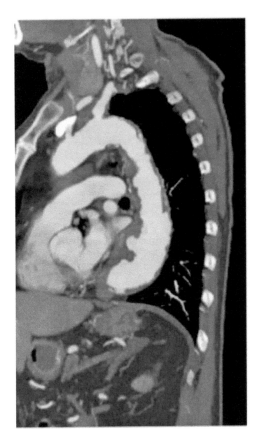

Figure 4 Multiple PAU extending from the left common carotid artery to the celiac trunk.

surgical treatment was deemed high risk. Numeric EuroSCORE was 13 and logistic EuroSCORE was 45. By imaging via gated 64-row CT scanning, a small atherosclerotic plaque could be identified as the primary entry site at the concavity of the distal arch.

Therefore an endovascular approach was chosen. After induction of general anesthesia as well as standard insertion of catheters and guidewires, three stent grafts (Medtronic, Valiant, Santa Rosa, CA) were inserted from the offspring of the left common carotid artery to the distal third of the descending aorta. The left subclavian artery had to be covered in this situation. Afterwards, the hemodynamically significant pericardial effusion was treated by subxyphoidal drainage. The patient recovered uneventfully and the CT scan showed complete resorption of the IMH in the ascending aorta as well as complete remodeling of the entire thoracic aorta so far within a two-year follow-up period (Fig. 9).

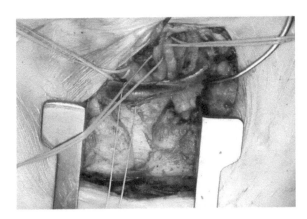

Figure 5 Intraoperative situs before double transposition.

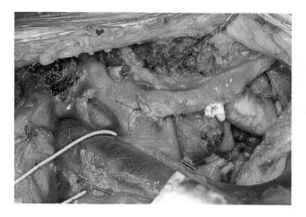

Figure 6 Intraoperative situs after double transposition.

The complexity in this case lies in the multisegmental affection of the aorta by this acute aortic syndrome with a high risk of rupture into the pericardium such as in classical type A aortic dissection. To date rupture of vasa vasorum was held responsible for the mechanism of IMH development. We strongly encourage every physician dealing with this entity to carefully look for a small entry tear such as the plaque in that very case. By defining such an entry tear, treatment can be performed by TEVAR and results may be favorable.

SUMMARY OF THE KEY ISSUES

In summary, a combined vascular and endovascular approach for the treatment of thoracic aortic pathology has emerged as an established procedure with excellent long-term results. Vascular transposition is safe and—by avoiding cardiopulmonary bypass as well as hypothermic circulatory arrest—the method proofs its less invasiveness.

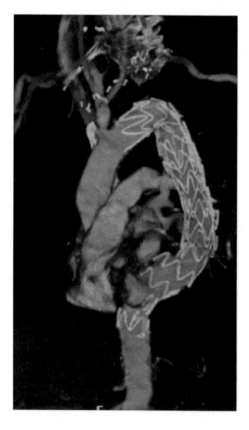

Figure 7 Completion CT scan after stent-graft placement.

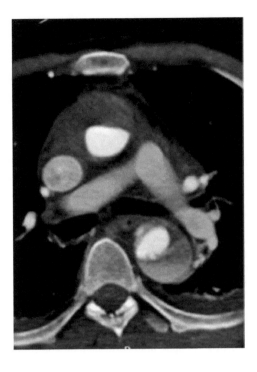

Figure 8 IMH of the entire thoracic aorta at the time of diagnosis.

By adhering to the principle of a long landing zone, a sufficient overlap as well as a low number of prostheses, the rate of early and late endoleak formation can be kept very low.

A broader application of these techniques will enable treatment of a patient group who a few years ago would have been sent home with mere antihypertensive therapy.

Perforating ulcers have to be regarded as a distinct clinical entity being the result of a very aggressive underlying obliterative disease. Indication for treatment is not based on the maximum diameter of the lesion but on morphology, dynamics as well as clinical symptoms.

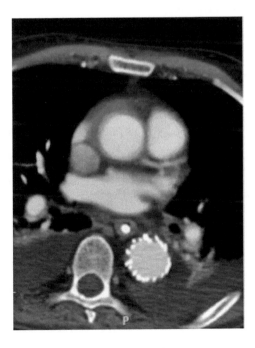

Figure 9 Complete resorption of IMH in the ascending aorta after stent-graft placement into the distal aortic arch.

Complicated type B dissections have become a domain of endovascular therapy and show excellent midterm results. Aneurysm development in downstream segments remains an unsolved issue and requires continuous follow-up in patients with chronic type B dissections irrespective of if after TEVAR or with best medical therapy.

IMH may be the result of plaque rupture in many cases and may therefore turn out to be a suitable target for TEVAR. If the mechanism of plaque rupture cannot be retraced, surgery should remain the mainstay of therapy.

REFERENCES

1. Czerny M, Fleck T, Zimpfer D, et al. Combined repair of an aortic arch aneurysm by sequential transposition of the supra-aortic branches and endovascular stent-graft placement. J Thorac Cardiovasc Surg 2003; 126:916–918.
2. Czerny M, Zimpfer D, Fleck T, et al. Initial results after combined repair of aortic arch aneurysms by sequential transposition of the supra-aortic branches and consecutive endovascular stent-graft placement. Ann Thorac Surg 2004; 78:1256–1260.
3. Czerny M, Gottardi R, Zimpfer D, et al. Transposition of the supraaortic branches for extended endovascular arch repair. Eur J Cardiothorac Surg 2006; 29:709–713.
4. Czerny M, Gottardi R, Zimpfer D, et al. Mid-term results of supraaortic transpositions for extended endovascular repair of aortic arch pathologies. Eur J Cardiothorac Surg 2007; 31:623–1627.
5. Gottardi R, Funovics M, Eggers N, et al. Supra-aortic transposition for combined vascular and endovascular repair of aortic arch pathology. Ann Thorac Surg 2008; 86:1524–1529.
6. Brinkman WT, Szeto WY, Bavaria JE. Stent graft treatment for transverse arch and descending thoracic aorta aneurysms. Curr Opin Cardiol 2007; 22:510–516.
7. Weigang E, Parker J, Czerny M, et al. Endovascular aortic arch repair after aortic arch de-branching. Ann Thorac Surg 2009; 87:603–607.
8. Gottardi R, Zimpfer D, Funovics M, et al. Mid-term results after endovascular stent-graft placement due to penetrating atherosclerotic ulcers of the thoracic aorta. Eur J Cardiothorac Surg 2008; 33:1019–1024.
9. Szeto WY, McGarvey M, Pochettino A, et al. Results of a new surgical paradigm: endovascular repair for acute complicated type B aortic dissection. Ann Thorac Surg 2008; 86:87–93.
10. Schoder M, Czerny M, Cejna M, et al. Endovascular repair of acute type B aortic dissection: long-term follow-up of true and false lumen diameter changes. Ann Thorac Surg 2007; 83:1059–1066.
11. Grimm M, Loewe C, Gottardi R, et al. Novel insights into the mechanisms and treatment of intramural hematoma affecting the entire thoracic aorta. Ann Thorac Surg 2008;86:453–456.
12. Czerny M, Cejna M, Hutschala D, et al. Stent-graft placement in atherosclerotic descending thoracic aortic aneurysms: midterm results. J Endovasc Ther 2004; 11:26–32.
13. Czerny M, Grimm M, Zimpfer D, et al. Results after endovascular stent graft placement in atherosclerotic aneurysms involving the descending aorta. Ann Thorac Surg 2007; 83:450–455.
14. Donas KP, Czerny M, Guber I, et al. Hybrid open-endovascular repair for thoracoabdominal aortic aneurysms: current status and level of evidence. Eur J Vasc Endovasc Surg 2007; 34:528–533.
15. Coselli JS, Bozinovski J, LeMaire SA. Open surgical repair of 2286 thoracoabdominal aortic aneurysms. Ann Thorac Surg 2007; 83:S862–S864.
16. Erbel R, Alfonso F, Boileau C, et al. Task force on aortic dissection, European Society for Cardiology. Diagnosis and management of aortic dissection. Eur Heart J 2001; 1642–1681.
17. Sundt TM. Intramural hematoma and penetrating atherosclerotic ulcer of the aorta. Ann Thorac Surg 2007; 83:S835–S841.
18. Cho KR, Stanson AW, Potter DD, et al. Penetrating atherosclerotic ulcer of the descending thoracic aorta and arch. J Thorac Cardiovasc Surg 2004; 127:1393–1401.
19. Verhoye JP, Miller DC, Sze D, et al. Complicated acute type B aortic dissection: midterm results of emergency endovascular stent-grafting. J Thorac Cardiovasc Surg 2008; 136:424–430.
20. Evangelista, A, Mukherjee, D, Mehta RH, et al; International Registry of Aortic Dissection (IRAD) Investigator. Acute intramural hematoma of the aorta: a mystery in evolution. Circulation 2005; 111:1063.
21. Tsai TT, Nienaber CA, Eagle KA. Acute aortic syndromes. Circulation 2005; 112:3802.
22. Czerny M, Zimpfer D, Rodler S, et al. Endovascular stent-graft placement of aneurysms involving the descending aorta originating from chronic type B dissections. Ann Thorac Surg 2007; 83:1635–1639.
23. Schuster I, Dorfmeister M, Scheuter- Mlaker S, et al. Endovascular and conventional treatment of thoracic aortic Aneurysms: a comparison of costs. Ann Thorac Surg 2009; 87:1801–1805.

10 | Abdominal Aortic Disease

Yuji Kanaoka and Takao Ohki

Department of Surgery, Jikei University School of Medicine, Nishishimbashi, Minatoku, Tokyo, Japan

Frank J. Veith

The Cleveland Clinic, Cleveland, Ohio, and New York University, New York, New York, U.S.A.

PART 1: INTRODUCTION

The majority of endovascular treatment for the abdominal aorta is for abdominal aortic aneurysms (AAAs). Endovascular aortic aneurysm repair (EVAR) has gained wide acceptance, and there has been a significant increase in the number of AAAs treated by EVAR (1,2). However, not all AAA cases are indicated to undergo EVAR. Patient selection of EVAR involves careful assessment of the anatomical features of aneurysm. The indications vary according to device; however, to summarize the preferable anatomy for EVAR (3,4), (*i*) the proximal neck's length should be long enough (15 mm or longer), orientation should be relatively straight (60° or less), and diameter should be 28 mm or less; (*ii*) as an access route, the iliac artery should be large enough (6–7 mm or more) without extreme tortuosity, bending, or calcification; and (*iii*) the distal neck should be 10 mm or longer. Conversely, it can be said that cases that do not include these anatomical criteria involve factors that make EVAR difficult. In addition, the presence of neck thrombus and calcification is known to affect the ability to achieve adequate seal between the device and the aortic wall.

Indications for an endovascular treatment of even complex, potentially complication-associated lesions are summarized in Table 1. The potential to eliminate the majority of open surgical aneurysm repairs, limit procedural mortality, and offer a treatment option to patients who have long been deemed inoperable is enormous.

The *potential risks* of endovascular treatment of complex abdominal aortic lesions are listed in Table 2.

Preinterventional diagnostic workup of patients with complex AAAs consists primarily of computed tomography angiography (CTA). When considering EVAR, preoperative evaluation and treatment strategies are very important to get good results. Treatment strategies with preoperative CTA can prevent various intraoperative complications. Otherwise, it may lead to occlusion of the abdominal branches, embolism, a type I endoleak, a damaged aorta, or an injury of access route, which may result in open conversion in some cases. Moreover, if EVAR is performed for cases that are not anatomically preferable, initial complications as well as chronic stent-graft migration and endoleak may be expected to increase (3,4), so a careful follow-up is required. One important matter in establishing a treatment strategy is the selection of a device. Several devices for treating AAAs are currently available (Table 3) and are further being developed (6,7). Among them, the Zenith (Cook Medical, Bloomington, IN) and the Excluder (Gore & Associates, Flagstaff, AZ) are popular and are frequently used, so it is important to become fully acquainted with their respective features and disadvantages.

First, the best feature of a Zenith stent graft is the minimal migration because of a suprarenal stent (4). Therefore, a Zenith is better for cases with a short and/or flare proximal neck. In addition, the Zenith has a wide range of iliac diameter and infrarenal aortic length, allowing treatment of AAAs with large iliac arteries and/or short infrarenal aorta. On the other hand, it has a disadvantage in that it has a Z stent base and is less responsive to flexure. In addition, the suprarenal stent is very effective for the endograft fixation, although it is difficult to apply in cases with a mural thrombus in the suprarenal aorta, cases with an angulated suprarenal aorta, or cases that involve aortic dissection. Moreover, because the tip of the Zenith device reaches the thoracic descending aorta, the appearance of the thoracic descending aorta should always be checked. On the other hand, because the Excluder is small in all the sizes, with the main body being 18-F and leg being 12-F, it is useful for cases with small access vessels and

Table 1 Indications for Complex Abdominal Aortic Intervention

Patients of poor health status considered unfit for open repair under general anesthesia
Patients who have severe COPD with forced expiratory volume in 1 minute (%FEV1.0) of less than 70%, congestive heart failure, unstable angina, coagulopathy, and cerebral vascular disease
Patients who have a history of abdominal aortic surgery
Patients who have hostile abdomen
Patients who have malignancy that needs treatment (operation and/or chemotherapy) (5)

with stenosis. In addition, because the stent graft is flexible, it can be advanced in cases with extremely tortuous access route and cases with significant angulation of the aneurysm neck.

After a device has been selected, further detailed treatment strategies will be established with a preoperative computed tomography (CT). Most complications of EVAR commonly result from the access route, and it should especially be carefully checked as to whether the access route is adequate. The judgment regarding the side from which the main body should be inserted is made based on the feature of the iliac artery. The main body should be inserted from the side without advanced tortuosity, stenosis, and calcification. If the access routes on the left and right are the same, the access route should be decided based on the angle of the neck. The side on which the guidewire is nearly parallel to the angle of the neck is preferable. If one renal artery is clearly lower, insertion of the main body via the femoral artery opposite to the lower renal artery makes alignment easier. In addition, in the case of the Zenith, because overlapping of the leg on the ipsilateral side is wide from 1 to 3 stents, it is easier to insert the main body from the side on which alignment of the iliac artery is difficult. On the other hand, it is easier for the Excluder to access the side with a more difficult alignment of the iliac artery than the contralateral leg. In addition, it is also useful to check the angle of the proximal neck, the clock position of the renal arteries, the angle of the hypogastric and external iliac arteries, and so on in a preoperative CT to estimate the cranial–caudal and lateral angle of the C-arm in each situation in EVAR. Information obtained via fluoroscopy is only two-dimensional, and all three dimensions should always be considered. We have created a schematic image (diagram) from this information obtained via a CT and have also recorded points to be noted (Fig. 1). Therefore, the possibilities that can occur during EVAR may be predicted before the EVAR as much as possible. The device is introduced without arterial clamping and creating an arteriotomy. One may encounter difficulties while introducing the device. This can be caused by several reasons. First, the iliac artery may be diseased or too small. In such cases, balloon angioplasty of the lesion may be helpful. Stenting should be avoided, as insertion of the endograft may dislodge the stent, and also because the stent may damage the delivery system.

If the difficulty is related to tortuousity, the push-and-pull technique should be used. This is done by simultaneously pulling on the super stiff wire while introducing the endograft.

Table 2 Potential Risks of Endovascular Treatment of Complex Abdominal Aortic Lesions

Clinical and anatomical presentation	Potential complication
Small and/or calcified iliac access	Injury of the access vessels (perforation, rupture, dissection, surgical conversion)
Diffuse iliac stenosis	
Extremely tortuous iliac access	Kinking and occlusion of endograft limbs
Inadequate proximal neck	
Short and/or flare	Type I endoleak, graft migration
Mural thrombus	Embolization
Angulated and/or crooked neck	Type I endoleak, cover the visceral arteries
Shaggy aorta	Embolization
Visceral artery stenosis	Occlusion of the visceral arteries
Horseshoe kidney	Kidney infarction
Accessory renal artery	
AAA and/or iliac aneurysm with an A-V fistel	Pulmonary thromboembolism
Borderline renal dysfunction	End stage renal insufficiency, contrast-induced nephropathy or embolism

Table 3 Commercially Available AAA Endografts

Device (company)	Material	Main body delivery system profile (F)	Iliac leg delivery system profile(F)	Features
Zenith Flex (Cook Medical)	Stainless steel Woven polyester	18,20-F sheath 20,22 OD	14,16-F	Modular Suprarenal fixation (suprarenal stent with 16 barbs) Various sizes Fenestrated and branched stentgraft
Excluder (Gore & Associates)	Nitinol ePTFE	18-F Sheath 20 OD 18-F Sheath 20 OD	12-F	Modular Smaller crossing profile Flexible Simple deployment sysytem
Powerlink (Endologix)	Cobalt-chromium alloy ePTFE	21 OD	Unibody	Unibody
AneuRx AAAdvantage (Medtronic)	Nitinol Woven polyester	21 OD		Modular Versatile

Having maximum purchase of wire, distally, should help the operator perform this maneuver. Alternatively, one may stabilize the tortuous vessel by applying external pressure onto the access vessel of the aneurysm. If such maneuvers are ineffective, pull-through method may be effective. This method is applied after placing 4Fr short sheath at right brachial artery; the radifocus guidewire is inserted into aneurysm from this sheath. Similarly, a 6Fr EN Snare is inserted from the ipsilateral side into aneurysm. After the Snare is used to catch the guidewire, pull it from the ipsilateral side, so that it can pass the guidewire from the right brachial artery to the ipsilateral artery, and do the push-and-pull technique, one may obtain better purchase (Table 4).

Finally, a limited retroperitoneal exposure of the common iliac artery may be made to bypass the diseased external iliac artery. A temporary conduit may be made by anastomosing a vascular graft to the common iliac artery, or an arteriotomy may be made in the iliac artery, for direct insertion. One should also consider the option of performing a standard, open repair, if difficulties are encountered and if the patient is a reasonable candidate for open surgery. Because it would be worse to damage the access route or exacerbate the aneurysm, thus leading to an emergent conversion to a surgical operation. When the main body can be inserted and the contralateral leg cannot be advanced, conversion to the aorto-uni-iliac (AUI) should be considered. For AUI, a converter is used in the case of the Zenith, but two aortic cuffs of the same size are used in the case of the Excluder.

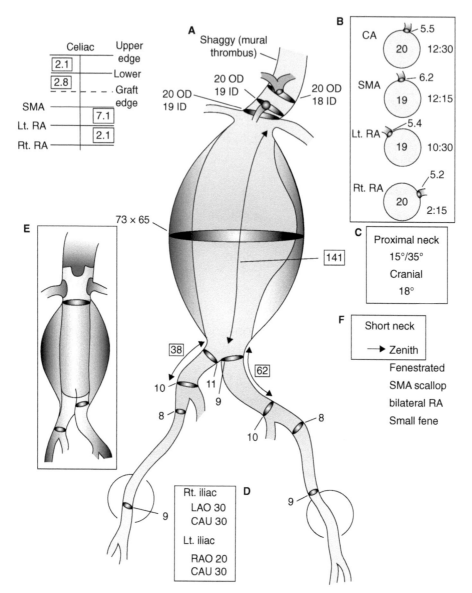

Figure 1 Preoperative schema (this schema is for case 3 of this chapter) (**A**) Main image of AAA. OD means outer diameter of aorta (mm). ID means inner diameter of aorta (mm). Numbers in the quadrilateral show length (mm). (**B**) Clock position of visceral branches. Diameter of the aorta and visceral branches. (**C**) Proximal neck angulation. (**D**) C arm angle when hypogastric artery is well identified. (**E**) Image of EVAR. (**F**) The reason why this device was chosen.

PART 2: TEACHING CASES

Case 1: Extremely tortuous iliac arteries and acute angle of the proximal neck

a. What made the lesion "complex" in this specific case? The complexity of the case results in the excessive tortuosity of the proximal aortic neck. Tortuosity of the proximal neck is not uncommon, and is more often seen in patients with a huge aneurysm.

b. What was the clinical indication for treatment of this specific case? The indication for the treatment was a large AAA greater than 10 cm. Unfortunately, the patient was unfit for open repair due to severe COPD with forced expiratory volume in 1 minute (FEV1.0) of less than 500 ml and was given up by other doctors as an inoperable patient.

Table 4 Recommended Devices for Complex Abdominal Aortic Interventions

Special situation	Tool	Device example(s)
Tortuous access	Stiff type guidewire	Asmplatz Super Stiff (Boston Scientific Corp.) Amplatz Ultra Stiff (Cook Medical) Lunderquist (Cook Medical)
	push- and- pull technique external pressure pull-through wire	Glidewire (TERUMO) 260 cm EN Snare (Angiotech)
	Flexible endograft	Excluder (Gore & Associates)
Segmental stenosis of iliac access	PTA balloon Iliac approach	
Short and/or flare proximal neck	Suprarenal fixation device Balloon expandable stent	Zenith (Cook Medical) Palmaz P4010 + Maxi LD PTA balloon (Cordis)
	Fenestrated and branched endograft	Zenith (Cook Medical) 7-F Flexor Check-Flo introducers, Ansel modification (Cook) Palmaz stent (Cordis) Advanta V12 covered stent (Atrium Medical) iCAST covered stent (Atrium Medical)
Angulated proximal neck	Flexible endograft Balloon expandable stent	Excluder (W.L. Gore) Palmaz P4010 + MAXI LD 25 mm (Cordis)
Difficulty to cannulate the contralateral gate	Brachial wire Ipsilateral wire with SH catheter	
	Snare wire	EN Snare (Angiotech) Goose Neck Snare (ev3, Inc)
	Aorto-uni-iliac	Zenith Converter and Occluder (Cook) Main body extension (Aortic cuff) (Gore)
Small terminal aorta	Kissing balloon	Equalizer (Boston Scientfic), Maxi LD (Cordis)
	Self-expandable stent	Luminexx (BARD)

c. What were the potential hazards of treating this specific patient and this lesion? The potential hazards were, first, incomplete exclusion of the aneurysm sac with type I endoleak And, second, the risk of aortic wall injury and embolism caused by extensive wire and catheter manipulations. Moreover, stent migration or stent-graft kinking had to be taken into consideration.

d. Which interventional strategies were considered and which interventional tools were used to handle this lesion? The procedure was performed in an operating room equipped with a fixed Flat Panel Detector C-arm system (Innova 4100, GE Healthcare, Waukesha, WI). The procedure was performed under epidural anesthesia. Bilateral common femoral arteries were exposed with oblique groin incision just below the inguinal ligament. Aortography showed an extremely tortuous AAA and left common iliac aneurysm [Fig. 2(A)]. Prior to the endograft deployment, coil embolization of the left hypogastric artery was performed with IDC coil [Fig. 2(B)]. Right brachial access was established percutaneously using a 6-F sheath. A 0.035-in. glidewire was inserted through the right femoral artery to the ascending aorta, and the tip of the wire was caught and pulled by the snare wire inserted via the right brachial artery to straighten the guidewire [pull through snare wire; Fig. 2(C) and 2(D)]. Heparin (100 U/kg) was injected intravenously. An 18-F sheath was inserted via the right femoral artery pulling both sides of the glidewire. A 26-mm Excluder

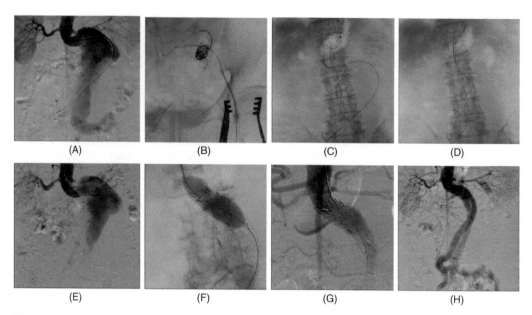

(A)   (B)   (C)   (D)

(E)   (F)   (G)   (H)

Figure 2

trunk-ipsilateral device (main body) was inserted through the right femoral artery sheath and was deployed at appropriate position in the infrarenal abdominal aorta [Fig. 2(E)]. Because of the tortuosity of the proximal neck, precise deployment was difficult. Therefore, compromised deployment of the main body device should be performed. An iliac extender was deployed via the right femoral artery not to cover the right hypogastric artery. After that, the aortic extender was precisely deployed at the proximal neck via the right femoral artery. At that time, appropriate cranial and Left Anterior Oblique (LAO) angulation of the C-arm provided best visualization of the neck. Furthermore, the extra large Palmaz stent (P4010) with a Maxi LD balloon (25 × 40 mm) was deployed to straighten the proximal neck and to reinforce the proximal fixation [Fig. 2(F)]. Because tortuosity and huge aneurysm sac made it difficult to cannulate the contralateral gate, the glidewire via the brachial artery was advanced to the left femoral artery [Fig. 2(G)], which was changed for a 0.035″ Amplaz Super Stiff Wire Guide (Boston Scientific) under fluoroscopic guidance. A 12-F sheath was inserted via the left femoral artery and subsequently a contralateral iliac limb and two iliac extenders were deployed through the left femoral artery. After touch-up balloon inflation to the attachment site and junction, completion angiography showed successful exclusion of the aneurysm sac without type I and III endoleaks [Fig. 2(H)]. The sheaths were removed from the femoral arteries, and femoral access site was closed with 5-0 polypropylene sutures.

e. Summary: How was the case managed, is there anything that could have been improved, what was the immediate and long-term outcome? The Excluder device is low profile and flexible and can track the tortuous aneurysm. When a main body device is deployed, appropriate cranial and LAO angulation of the C-arm provides best visualization of the proximal neck perpendicularly. Furthermore, deployment of the extra large Palmaz stent (P4010) with a Maxi LD balloon is quite effective to straighten the proximal neck and to reinforce the proximal fixation. Because tortuosity and huge aneurysm sac make it difficult to cannulate the contralateral gate, the glidewire via the brachial artery is easy access to advance the left femoral artery. A completion angiography showed successful exclusion of the aneurysm sac without endoleak. Six months after EVAR, CT revealed shrinking aneurysm sac with no evidence of an endoleak.

f. List of contemporary equipments that should be used in this case:
    o Interlock™ Fibered IDC Occlusion System (Boston Scientific)
    o Renegade HI-FLO Microcatheter (Boston Scientific)
    o Excluder (Gore & Associates)

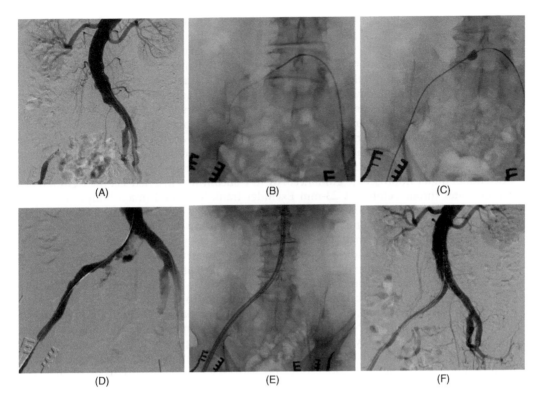

(A)   (B)   (C)

(D)   (E)   (F)

Figure 3

- ○ Glidewire 0.035″ (TERUMO)
- ○ Amplaz Super Stiff Wire Guide 0.035″ (Boston Scientific)
- ○ Amplatz GOOSE NECK Snare (ev3)
- ○ Equalizer balloon catheter (Boston Scientific)
- ○ Maxi LD PTA dilatation catheter (Cordis)
- ○ Palmaz XL P4010 (Cordis)

g. Key learning issues of this specific case: If the difficulty of device insertion is related to tortuousity, pull-through method may be effective. Even though flexible Gore Excluder device does not fit a tortuous proximal neck, Palmaz XL with Maxi LD balloon can provide the complete exclusion of the aneurysm sac.

Case 2: Total occlusion of iliac vessel: EVAR after thrombectomy of iliac access

a. What made the lesion "complex" in this specific case? The right iliac artery was totally occluded [Fig. 3(A)]. Therefore, the patient complained about a severe intermittent claudication (50 m). Usually the AUI device should be indicated; however, the Gore Excluder bifurcated endoprosthesis was applied.

b. What was the clinical indication for treatment of this specific case? The patient with a 5.0-cm AAA complained about a 50-m claudication. He was unfit for open repair because he also had a COPD and an uncontrolled angina pectoris.

c. What were the potential hazards of treating this specific patient and this lesion? The major hazard was to injure an iliac access and embolization.

d. Which interventional strategies were considered and which interventional tools were used to handle this lesion? The procedure was performed in an operating room equipped with a fixed Flat Panel Detector C-arm system (Innova 4100, GE Healthcare, Waukesha, WI). The procedure was performed under epidural anesthesia. Bilateral common femoral arteries were exposed with oblique groin incision just below the inguinal ligament. Heparin (100 U/kg) was injected intravenously. First, right femoral artery was punctured and 0.035″

glidewire was tried to advance into the aorta. It seemed to be impossible to cross the occlusive iliac artery. After a 9-F sheath was inserted via the left femoral artery, angiography was performed through the 9-F sheath. An angiography revealed the AAA with occlusion of the right common iliac artery [Fig. 3(A)]. After the right femoral approach was abandoned, a pigtail catheter through the left femoral artery was changed to the RIM catheter. Using the RIM catheter, the glidewire was passed down to the right femoral artery [Fig. 3(B)]. It could be retrieved in the right femoral artery through a small arteriotomy. Thrombectomy of right iliac access was performed using a 5.5-F Fogarty over-the-wire catheter [Fig. 3(C) and 3(D)]. A KMP catheter was then passed up the wire on the right iliac access and as this was done the wire on the left iliac side was released so that it flicked up into the aorta. A glidewire was changed for a 0.035-in. Amplaz Super Stiff Wire Guide (Boston Scientific) under fluoroscopic guidance. An 18-F sheath was inserted via the right femoral artery after thrombectomy. A 23-mm Excluder trank-ipsilateral (main body) device was inserted through the right femoral artery sheath [Fig. 3(E)] and was deployed at appropriate position in the infrarenal abdominal aorta. If a main body device is completely deployed, occupying ipsilateral leg makes it difficult to cannulate the contralateral gate in the case that has a small terminal aorta. Therefore, a deployment knob was pulled about 40 cm until the contralateral gate was open in this case. After halfway deployment of the trank-ipsilateral device, cannulation to the contralateral gate was conducted with a KMP catheter and a glidewire. After the contralateral gate cannulation, appropriate exchanges were made for Super Stiff Wire Guide, and a 12-F sheath was then passed through the contralateral limb. Once the sheath was placed, the contralateral log was positioned and the contralateral limb was deployed. Finally, the ipsilateral limb was completely deployed. An Equalizer balloon and a 15-mm Maxi LD were used to seal the attachment sites and junction. After the procedure was completed, angiography was performed to confirm exclusion of aneurysm [Fig. 3(F)]. Arterial access sites were closed according to standard manner. Angiography of the right leg was performed to confirm that no embolization had occurred to his leg.

e. Summary: How was the case managed, is there anything that could have been improved, what was the immediate and long-term outcome? An 18-F sheath was inserted via the femoral artery after thrombectomy with Fogarty catheter because of occluded iliac access in this case. When the patient has a segmental stenosis of access vessels, balloon angioplasty with 6 to 7 mm diameter balloon will be helpful to insert the device. A deployment of stent should be avoided, as insertion of the device may dislodge the stent, and also because the stent may damage the device. If there is a residual stenosis at the access vessels, stenting should be performed after deployment of endograft. If a trank-ipsilateral device is completely deployed, occupying ipsilateral leg makes it difficult to cannulate the contralateral gate in the case that has a small terminal aorta. Therefore, a deployment knob was pulled about 40 cm until the contralateral gate is open (two-stage deployment). In the case of small or diseased access vessels, placement of a 9-F sheath into the femoral artery should be performed prior to removing the guidewire to perform a retrograded arteriography. If dissection or perforation is detected, self-expandable stent or covered stent may treat these troubles. In the case of prior thrombectomy, final angiography of the leg should be performed to check embolization. The short-term outcome of this case was excellent, with an evanescence of 50 m-claudication. He had a good DP pulse and remained stable during the follow-up period.

f. List of contemporary equipments that should be used in this case:
   ○ RIM catheter
   ○ 5.5-F Fogarty catheter
   ○ 0.035″ Amplatz Super Stiff Wire Guide (Boston Scientific)
   ○ Excluder (Gore & Associates)
   ○ Equalizer balloon catheter (Boston Scientific)
   ○ Maxi LD PTA dilatation catheter (Cordis)

g. Key learning issues of this specific case: When terminal aorta is small, the ipsilateral leg should be deployed after contralateral gate cannulation is completed. It seems to be difficult to cannulate the contralateral gate after the ipsilateral leg occupies a terminal aorta. Kissing balloon technique can be used for optimizing vessel wall apposition of the stent.

Case 3: No proximal neck aneurysm involving visceral arteries

a. What made the lesion "complex" in this specific case? Proximal seal is dependent on a suitable infrarenal neck with straight parallel wall that is long enough to allow an adequate area for a complete and durable seal. The most unfavorable feature of proximal neck is a short neck. The complexity of this case results in the AAA involving with visceral arteries.

b. What was the clinical indication for treatment of this specific case? The patient had a large AAA greater than 7 cm that was expanding 1 cm/yr. He had a history of thoracoplasty due to tuberculosis. Therefore, he was suffering from dyspnea despite the home oxygen therapy.

c. What were the potential hazards of treating this specific patient and this lesion? The potential hazards were as follows: first, incomplete exclusion of aneurysm sac with type I endoleak and, second, the risk of visceral ischemia and acute renal failure caused by covering visceral arteries and/or embolism including renal arteries. Moreover, stent migration had to be taken into consideration.

d. Which interventional strategies were considered for this lesion? The problem of inadequate short neck can be solved by custom-made grafts with fenestrations or branches (8). Repair with fenestrated or branched grafts serves two purposes: exclusion of aneurysm sac and maintenance of blood flow to the aortic branches.

e. Which interventional tools were used to handle this lesion? Prior to the EVAR, a graft with a scallop for the superior mesenteric artery (SMA) and fenestrations for the bilateral renal arteries (RAs) was designed according to the preoperative CT (Cook Medical) [Fig. 1 & Fig. 4(A)]. Accurate planning and construction requires high-quality 3D-CT.

The procedure was performed in an operating room equipped with a fixed Flat Panel Detector C-arm system (Innova 4100, GE Healthcare, Waukesha, WI). The procedure was performed under epidural anesthesia. Bilateral common femoral arteries were exposed with oblique groin incision just below the inguinal ligament. Right brachial access was established percutaneously using a 5-F sheath for an angiographic catheter. Angiography showed a large AAA involved with RAs as the preoperative CT showed [Fig. 4(B)]. Heparin (100 U/kg) was injected intravenously. First, we tried to insert the Zenith endograft with a scallop and two fenestrations (proximal body) via the left femoral artery over the Amplaz Super Stiff Wire Guide. However, it was impossible to reach the proximal neck because of iliac angulation. Subsequently, a proximal body was inserted from the right femoral artery [Fig. 4(C)], and a short 20-F sheath was inserted from the left femoral artery to advance 7-F Ansel sheaths (Cook Medical, Bloomington, IN). To facilitate intervention, three 7-F Ansel sheaths were then placed over the aortic bifurcation. The use of fenestration required controlled and accurate deployment, especially rotational maneuverability, to allow exact positioning of the fenestration over the target orifice. Controlled and accurate positioning of the fenestrated device was based on partial deployment of the graft to allow fine adjustment to position the fenestrations over the orifice of the visceral arteries [Fig. 4(D)]. According to angiography, the device was positioned and partially deployed; the vessels were cannulated from inside the graft through the fenestration to the vessels with shepherd hook (SH) catheter and glidewire via 7-F Ansel sheaths. The left RA was catheterized, and a 7-F Ansel 2 introducer sheath was inserted. At that time, the patient complained of abdominal discomfort and nausea. Angiography revealed that a SMA had disappeared, consequently covering a SMA, or embolic occlusion was highly suspected. The remaining procedure of EVAR was performed at a quick pace. A proximal body was completely deployed including suprarenal stent deployment. A left renal stent (Palmaz P1506) was deployed through the fenestration via 7-F Ansel introducer sheath [Fig. 4(E)]. After that distal bifurcated body was deployed, the contralateral limb was deployed in a similar manner. Following touch-up ballooning for the attachment sites and every junction, angiography showed successful exclusion of aneurysm without a SMA flow [Fig. 4(F)]. The sheaths were removed from the femoral arteries, and the femoral access site was closed with 5-0 polypropylene sutures.

We decided to save SMA with retrograde SMA stenting. After the patient was sedated, midline laparotomy was performed. The intestine was pale, and a distal SMA that had no pulsation was exposed. The distal SMA was punctured with micropuncture kit and a 6-F sheath was inserted toward the aorta. Contrast injection from the SMA sheath revealed that the distal SMA was covered by the endograft fabric [Fig. 4(G) and 4(H)]. A 0.035″ glidewire was easily

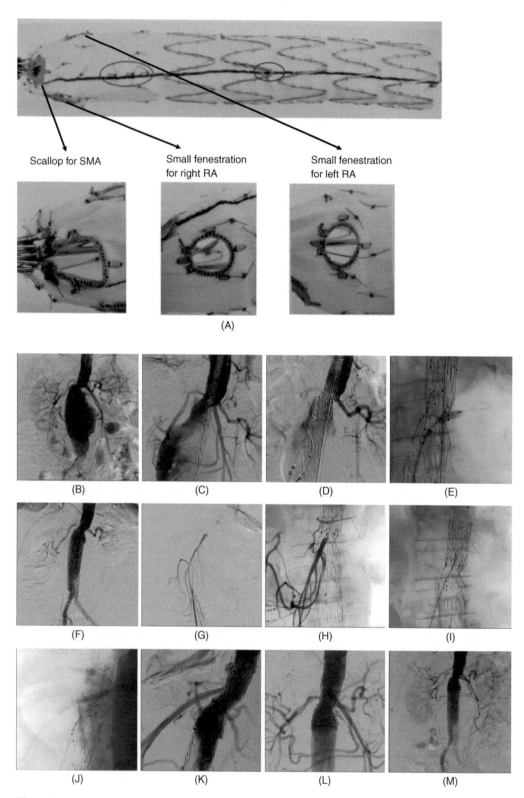

Scallop for SMA

Small fenestration
for right RA

Small fenestration
for left RA

(A)

(B)

(C)

(D)

(E)

(F)

(G)

(H)

(I)

(J)

(K)

(L)

(M)

Figure 4

advanced to the aorta [Fig. 4(I)], and Palmaz stent (P2006) was deployed as a final procedure [Fig. 4(J)]. The SMA stent made an intestine color vital, and an angiography showed successful exclusion of aneurysm with a good SMA flow [Fig. 4(K)–4(M)]. The laparotomy was closed in a multilayer fashion. The patient was discharged from hospital without any complication 10 days after the procedure.

f. Summary: How was the case managed, is there anything that could have been improved, what was the immediate and long-term outcome? EVAR with stented fenestrated graft is feasible, and good short-term and midterm results are reported. Despite the preoperative precise evaluation of aneurysm and branches, loss of visceral artery patency is one of the most important complications. When visceral artery was covered and lost, this retrograde stenting may be one of the ultimate troubleshooting. This retrograde stenting technique may be applied to TEVAR for aortic arch aneurysm.

g. List of contemporary equipments that should be used in this case:
    o 9-F, 7-F, 6-F, and 5-F sheaths
    o Zenith fenestrated graft (Cook Medical)
    o Flexor Check-Flo introducer Ansel Modification (Cook Medical)
    o Palmaz stent (P1506 for RA) (P2006 for SMA)
    o Micropuncture set (Cook Medical)

h. Key learning issues of this specific case: Fenestrated and branched endografts expand the application of EVAR to a wider range of patients. However, these new devices present new complications. Important requirements for successful fenestrated EVAR are careful planning, precise measurement, appropriate device making, and extremely experienced deployment technique. Fenestrated and branched endografts are associated with relatively high risks of visceral branch loss and renal complications. When visceral artery was covered and lost, this retrograde stenting may quickly recover the visceral ischemia.

PART 3: AUTHOR'S SUMMARY OF KEY ISSUES FOR SUCCESSFUL AND SAFE TREATMENT OF COMPLEX LESIONS IN THIS VESSEL AREA

Basis for a successful and safe treatment of complex abdominal aortic lesions is to understand the features of some endografts. In order to avoid EVAR complications, the important issue is patient selection. Successful EVAR mandates precise measurement and evaluation prior to procedure so that an appropriate endograft can be chosen. Key features to avoid complications are as follows:

- Patient selection involves careful assessment of anatomical features of the aneurysm.
    - Proximal neck length, diameter, angulation, shape, presence of mural thrombus, calcification, etc.
    - Access vessels diameter, tortuosity, stenosis, thrombus, calcification, etc.
- Precise measurement and device selection.
- Preoperative determination of the cranial–caudal and lateral angle of the C-arm in each situation in EVAR and execution.
- Withdrawal should be considered in some cases. Perfect is enemy of good.
- Confirm the access route before the guidewire is removed. In the case of small or diseased access vessels, placement of a 9-F sheath into the femoral artery is highly recommended prior to removing the guidewire to perform a retrograded arteriography.
- Avoid unnecessary interventional steps. Every step makes sense.
- Reduce the amount of contrast.
- Check the patient status. Vital sign, consciousness, pain, etc.

REFERENCES

1. McPhee JT, Hill JS, Eslami MH. The impact of gender on presentation, therapy and mortality of abdominal aortic aneurysm in the US, 2001–2004. J Vasc Surg 2007; 45:891–899.
2. Anderson PL, Arons RR, Moskowitz AJ, et al. A statewide experience with endovascular abdominal aortic aneurysm repair: rapid diffusion with excellent early results. J Vasc Surg 2004; 39(1):10–19.

3. Stanley BM, Semmens JB, Mai Q, et al. Evaluation of patient selection guidelines for endoluminal AAA repair with the Zenith Stent-Graft: the Australasian experience. J Endovasc Ther 2001; 8(5):457–464.
4. Abbruzzese TA, Kwolek CJ, Brewaster DC, et al. Outcomes following endovascular abdominal aortic aneurysm repair (EVAR): an anatomic and device-specific analysis [published online ahead of print April 25, 2008]. J Vasc Surg. 2008; 48(1):19–28.
5. Porcellini M, Nastro P, Bracale U, et al. Endovascular versus open surgical repair of abdominal aortic aneurysm with concomitant malignancy. J Vasc Surg 2007; 46(1):16–23.
6. Ohki T, Deaton DH, Condado JA. Aptus Endovascular AAA Repair System: report of the 1-year follow-up in a first-in-man study. Endovascular Today. 2006:29–36.
7. Saratzis N, Melas N, Saratzis A, et al. Anaconda aortic stent-graft: single-center experience of a new commercially available device for abdominal aortic aneurysms. J Endovasc Ther 2008; 15(1):33–41.
8. O'Neill S, Greenberg RK, Haddad F, et al. A prospective analysis of fenestrated endovascular grafting: intermediate-term outcomes. Eur J Vasc Endovasc Surg 2006; 32(2):115–123.

11 | Renal Arteries

Thomas Zeller

Department of Angiology, Herz-Zentrum Bad Krozingen, Bad Krozingen, Germany

PART 1: INTRODUCTION

What Makes a Lesion "Complex" in Renal Interventions?

In the past decade, stent-supported angioplasty of atherosclerotic renal artery stenosis (RAS) became the treatment of choice and replaced surgery in most cardiovascular centers (1). Recent advances in catheter technology have made the procedure a supposed simple procedure (2). However, anatomical variations and concomitant aortic–pelvic disease can translate the intervention into a challenging procedure.

Clinical Indications for Treatment of Complex Lesions in Renal Interventions

Indications for an endovascular treatment of even complex, potentially complication-associated lesions are summarized in Table 1.

Hazards and Complications

The *potential risks* of endovascular treatment of complex renal artery lesions are listed in Table 2.

Interventional Strategies

Preinterventional diagnostic workup of patients with RAS consists primarily of color duplex ultrasound. In experienced hands, this technology allows the reliable diagnosis of a severe RAS, defined as at least 70% stenosis (3). Furthermore, it is the ideal diagnostic tool to examine the morphology of the abdominal aorta in terms of detecting aneurysm formation and plaque burden. However, this technology frequently misses atypically located accessory renal arteries and usually does not allow visualizing the course of the renal artery in detail and the division into the side branches. For these purposes, magnetic resonance angiography (MRA) or computed tomography angiography (CTA) are the diagnostic tools of choice. These methods allow the three-dimensional reconstruction of the renal artery anatomy and in case of CTA the evaluation of the plaque composition. This can be helpful for planning the interventional access route even if nowadays the majority of the renal interventions can be managed from the femoral access.

The most frequently used access routes are the femoral and brachial *access*, few physicians prefer the radial access. The main indication for a brachial or—if preferred a radial access—is an acute angle of the off-take of the renal artery (Fig. 1). Another more rare indication is an untreated total occlusion of the infrarenal aorta (Fig. 2). The most frequently used guiding catheter configuration for this approach is the multipurpose shape; alternative shapes are the right "Amplatz 1" and "Judkins right 4" configurations.

In particular cases of ulcerated and bended course of the renal artery in which the guidewire—usually a 0.014″ stiff uncoated type—the telescoping technique can manage to cross the lesion with wire. And at least 125-cm long 4-F angled diagnostic catheter (e.g., "Multipurpose") has to be introduced through the 6-F guiding catheter (100 cm in length) to navigate the guidewire through the lesion (Fig. 3).

In the majority of the cases, the femoral approach is feasible even in unfavorable anatomic situations, as shown in Figure 4 using the telescoping technique.

Usually, a 6-F guiding catheter is large enough to introduce stent devices up to a diameter of 7 mm. However, in bifurcation lesions requiring kissing balloon angioplasty or kissing stenting, 8-F guiding catheters might be indicated. In small aortic diameters, the "IMA" or "Judkins right" configuration is appropriate, whereas in larger diameters (>20 mm) the "Renal Double Curve" or the "Hockey Stick" configuration fits the best. In extremely caudal angulated off-takes of the

Table 1 Indications for Complex Renal Artery Interventions

Every patient with an absolute indication for renal artery revascularization with contraindications for surgical revascularization
Insufficient medical blood pressure associated with a RAS > 70%
Recurrent flush pulmonary edema associated with (bilateral) RAS
Decreasing renal function associated with either unilateral RAS of a functional single kidney or bilateral RAS
Recurrent unstable angina in severe coronary artery disease associated with hypertensive crises not manageable with coronary revascularization procedures or medication

renal artery the telescoping technique must be used to introduce the guidewire: a 5-F "Simmonds (SIM) 1" or "SOS Omni" diagnostic catheter has to be introduced through a 6-F guiding catheter such as an "IMA" shaped one to engage the renal artery origin with the guidewire. Once the wire is in place, the guiding catheter is advanced over the diagnostic catheter close to the ostium of the renal artery and the diagnostic catheter can be withdrawn (Fig. 4). The standard guidewire is a 0.014" extra support wire with a floppy radio opaque tip, such as Galeo ES™ (Biotronik, Berlin, Germany). Hydrophilic-coated wires should only be used in difficult-to-pass lesions because of the increased risk of perforation using such types of wire. Predilation is only indicated in subtotal occlusions or highly calcified lesions when it is uncertain if the stenosis can be dilated with a balloon. In situations of a nondilatable stenosis, a Cutting Balloon™ (Boston Scientific, Rangendingen, Germany) or a Scoring Balloon™ (Biotronik, Berlin, Germany) might be indicated.

Interventional Tools

In bended arteries, dedicated renal stent devices with a long so-called "anti-flip-tip" of the balloon catheter facilitate the introduction of the stent into the lesion even without predilation. The Hippocampus™ 0.014 Balloon Expanding Rapid Exchange Renal Stent System (Invatec Corp., Concesio, Brescia, Italy) device consists of a long "non-flip-tip" with progressive flexibility and minimal entry profile. Since the system shows a progressive flexibility, coming from the long tip, followed by the long balloon cone, the guidewire will not be straightened and possibly flipped out of the origin (Fig. 5). As soon as the balloon segment with the crimped stent is advanced through the curve of the guiding catheter or introducer sheath, the long tip is already inserted in the renal artery origin so that the position cannot be lost again.

Currently, no dedicated distal protection devices for renal use are on the market. Therefore, their general use cannot yet be recommended. The most important step potentially leading to renal embolism is the engagement of the renal artery with the guiding catheter. During this manipulation, a lot of debris can be collected from the aortic wall at the tip of the guiding catheter. With the first selective contrast agent injection into the renal artery, all this captured

Table 2 Potential Risks of Endovascular Treatment of Complex Lesions

Clinical and anatomical presentation	Potential complication	Frequency of complication
AAA	Micro- and macro embolism	Up to 4%
	Aortic wall dissection	anecdotic
Diffuse atherosclerotic plaques of abdominal aorta	Micro- and macro embolism Cholesterol embolism	Up to 4%
Acute angle of renal artery off-take	Wire-induced dissection or perforation Stent misplacement	Up to 1% each
Early renal artery bifurcation	Stenosis or occlusion of one of the side branches	No reports
Common renal artery trunk	Plaque shift into one of the side branches	No reports
Accessory renal artery	Lesion can be overseen, dissection, plaque shift	No reports
Borderline renal function	End-stage renal insufficiency > contrast-induced nephropathy or embolism	Up to 0.5%
Stent protrusion into the aorta	Stent dislocation when passing the abdominal aorta with wires or catheters	Case reports

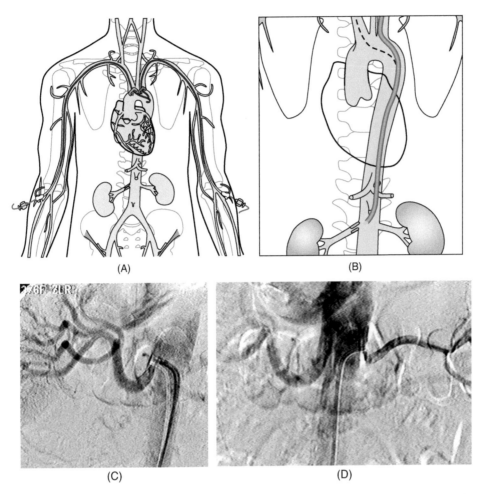

Figure 1 (A,B) Drawing of brachial access to an acutely angled off-take of a right renal artery. (C–E) Acute angle of the right and the left cranial RA, regular origin of the left caudal RA. (F–H) Transbrachial angioplasty of the left cranial renal artery (6-F multipurpose guiding catheter).

(*Continued on page 146*)

debris is already dislodged into the kidney before any distal protection device works. To avoid embolism during this crucial step of the intervention the "no-touch" technique (4; Fig. 6) should be used or at least before the first dye injection, the catheter should be cleaned from debris by aspirating blood through a Y-connector (Fig. 7).

In ostial atherosclerotic RAS balloon, expandable stents are mandatory to resist the vessel recoil at the origin. Several stents show a progressive radial strength toward the proximal end, which covers the renal artery origin (e.g., Hippocampus ™). In more distally located lesion, low-profile self-expanding stents fitting through a 6-F guiding catheter (e.g., Xpert™, Abbott Vascular, Diegem, Belgium or Maris deep™, Invatec) should be used because of the high mechanical forces that are applied to the renal artery trunk by respiration synchronic vessel bending, which can lead to stent fracture in rigid balloon expandable stents with consecutive abrupt vessel occlusion resulting in functional kidney loss. Neither passive stent coating (5,6) nor drug-eluting stent technology (7) could yet prove superior technical outcome compared to bare metal stent technology.

Summary of Outcomes

Overall, including complex lesions, in experienced hands technical success rates of endovascular renal artery interventions are close to 100% and one-year restenosis rates reported, depending

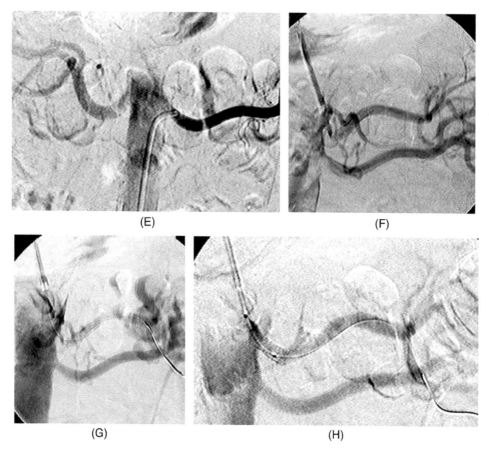

(E) (F)

(G) (H)

Figure 1 (*Continued*)

on the definition of restenosis, are ranging from 5% to 20% using current stent devices (Table 3). Restenosis rate inversely correlates with the vessel or stent diameter, respectively (5,6).

Restenosis can become a challenging situation especially in those cases where the stent protrudes more than 1 mm into the aortic lumen. The engagement of the proximal stent lumen can become time consuming and might need several attempts with different kinds of diagnostic or guiding catheters. There are two major signs that predict the correct position of the wire: The first is when the diagnostic or guiding catheter easily slips into the proximal stent segment

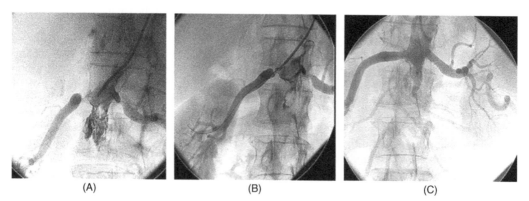

(A) (B) (C)

Figure 2 (A–C) Bilateral severe RAS and infrarenal occlusion of abdominal aorta before and after transbrachial stenting.

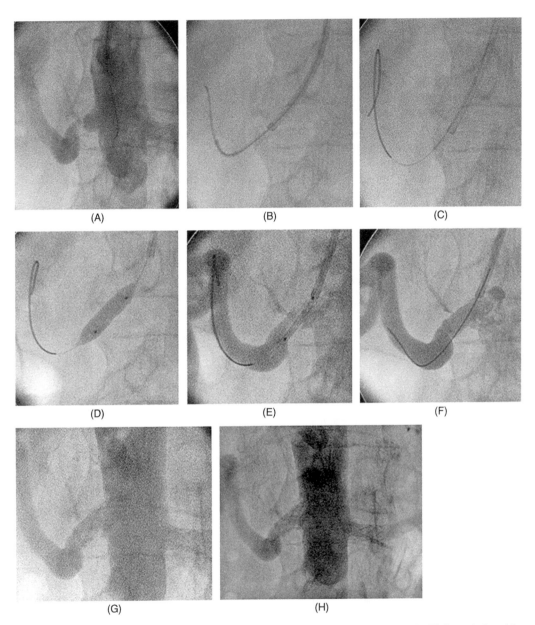

Figure 3 (A) Right RAS, unfavorable angle of the origin and bended course of the trunk. (B) Cannulation of the ostium with a 5-F JR 4 125-cm long diagnostic catheter to place the guidewire. (C) Guiding sheath pushed into the origin, diagnostic catheter withdrawn. (D) Predilation with a 5/20 mm balloon. (E) Positioning of the stent. (F) Result after 5/13 mm Multilink ultra stent. (G and H) Final result after bilateral RA stenting.

after the lesion is passed with wire. If this is not possible, the wire went through the stent mashes from outside. The second sign is, when the balloon catheter or in case of intended direct stenting the stent device can easily be placed in the restenosed stent. In some rare cases, it can be helpful to use an orthogonal view for the engagement of the stent. Rare data are available about the appropriate treatment strategy of restenosis. It seems that plain balloon angioplasty, cutting balloon angioplasty, and restenting are associated with recurrent restenosis rates of about 30%. Covered stents (Jostentgraft™, Abbott Vascular) or drug-eluting stents (Taxus™, Boston Scientific) seem to considerably reduce this recurrence rate (17). However, no randomized data are yet available to proof this concept.

Equipment Checklist

Table 4 summarizes access and lesion-specific tools that should be available on stock for complex renal interventions.

PART 2: TEACHING CASES

Case 1: Telescoping technique (Fig. 4): This case shows an acute angle of the off-take of the left renal artery of approximately 180° with an origin near subtotal eccentric RAS.

a. What made the lesion "complex" in this specific case? The complexity of the case results in the difficult angulations of the course of the renal artery associated with the eccentric subtotal stenosis making it nearly impossible to cross the lesion with the wire guided simply through a guiding catheter [Fig. 4(E)]. The second challenge was the navigation of the stent into the stenosis.

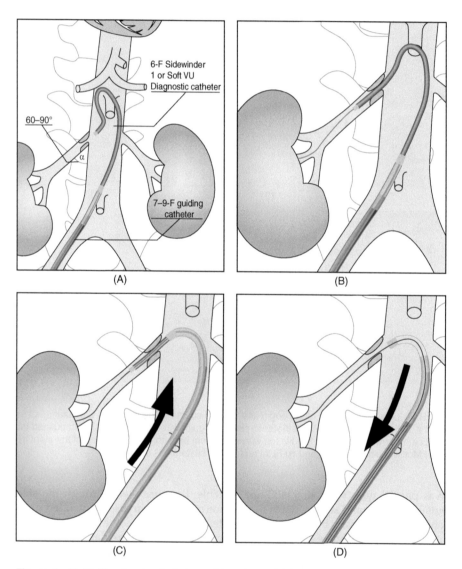

Figure 4 (A–D) Step by step technique of transfemoral telescoping technique for engagement of an acutely angled off-take of a right renal artery. (E) Tight stenosis of the left RA, RDC guiding catheter. (F) SOS omni catheter through RDC guiding catheter. (G) Guiding catheter advanced over the diagnostic catheter. (H) Left RA after first stent. (I) Final result after second stent.

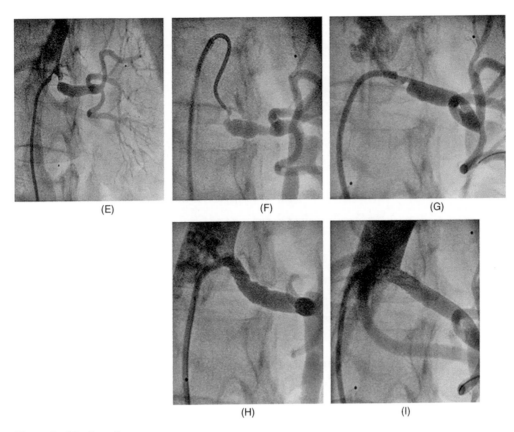

(E) (F) (G)

(H) (I)

Figure 4 (*Continued*)

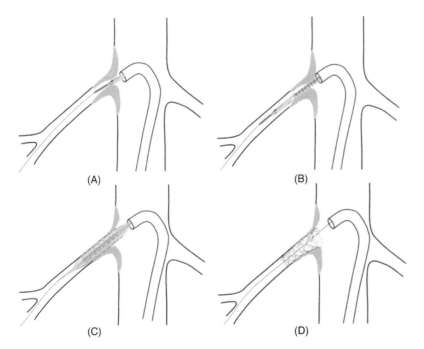

(A) (B)

(C) (D)

Figure 5 Unique crossing design of the Hippocampus™ stent system: The long anti-flip tip (A) with progressive flexibility and minimal entry profile. As soon as the balloon segment with the crimped stent is advanced through the curve of the guiding catheter the long tip is already inserted in the ostium. Thus the device cannot flip out the renal artery (B). Figure (C) and (D) show the release of the stent slightly protruding into the aortic lumen.

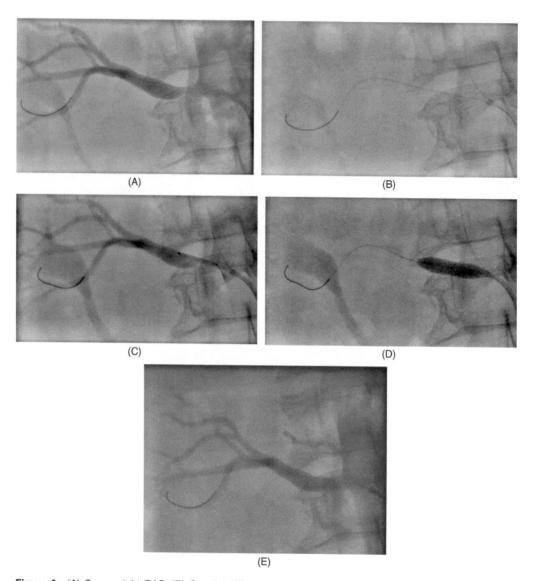

Figure 6 (A) Severe right RAS. (B) One 0.014″ wire each in the renal artery and the suprarenal aorta. (C) Placement of the stent. (D) Release of the stent, aortic wire still in place. (E) Final result.

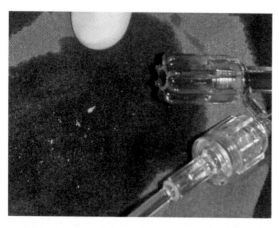

Figure 7 Atheromatous debris after back-bleeding through the guiding catheter following cannulation of the renal artery ostium in a patient with diffusely diseased aorta.

Table 3 Restenosis Rates for Ostial Stent Angioplasty, Literature Review

References	*n* pts	Stent type	Technique and definition of restenosis	Restenosis rate and follow-up period
8	68	Palmaz	Duplex; PSV > 2.0 m/sec + dRI > 0.05 followed by angiography (> 50%)	11% (mean FU 27 months)
9	29	Palmaz	Angiography, ≥ 50%	16% (mean FU 6.7 months)
10	100	Mixed	Angiography, > 50%	19% (mean FU 8.7 months)
11	30	Palmaz, InFlow, beStent	Angiography, not defined	12.5% (6 months)
12	42	Palmaz	Angiography; ≥ 50%	14% (6 months)
13	63	Not documented	Angiography, ≥ 50%	30% (median FU 23 months)
14	300	Mixed	Angiography, ≥ 50%	21% (median 16 months)
15	51	Palmaz	Duplex; ≥ 60% (PSV > 2 m/sec, RAR > 3.5) or angiography (≥ 50%)	14.3% (mean FU 13.1 months)
16	215	Mixed	Duplex; ≥ 70% (RAR > 3.5 + dRI > 0.05)	11.2% (1 year)
5	143	Palmaz Genesis, Radix	Duplex; ≥ 70% (RAR > 3.5 + dRI > 0.05)	6.4% (mean FU 22 months)

b. What was the clinical indication for treatment of this specific case? The indication for the treatment was a poorly controlled hypertension despite five antihypertensive drugs. The patient presented with a diffuse type of atherosclerosis including coronary artery disease with already twice done percutaneous coronary intervention and peripheral artery disease with no lifestyle-limiting claudication of the left leg. Baseline creatinine concentration was slightly elevated to 1.5 mg/dl. Risk factors besides arterial hypertension included all aspects of a metabolic syndrome.

c. What were the potential hazards of treating this specific patient and this lesion? The potential hazards were first inducing a dissection during the crossing attempt of the lesion with the wire potentially leading to acute vessel occlusion and second the risk of embolism caused by extensive wire and catheter manipulations. Moreover, stent loss or misplacement had to be taken into consideration.

Table 4 Recommended Devices for Complex Renal Interventions

Special situation	Tool	Device example(s)
Brachial access	Diagnostic (4/5-F) or guiding catheter (6-F)	Multipurpose, Amplatz right, Judkins right
Femoral access	• Diagnostic (4/5-F) • Guiding catheter (6-F)	SIM 1 or SOS Omni (diagnostic catheter) IMA, Judkins right, Hockey Stick, RDC (guiding catheter)
Subtotal occlusion	Guidewire	Hydrophilic-coated 0.014″ extra support guide-wire (e.g., Pilot™ 150, Abbott Vascular)
"Undilatable" lesion	Plaque modulation device	Scoring Balloon (Biotronic) Cutting Balloon (Boston Scientific)
Acute angle of the renal artery origin	"Anti-flip-tip" balloon/stent device	Hippocampus™ stent (Invatec)
In-stent restenosis	• Drug-eluting stent • Covered stent	Taxus™ (Boston Scientific) Graftmaster (Abbott Vascular)
Chronic total occlusion	Crossing device	Excimer laser (Spectranetics)
Thrombus containing lesion	Distal protection devices	Filters (e.g., Emboshield pro™, Abbott Vascular, Fibernet™, Lumen Biomedical, Plymouth, MN) Distal occlusion balloon (Percusurge™, Medtronic)
Renal artery perforation	• Main artery • Segmental artery	Covered stent (Graftmaster™) Microcoils (e.g., Trufill, Cordis J&J)

d. Which interventional strategies were considered and which interventional tools were used to handle this lesion? The easiest approach would have been the brachial access using a "Multipurpose"-shaped guiding catheter. However, at the time this intervention was performed, stents had to be crimped onto the balloon by hand and 8-F guiding catheters had to be used. The risk of an access site complication inserting an 8-F sheath into the brachial artery was considered to be high. Therefore, the femoral approach was chosen. Because no 0.014″ wire compatible devices were available at the time of the intervention, a stiff uncoated 0.018″ guidewire had to be used. This wire was unable to cross the lesion navigated through the guiding catheter. This lead to the decision for a selective engagement of the renal artery origin using a 5-F SOS Omni diagnostic catheter, which was introduced through the 55-cm long 8-F "RDC" guiding catheter [Fig. 4(A, B, and F)]. Once the origin was cannulated with the diagnostic catheter with its soft atraumatic tip, the 0.018″ guidewire could be easily passed through the lesion and the guiding catheter was advanced across the diagnostic catheter and positioned at the origin of the renal artery [Fig. 4(C, D, and G)]. Following predilation with a 3/20-mm balloon catheter, a 6/17-mm AVE bridge^{TM} stent was placed [Fig. 4(H)]. However, this stent did not cover the renal artery origin, which was also diseased. Therefore, a second 6/10 mm stent was placed without leaving a residual stenosis [Fig. 4(I)].

e. Summary: How was the case managed, is there anything that could have been improved, what was the immediate and long-term outcome? The first stent was placed slightly too far distal. Either, this stent should have been placed 3 mm more proximal or a longer (20 mm) stent should have been used to avoid the placement of a second stent. The long-term outcome in this particular patient was favorable; the stents are still patent after nine years of serial annual duplex ultrasound follow-up. Renal function slightly improved with serum creatinine values dropping to 1.0 mg/dl immediately after the intervention and being stable during follow-up with 1.1 mg/dl after nine years. Blood pressure control persistently improved by a reduction of two antihypertensive drugs.

f. List of contemporary equipments that should be used in this case:
    *   Guiding catheter 6-F (RDC-1 or IMA)
    *   Diagnostic catheter 5-F (SOS Omni or SIM-1)
    *   Guidewire 0.014″ hydrophilic coated (Pilot^{TM} 150) or uncoated (Galeo ES^{TM})
    *   Coronary balloon catheter 3/20 mm (e.g., Maverick^{TM}) for predilation
    *   6/20 mm renal stent device (e.g., Hippocampus^{TM})

g. Key learning issues of this specific case: Even if appropriately angled guiding catheters are not available to engage a renal artery origin due to an acute angle of the renal artery off-take, the telescoping technique can avoid the need of an additional brachial approach.

Case 2: Bifurcation lesion: Early bifurcation of the renal artery, kissing balloon technique.

a. What made the lesion "complex" in this specific case? The right renal artery was acutely occluded one year before the index procedure by a cardioembolic event and there was only 6% residual function despite successful, but delayed stent recanalization [Fig. 8(A)]. Therefore, the patient presented with a functional single kidney (the left one) and a stenosis of the left renal artery, which presented with a short trunk of about 8 mm length before the division in the two major side branches [Fig. 8(B) and 8(D)]. Because of the functional single kidney situation, none of the both side branches should have been compromised by the intervention. Interestingly, the left renal artery was unsuspicious for stenosis one year before during the recanalization of the acutely occluded right renal artery.

b. What was the clinical indication for treatment of this specific case? The patient presented with deterioration in blood pressure control and decrease of glomerular filtration rate (GFR) of 15 mL/min within one year. Major concomitant diseases were moderate coronary 1-vessel disease, intermittent atrial fibrillation, and nonsignificant peripheral artery disease (Fontaine class I, Rutherford category 1). Risk factors besides arterial hypertension were history of smoking and hypercholesterolemia.

c. What were the potential hazards of treating this specific patient and this lesion? The major hazard was to compromise one of the side branches by plaque shift. Moreover, the large vessel diameter made the use of a noncoronary stent device, in this case a Palmaz stent

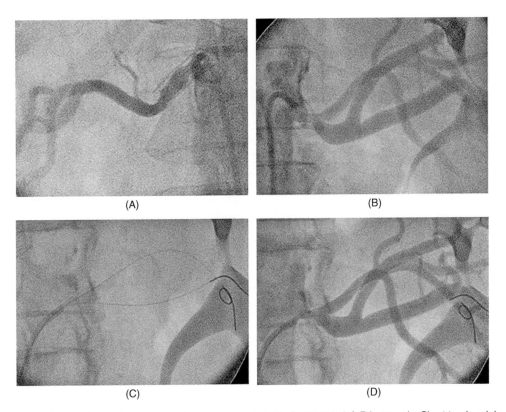

Figure 8 (A) Right RA 12 months after recanalization. (B) Ostial 75% left RA stenosis. Short trunk, origin near bifurcation. (C and D) One 0.014″ Galeo ES guidewire in each side branch. (E) Stent positioning, two wires stent PTRA of the RA trunk. (F) Result after stent placement. (G) Additional double balloon angioplasty. (H) Final result after Palmaz P 104 stent.

(*Continued on page 154*)

necessary. Covering one of the side branches with this stent type it would have been impossible to dilate the connections between the struts performing kissing balloon angioplasty after stent deployment.

d. Which interventional strategies were considered for this lesion? First, one 0.014″ extra support guidewire had to be placed into each main side branch [Fig. 8(C) and 8(D)]. Thereafter, the shortest available stent (Palmaz P 104) had to be positioned with the distal stent end reaching into the bifurcation but not covering completely the cranial side branch to enable flaring the distal stent end into both side branches using kissing balloon technique following stent placement [Fig. 8(E) and (8F)].

e. Which interventional tools were used to handle this lesion? The intervention was performed via an 8-F "RDC" guiding catheter using two 0.014″ Galeo ES™ guidewires. The Palmaz P 104™ stent was hand crimped onto a 6/20-mm Bypass Speedy™ balloon and positioned into the short common renal artery trunk covering the dummy wire that was placed into the cranial side branch [Fig. 8(E) and (8F)]. After repositioning the guidewire through the stent into the cranial side branch [Fig. 8(F)], a 3.5/20-mm coronary balloon was positioned reaching from the main trunk into the cranial side branch and a 6/12-mm balloon from the common trunk into the caudal main side branch. Performing prolonged kissing balloon angioplasty for one minute [Fig. 8(G)], the distal stent ends were flared into both side branches to achieve an optimized vessel wall apposition [Fig. 8(H)].

f. Summary: How was the case managed, is there anything that could have been improved, what was the immediate and long-term outcome? The immediate and long-term technical outcome was excellent with a patent vessel for more than eight years. Clinically, GFR increased immediately after the intervention by 12 mL/min and remained stable during

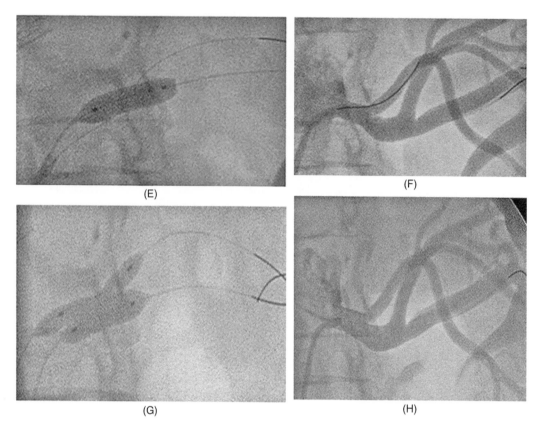

Figure 8 (*Continued*)

the follow-up period. Blood pressure is well controlled under a dual drug therapy including a ß-blocker and an angiotensin receptor blocker.

g. List of contemporary equipments that should be used in this case:
  - Guiding catheter 7-F (RDC-1 or IMA)
  - Two uncoated 0.014″ extra support guidewires (Galeo ES™)
  - Rapid exchange balloon catheters 3.5/20 mm and 6/12 mm (e.g., Maverick™, Submarine rapido™ (Invatec)) for postdilation
  - 6/10 mm renal stent device (e.g., Hippocampus™, Palmaz blue™, etc.)

h. Key learning issues of this specific case: Even a short common renal artery trunk can be treated with appropriate tools selectively without the need to cover one of the major side branches with the stent. Kissing balloon technique can be used for optimizing vessel wall apposition of the stent.

Case 3: Laser-assisted recanalization of a chronic total renal artery occlusion and of restenosis 6 months after vessel recanalization.

a. What made the lesion "complex" in this specific case? The left renal artery was chronically occluded presenting only with a short stump [Fig. 9(A)]. Usually, support to cross a renal CTO is limited.

b. What was the clinical indication for treatment of this specific case? A still preserved but in length by 2 cm reduced kidney compared to the contralateral side with a residual excretory function of 15% relative to global renal function by scintigraphy. The patient was hypertensive and had mild renal dysfunction (serum creatinine 1.5 mg/dl, eGFR 37.6 mL/min). The patient also suffered from mild coronary artery disease and peripheral artery disease with a history of percutaneous superficial artery recanalization of the left side. Risk factors—besides arterial hypertension—were smoking and hypercholesterolemia.

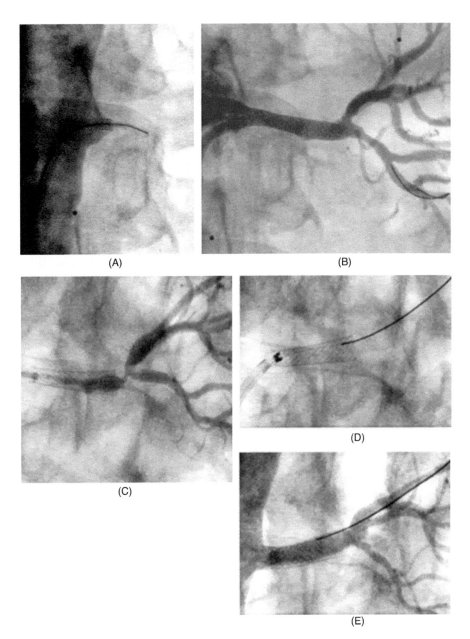

Figure 9 (A) Left renal artery 100%. (B) Result after laser recanalization and implantation of a Magic Wallstent. (C) In-stent restenosis after six months after the index procedure. (D) Two-millimeter eccentric excimer laser catheter, 8-F RDC guiding catheter. (E) Left RA after laser, 6 mm balloon angioplasty, and Palmaz P 104 at the origin.

c. What were the potential hazards of treating this specific patient and this lesion? Major risks of recanalization of renal artery CTOs are dissections of the aorta and renal artery, perforation, and embolism (renal and lower limbs).

d. Which interventional strategies were considered for this lesion? Most important was the choice of the appropriate guiding catheter or diagnostic catheter configuration to guarantee a stable catheter position for sufficient wire backup. As guiding catheter, the "RDC" configuration or "Hockey Stick" shape would offer the best support. Alternatively, the telescoping technique using a "SIM-1" or "SOS Omni" diagnostic catheter introduced through the guiding catheter would offer adequate wire support to cross the lesion.

e. Which interventional tools were used to handle this lesion? To facilitate the passage of the CTO and for debulking of potentially embolic occlusive material, an excimer laser catheter was used. Because of the length of the lesion, a self-expanding stent was chosen, even though the origin of the renal artery was also affected.

f. Summary: How was the case managed, is there anything that could have been improved, what was the immediate and long-term outcome? The recanalization procedure was performed via an 8-F "RDC" guiding catheter. The lesion could be penetrated with a 0.014″ hydrophilic-coated coronary guidewire. Using the step-by-step technique, a 2-mm eccentric laser probe was passed through the lesion with reconnection of the wire to the perfused lumen at the level of the division of the renal artery trunk into the segmental arteries. A 6/24-mm Easy Wallstent™ was placed covering the whole length of the former occlusion [Fig. 9(B)]. Postdilation was performed with a 6/20-mm coronary balloon catheter. Six months later, severe restenosis was detected by duplex ultrasound and confirmed by angiography [Fig. 9(C)]. Restenosis included the origin with incomplete expansion of the proximal stent end, diffuse in-stent neointima hyperproliferation, and restenosis at the division of the segmental arteries. Using again an 8-F "RDC" guiding catheter, four passes with an eccentric 2-mm excimer laser probe were performed [Fig. 9(D)], followed by postdilation with a 6/20-mm monorail balloon catheter and the placement of a 10-mm long balloon expandable stent into the renal artery origin without residual stenosis [Fig. 9(E)]. Nine years later, the artery is still patent as shown by duplex ultrasound. To avoid restenosis at least at the origin, a balloon expandable stent should have been placed already during the index procedure. Nowadays, a self-expanding low-profile nitinol stent device should be preferred fitting through a 6-F guiding catheter.

Clinically, even after nine years, renal function was preserved with a serum creatinine concentration of 1.0 mg/dl and blood pressure is well controlled with an angiotensin converting enzyme blocker only.

g. List of contemporary equipments that should be used in this case:
- Guiding catheter 7-F ("RDC"-1 or "Hockey Stick")
- Hydrophilic-coated 0.014″ extra support guidewire (Pilot™ or Choice PT™)
- 1.4 or 1.7 mm Turbo elite™ laser catheter (Spectranetics)
- For occasional predilation, RX balloon catheter 3/20 mm (e.g., Maverick™)
- 6/20 mm or 7/20 mm low-profile nitinol stent device, for example, Xpert™ (Abbott Vascular), Astron pulsar™ (Biotronik) for the renal artery trunk
- 6/20 mm RX balloon catheter for postdilation of the nitinol stent (e.g., Submarine rapido™)
- 6/10 mm balloon expandable stent for the renal artery origin (e.g., Hippocampus™)

h. Key learning issues of this specific case: Recanalization of even chronic total renal artery occlusions is feasible provided a renal artery stump can be identified. Photoablation for debulking with the excimer laser can facilitate the recanalization procedure and potentially prevent distal embolism during the recanalization attempt. Excimer laser technology can also be used for debulking of in-stent restenosis. In long lesions, self-expanding stents can be used to cover the renal artery trunk. However, if the origin is involved into the occlusion, radial strength of the self-expanding stent might be insufficient to keep the proximal stent segment fully expanded. The overlapping additional placement of a balloon expandable should be considered.

PART 3: KEY ISSUES FOR SUCCESSFUL AND SAFE TREATMENT OF COMPLEX RENAL LESIONS

The basis for a successful and safe treatment of complex renal artery lesions is the exact knowledge of the pathoanatomy and the presence of a predefined treatment strategy. If not all needed tools are on the shelf, reschedule the patient for a later date. Because complex interventions incorporate an increased periinterventional risk, the indication for the intervention must be undisputed. Key features to avoid complications are as follows:

- No guiding catheter manipulation along the aortic wall without aspiration of potentially trapped debris.

- Use the appropriate access to the lesion. If indicated change from a femoral to a brachial approach.
- Avoid unnecessary interventional steps. Every additional interventional step increases the risk of complication.
- Reduce the amount of contrast agent to what is absolutely necessary.
- Use the whole cardiovascular–endovascular toolbox and techniques. In doubt, ask a colleague of another specialty for support.

REFERENCES

1. Safian RD, Textor SC. Renal-artery stenosis. N Engl J Med 2001; 344:431–442.
2. Zeller T, Frank U, Müller C, et al. Technological advances in the design of catheters and devices used in renal artery interventions: impact on complications. J Endovasc Ther 2003; 10:1006–1014.
3. Zeller T, Bonvini RF, Rastan A, et al. Colour-coded duplex ultrasound for diagnosis of renal artery stenosis and as follow-up examination after revascularization. Catheter Cardiovasc Interv 2008; 71:995–999.
4. Feldman RL, Wargovich TJ, Bittl JA. No-touch technique for reducing aortic wall trauma during renal artery stenting. Catheter Cardiovasc Interv 1999; 46:245–248.
5. Zeller T, Rastan A, Kliem M, et al. Impact of carbon coating on restenosis rate after stenting of atherosclerotic renal artery stenosis. J Endovasc Ther 2005; 12:605–611.
6. Zeller T, Müller C, Frank U, et al. Gold-coating and restenosis after primary stenting of ostial renal artery stenosis. Catheter Cardiovasc Interv 2003; 60:1–6.
7. Zähringer M, Sapoval M, Pattynama PM, et al. Sirolimus-eluting versus bare-metal low-profile stent for renal artery treatment (GREAT Trial): angiographic follow-up after 6 months and clinical outcome up to 2 years. J Endovasc Ther 2007; 14(4):460–468.
8. Blum U, Krumme B, Flügel P, et al. Treatment of ostial renal-artery stenoses with vascular endoprotheses after unsuccessful balloon angioplasty. N Engl J Med 1997; 336:459–465.
9. Taylor A, Sheppard D, MacLeod MJ, et al. Renal artery stent placement in renal artery stenosis: Technical and early clinical results. Clin Radiology 1997; 52:451–457.
10. White CJ, Ramee SR, Collins TJ, et al. Renal artery stent placement: utility in lesions difficult to treat with balloon angioplasty. J Am Coll Cardiol 1999; 30:1445–1450.
11. Gross CM, Krämer J, Waigand J, et al. Ostial renal artery stent placement for atherosclerotic renal artery stenosis in patients with coronary artery disease. Cathet Cardiovasc Diagn 1998; 45:1–8.
12. Van de Ven PJG, Kaatee R, Beutler JJ, et al. Arterial stenting and balloon angioplasty in ostial atherosclerotic renovascular disease: a randomised trail. Lancet 1999; 353:282–286.
13. Beutler JJ, van Ampting JM, van de Ven PJ, et al. Long-term effects of renal artery stenting on kidney function for patients with ostial atherosclerotic renal artery stenosis and renal insufficiency. J Am Soc Nephrol 2001; 1475–1481.
14. Lederman RJ, Mendelsohn FO, Santos R, et al. Primary renal artery stenting: characteristics and outcomes after 363 procedures. Am Heart J 2001; 142:314–323.
15. Rocha-Singh KJ, Ahuja RK, Sung CH, et al. Long-term renal function preservation after renal artery stenting in patients with progressive ischemic nephropathy. Catheter Cardiovasc Interv 2002; 57: 135–141.
16. Zeller T, Frank U, Müller C, et al. Predictors of improved renal function after primary stenting of severe atherosclerotic ostial renal artery stenosis. Circulation 2003; 108:2244–2249.
17. Zeller T, Rastan A, Schwarzwälder U, et al. Treatment of instent restenosis following stent-supported renal artery angioplasty. Catheter Cardiovasc Interv 2007; 70:454–459.

12 | Chronic Mesenteric Ischemia: Mesenteric Vascular Intervention

Rajan A. G. Patel, Stephen R. Ramee, and Christopher J. White

Department of Cardiology, Ochsner Heart and Vascular Institute, Ochsner Clinic Foundation, New Orleans, Louisiana, U.S.A.

PART 1: INTRODUCTION

Atherosclerosis of the mesenteric vessels may result in chronic mesenteric ischemia (CMI). This uncommon condition is often amenable to percutaneous intervention by experienced operators. Percutaneous endovascular procedures have been applied to the mesenteric arterial system since the early 1980s. In most symptomatic patients, at least two splanchnic vessels have severe stenosis. Moawad and Gewertz (1) report at least two-vessel disease in 91% of CMI patients and three-vessel disease in 55% of CMI patients. In this review, only 7% of CMI patients had an occluded superior mesenteric artery (SMA) and 2% had isolated celiac disease. Abrupt occlusion of mesenteric blood vessels can result in acute mesenteric ischemia. In a review of the topic, Oldenburg et al. (2) report the incidence of various etiologies of acute mesenteric ischemia as follows: arterial embolism 40% to 50%, arterial thrombosis 25%, nonocclusive arterial disease resulting in ischemia secondary to other factors such as low cardiac output or αadrenergic agonist use 20%, and venous thrombosis 10%. The patient with acute mesenteric ischemia has often developed infarcted bowel by the time of presentation. These patients generally require surgical treatment to remove necrotic tissue. Therefore, the focus of this chapter is the percutaneous treatment of CMI.

What Makes a Lesion "Complex" in Mesenteric Artery Interventions?

Endovascular treatment of mesenteric artery atherosclerotic lesions is made complex by the lesion location. These lesions are typically located near the aortic origin of the affected vessel. Furthermore, proximal segments of the mesenteric vessels frequently have an acute caudal orientation. The proximal location requires balloon expandable stents for precise positioning. The vessels are moderate in size usually 5 to 7 mm in diameter. These factors can make balloon expandable stent delivery from the femoral artery challenging. Additionally, angiographic imaging of mesenteric vessels, which arise from the anterior aspect of the aorta, requires steep lateral angulation with cranial or caudal orientation of the image intensifier. With steep angulation, X-rays must penetrate a larger volume of tissue that may decrease the image quality. Additionally, the patient is exposed to a higher dose of X-rays and the operators may be exposed to greater scatter radiation. Finally, the incidence of restenosis after stent placement in mesenteric arteries is higher than that reported for renal or coronary arteries.

Clinical Indications for Treatment of Complex Lesions in Mesenteric Artery Interventions

Atherosclerotic disease of the aorta with associated aorto-ostial stenosis of the mesenteric vessels is a common finding. Of 552 healthy Medicare beneficiaries that were screened with abdominal ultrasound, 17.5% had significant narrowing of a mesenteric vessel detected (3). However, less than 1% of patients with atherosclerotic narrowing of a mesenteric artery require revascularization (4). The most likely explanation for the infrequent occurrence of CMI in clinical practice is the redundancy of the splanchnic circulation with multiple interconnections (collaterals) between the visceral vessels.

Patients with CMI avoid food because of associated abdominal discomfort with eating and, therefore, almost always demonstrate significant weight loss. Abdominal pain in the absence of weight loss is more likely a result of a "functional" complaint, rather than bowel ischemia. Postprandial abdominal pain from CMI typically persists for one to three hours (5). However,

Table 1 Clinical Indications for Treatment of Mesenteric Artery Stenosis Are Defined by the Syndromes of Chronic Mesenteric Ischemia

Typical chronic mesenteric ischemia	Clinical triad: postprandial symptoms, pain or bloating
	Weight loss over time
	"Food fear"—avoidance of food due to abdominal pain associated with eating
Ischemic gastropathy	Nausea
	Vomiting
	Fullness
	Abdominal pain
	Weight loss
Ischemic colitis	Abdominal pain
	Gastrointestinal bleeding
	Hematochezia

patients with ischemic gastropathy may present with atypical symptoms, such as vomiting, diarrhea, constipation, ischemic colitis, and lower gastrointestinal bleeding. CMI may be very low on the list of differential diagnoses for patients with atypical symptoms. However, a high degree of suspicion for mesenteric ischemia is warranted for patients with other manifestations of atherosclerosis and unexplained weight loss. Table 1 summarizes the symptoms associated with CMI syndromes.

Among patients with the aforementioned symptoms and weight loss, the diagnosis of CMI is often delayed while evaluation for possible malignancy is conducted. Patients with functional bowel complaints rarely experience significant weight loss, which helps to differentiate them from CMI patients. Evidence of significant obstruction of two or more vessels is often found when classic symptoms and endoscopy suggest bowel ischemia (6). However, cases of single-vessel disease, usually of the SMA, have been described, particularly if collateral connections have been disrupted by prior abdominal surgery. When critical stenosis ($\geq$70%) is found in symptomatic patients with weight loss, revascularization is appropriate. Unfortunately, for patients with borderline lesions or atypical symptoms, there is no noninvasive stress test to elicit an ischemic response.

Hazards and Complications

Revascularization for CMI has traditionally been accomplished with open surgery using bypass grafting, endarterectomy, or aortic reimplantation of the SMA. This patient group has a high incidence of associated coronary artery disease. The reported perioperative mortality ranges from 3.5% to 15% (1,7–16). The highest incidence of complications during surgical revascularization reported is in the cohort of patients over the age of 70 (17).

At the Ochsner Clinic, we have reported the largest series of patients with CMI treated with endovascular techniques (18). A total of 79 vessels were treated in 59 patients. One patient in this series died from complications of multiorgan failure postprocedure. Table 2 lists the clinical event rates from this series. Two patients in this cohort experienced vascular access site complications. Both patients experienced brachial artery thombosis that was treated percutaneously. In another case series of 25 patients with CMI treated using stents, 2 (8%) cases of pseudoaneursym and 1 (4%) case of acute renal failure were reported (19).

Interventional Strategies

Atherosclerotic aorto-ostial obstructions of the visceral vessels are similar to those of the renal arteries and the technical considerations for percutaneous transluminal angioplasty (PTA) with stent placement are similar to those for renal artery intervention. As with renal artery interventions, stent placement offers superior patency compared to PTA alone (20). The endovascular approach circumvents the need for general anesthesia and the operative trauma associated with open surgery. Retrospective data suggest that the endovascular approach results in lower acute mortality and morbidity relative to surgical revascularization (6,16,18,20,21).

Table 2 Clinical Events in a Series of 58 Patients with CMI
Treated using Endovascular Techniques with Initial
Angiographic Success Followed for 14 ± 5 Months

Event	n (%)
Death	12 (21)
Myocardial infarction	6
Renal failure	1
Stroke	1
Symptom recurrence	10 (17)
Death or symptom recurrence	21 (36)
Event-free survival	37 (64)
Patients with restenosis	19 (37)

Source: From Ref. 18.

Noninvasive assessment of the mesenteric arteries can be accomplished with duplex ultrasound (DUS), computed tomographic angiography (CTA), or magnetic resonance angiography (MRA). There are no comparative studies comparing the accuracy of these three imaging modalities. Our experience at the Ochsner Clinic is that MRA is associated with a higher degree of false positives and that DUS often fails to identify lesions at the origin of the mesenteric vessels. Others have also reported a preference for CTA over MRA when imaging the visceral vessels due to the higher spatial and temporal resolution of the CTA (22). In addition to providing information regarding the presence or absence of atherosclerotic occlusive disease, MRA and CTA provide data regarding the orientation of the ostia of the mesenteric arteries, which may be useful in procedural planning and equipment selection.

Interventional Tools
The orientation of the ostia and proximal portion of the mesenteric arteries from the aorta dictate the vascular access site. The celiac and SMA trunks commonly arise in a caudal direction making arm access desirable. Brachial or radial artery access has been described when performing interventions on the celiac and SMA trunks. Percutaneous coronary interventions performed via the radial artery have a lower vascular complication rate than those performed via the brachial artery (23,24). When the origin of the mesenteric artery of interest is horizontal or cephalad in orientation, common femoral artery access is preferable.

Patients are premedicated with aspirin ($\geq$80 mg daily). There is no data to support the routine use of thienopyridine pretreatment or glycoprotein IIb/IIIA inhibitor use during mesenteric artery interventions. When deploying 5 to 7 mm balloon expandable stents, 6-French (Fr) coronary or renal guide catheters are utilized. Without clinical trial evidence, we would discourage the use of coronary artery drug-eluting stents for these mesenteric artery lesions. From the arm, a multipurpose-shaped catheter is favored. From the common femoral artery, a Hockey stick shape or renal double curve guiding catheter is our preference.

Summary of Outcomes
In our Ochsner Clinic series of 79 vessels in 59 patients, the angiographic success rate was 97% (77/79 vessels) and the procedural success rate was 96% (76/79 vessels) (18). Table 3 summarizes the acute angiographic results and late clinical outcomes. The five-year freedom from death was 72% and from symptom recurrence was 79%. The angiographic restenosis rate with stents was 29%. However, only 17% of patients required target vessel revascularization due to the development of recurrent symptoms. No cases of acute mesenteric ischemia or abdominal catastrophes were reported due to in-stent restenosis. Furthermore no cases of stent thrombosis were reported. In comparison, the reported recurrence rate from surgical revascularization ranges up to 26.5% (5).

Table 3 Acute Angiographic Results and Five-Year Clinical Outcomes from a Series of 59 Patients with CMI Treated with Endovascular Techniques Including Stent Placement

Angiographic findings:	
Reference vessel diameter, baseline (mm)	6.20 ± 1.1
Minimal luminal diameter, baseline (mm)	1.26 ± 0.4
Percent diameter stenosis, baseline (%)	80 ± 6
Reference vessel diameter, postintervention (mm)	6.21 ± 1.1
Minimal luminal diameter, postintervention (mm)	5.82 ± 1.0
Percent diameter stenosis, postintervention (%)	7 ± 15
5-year clinical outcomes:	
Freedom from death (%)	72
Freedom from symptom recurrence (%)	79
Freedom from death or symptom recurrence (%)	57

Source: From Ref. 18.

Equipment Checklist

Table 4 Equipment Checklist

Upper extremity access	
Guide catheter 6–8-Fr	Multipurpose/Hockey stick
Guidewire 0.014-in	Choice of moderate to extra-support
Stents	5–7 mm balloon expandable (off-label biliary) stents
Inflation device	
Rotating hemostatic valve	
Femoral access	
Guide catheter 6–8-Fr	Hockey stick/internal mammary
Guidewire 0.014-in	Extra-support 0.014-in guidewire
Stents	5–7 mm balloon expandable (off-label biliary) stents
Inflation device	
Rotating hemostatic valve	

PART 2: CASE PRESENTATIONS

Mesenteric Case #1

The patient is a 32-year-old female with a one-month history of postprandial abdominal pain. The abdominal pain is associated with abdominal bloating. Abdominal ultrasound showed a mildly enlarged liver and the abdominal DUS showed elevated velocities in the celiac trunk suggestive of a $\geq$70% stenosis. The patient underwent an abdominal aortogram with runoff that showed a 90% stenosis involving the celiac trunk. The patient was therefore referred for percutaneous intervention to the celiac stenosis.

On physical examination, blood pressure was 99/64 mm Hg and the heart rate was 72 bpm. The patient was in no acute distress. There was no jugular venous distention (JVD) or carotid bruit. The lungs were clear to auscultation bilaterally. Examination of the heart revealed a regular rate and rhythm with no murmurs. The abdomen was soft, mildly distended, and nontender. Bowel sounds were present. There was no hepatosplenomegaly. The extremities exam revealed no cyanosis, clubbing or edema. Peripheral pulses were as follows: femoral 2+ bilaterally, dorsalis pedis and posterior tibial 2+ bilaterally, brachial 2+ bilaterally, and radial pulses 2+ with her Allen's test was normal bilaterally. Laboratory results were normal.

What Made the Case "Complex"?

Diagnosing CMI in this 32-year-old woman was challenging in that CMI is not typically high on the list of differential diagnoses for vague abdominal symptoms among patients in this age group. Figures 1 and 2 show a 4-Fr multipurpose catheter selectively engaged at the origin of the celiac artery placed via the brachial artery. Note the steep downward angulation of the celiac

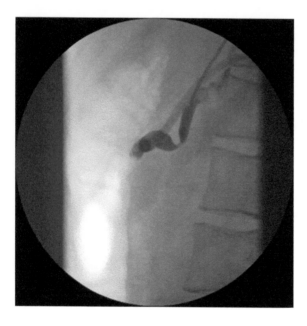

Figure 1 Selective (LAT) celiac trunk angio-gram showing a tight stenosis in the proximal portion of the vessel prior to the bifurcation of the splenic and hepatic arteries.

artery. This case could be performed via femoral access, but it would be much more difficult given the angle at which the celiac artery leaves the aorta. Choosing the upper extremity for arterial access, either the radial or brachial artery, is a key decision point in this case. If the procedure is performed via the radial artery, a 125-cm long guide catheter may be necessary depending on the height of the patient.

What Was the Clinical Indication for the Treatment of This Patient?

The clinical indication for the treatment of this patient was a history of postprandial pain and the finding of severe celiac trunk disease on noninvasive ultrasound imaging confirmed with invasive angiography. Interestingly, the SMA and inferior mesenteric arteries were patent. The patient was evaluated by both a gastroenterologist and a vascular surgeon who concurred in the diagnosis and agreed that endovascular therapy was the treatment modality of choice for this patient.

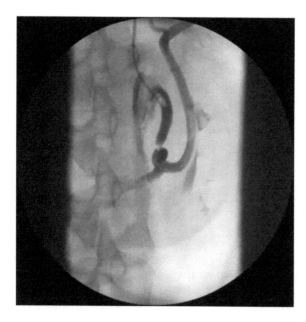

Figure 2 Selective (RAO cranial) celiac trunk angiogram with a 4-Fr multipurpose catheter showing an 80% stenosis in the celiac trunk, just proximal to the bifurcation of the hepatic and splenic arteries.

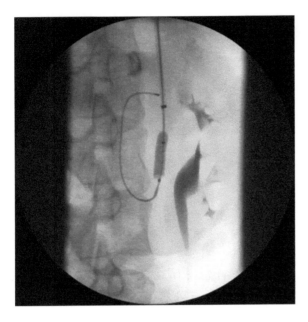

Figure 3 Placement of 6-Fr shuttle sheath (Cook, Bloomington, IN) over an 0.035-in. Wholey guidewire (Guidant, Santa Clara, CA), with predilation of the celiac artery stenosis with a 6-mm balloon at 6 atm.

What Were the Potential Hazards of Treating This Patient and Anatomy?

The primary potential hazards of treating this patient are vascular complications. First, the brachial artery access site must be appropriately managed. Once the procedure is complete, the sheath should be removed. Manual pressure should be held over the brachial artery. However, as the brachial artery is an end artery the pressure should not be occlusive. Second, performing PTA and stent placement at the aorto-ostial junction of the celiac trunk has the potential complication of vessel dissection at the celiac trunk and its branches as well as of the aorta itself. Atheroembilization is another potential complication and concern when treating bulky aorto-ostial plaques.

What Interventional Strategies Were Considered?

The interventional strategy considered was to first predilate the lesion using a 6-mm PTA balloon and then place a balloon expandable stent across the lesion. Prior to crossing the lesion with a guidewire, an intravenous heparin bolus was administered to maintain an activated clotting time (ACT) between 250 and 300 seconds.

Which Interventional Tools Were Used to Manage This Case?

Figure 3 shows a 6-Fr 90-cm long Shuttle sheath (Cook Incorporated, Bloomington, IN) exchanged over the diagnostic catheter, with a 0.035-in Wholey guidewire (Mallinckrodt Inc., Hazelwood, MO) across the lesion. Predilation of the lesion was performed with a 6 × 20 mm Opta 5 PTA balloon (Cordis, Warren, NJ). Figure 4 shows positioning of the 6 × 28 mm Omni-link balloon expandable stent (Guidant, Santa Clara, CA) across the celiac stenosis. Figure 5 shows the final result with the stent deployed and relief of the stenosis.

Summary

Procedural, angiographic, and clinical success were achieved in this case. The brachial sheath was removed after the case and manual pressure was held until hemostasis was achieved. An alternative to using heparin in this patient might have been to use bilvalirudin. However, bilvalirudin has not been studied during mesenteric intervention. The theoretical advantage of using bilvalirudin is that the ACT would not need to be monitored and the bilvalirudin infusion would not need to be adjusted during the procedure. Additionally, the sheath could be removed one hour after discontinuing the infusion.

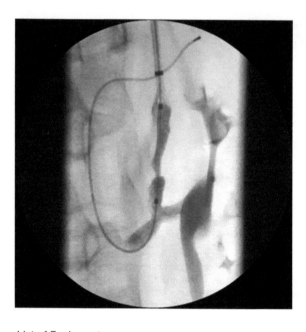

Figure 4   Placement of a 6 × 28 mm Omnilink (Guidant, Santa Clara, CA) stent at the lesion site in the celiac artery.

List of Equipment
6-French brachial artery sheath
6-French multipurpose diagnostic catheter
6-French 90-cm long Shuttle sheath (Cook Incorporated, Bloomington, IN)
0.035-in Wholey guidewire (Mallinckrodt Inc., Hazelwood, MO)
6 × 20 mm Opta 5 PTA balloon (Cordis, Warren, NJ)
6× 28 mm Omni-link balloon expandable stent (Guidant, Santa Clara, CA)

Key Learning Issues
The key learning issue in this case is recognition of the acute downward angle at which the celiac trunk originates from the aorta. Approaching the celiac trunk from above (i.e., arm access) facilitates engaging the vessel and delivering a stent. The vessel could have been treated via the femoral artery. However, the steep angle would have made crossing the lesion with a balloon or

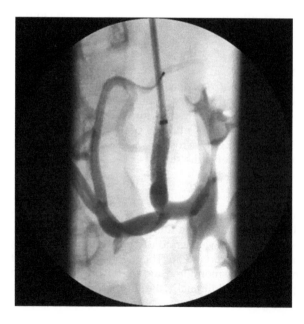

Figure 5   Final angiogram following stent placement to the celiac artery.

stent difficult and increased the risk of stent dislocation or embolization. When approaching a mesenteric vessel with downward angulation from the arm, the multipurpose-shaped catheter often provides an ideal curve.

Mesenteric Case #2
The patient is a 49-year-old female with history of chronic abdominal pain during the last three years. The abdominal pain was not temporally related to food intake, but was associated with nausea and vomiting. The patient lost 40 pounds over one year. Color flow Doppler studies were suggestive of celiac, superior mesenteric, and inferior mesenteric artery stenosis. The patient was referred for mesenteric angiography to establish the presence and severity of splanchnic vascular disease.

On examination, the patient's blood pressure was 100/70 mm Hg and her heart rate was 64 bpm. There was no JVD or carotid bruit. Her lungs were clear. Auscultation of the heart revealed normal S1 and S2 with no murmurs, gallop, rub, or heave. The patient had normal bowel sounds. Her abdomen was soft and nontender. Examination of her extremities demonstrated no clubbing or cyanosis. Peripheral pulses were as follows: femoral pulses 2+ bilaterally, dorsalis pedis and posterior tibial pulses 2+ bilaterally, brachial pulses 2+ bilaterally, and radial pulses 2+ bilaterally. Her Allen's test was normal bilaterally. The patient's medications included valsartan and lansoprazole.

What Made the Case "Complex"?
The diagnostic angiogram was performed from the right brachial artery with a 6-Fr multipurpose catheter. A critical narrowing [Fig. 6(A)] of the superior mesenteric artery was found. The celiac artery was also occluded. An exchange length 0.014-in extrasupport coronary guidewire (Spartacore, Guidant/Boston Scientific, Santa Clara, CA) was advanced into the SMA across the lesion. The 6-Fr multipurpose catheter was exchanged for a 6-Fr multipurpose coronary guide catheter, which engaged the ostium of the SMA. This case was made "complex" by the location of the lesion. In order to gain adequate guide catheter support to cross the lesion, a multipurpose catheter was utilized and the lesion was approached in antegrade manner via the arm.

What Was the Clinical Indication for the Treatment of This Patient?
The clinical indication for the treatment of this patient was a history of abdominal symptoms and weight loss in the context of an occluded celiac artery and a critically narrowed SMA without another explanation for her symptoms.

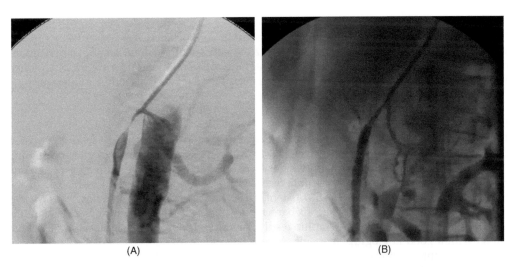

(A)   (B)

Figure 6 (**A**) Angiogram of superior mesenteric artery ostial stenosis with 6-Fr multipurpose angiographic catheter from the brachial access. (**B**) Angiogram after balloon expandable stent deployment.

What Were the Potential Hazards of Treating This Patient and Anatomy?
As this patient's celiac artery is occluded, perfusion of her small bowel is dependent on her SMA. A procedural complication such as SMA dissection resulting in cessation of SMA arterial flow could theoretically result in life-threatening bowel necrosis.

What Interventional Strategies Were Considered?
The keys to this case were engaging the SMA from above and crossing the lesion with adequate guide catheter support. The plan was to predilate the lesion with PTA, and then deploy a balloon expandable stent.

Which Interventional Tools Were Used to Manage This Case?
As stated above, after diagnostic angiography of the SMA, 2500 IU of heparin was administered intravenously and a 0.014-in extra-support coronary guidewire was advanced into the SMA and across the lesion. Then the 6-Fr multipurpose catheter was exchanged for a 6-Fr multipurpose coronary guide catheter. The ostium of the SMA was engaged with this catheter while using the coronary guidewire as a rail. The lesion was then predilated using a 3.0 × 20 mm Quantum Maverick balloon (Boston Scientific, Natick, MA). A 4.0 × 25 mm NIR balloon expandable stent (Boston Scientific, Natick, MA) was then placed into the lesion. The stent was deployed with the balloon inflated to 12 atm. A 5.0 × 20 Cross Sail balloon (Guidant, San Jose, Ca) was utilized to postdilate the stent. The final angiographic result is illustrated in Figure 6(B). The patient tolerated the procedure well.

Summary
Procedural, angiographic, and clinical success were achieved in this case. An alternative to using a multipurpose guide catheter in this case may have been to utilize a right coronary bypass graft guide catheter from the brachial artery. Both catheters provide support when working in vessels with inferior angulation.

List of Equipment
6-French brachial artery sheath
6-French multipurpose diagnostic catheter
6-French multipurpose guide catheter
0.014-in extra-support coronary guidewire (Spartacore, Guidant, Santa Clara, CA)
3.0 × 20 mm Quantum Maverick balloon (Boston Scientific, Natick, MA)
4.0 × 25 mm NIR balloon expandable stent (Boston Scientific, Natick, MA)
5.0 × 20 Cross Sail balloon (Guidant, San Jose, CA)

Key Learning Issues
The key learning issues in this case are to recognize the importance of guide catheter support from the arm to cross a critical stenosis as well as to successfully deliver angioplasty balloons and stents. Another key issue is an appreciation of the collateral blood flow via the SMA when the celiac artery is occluded and the potential for massive bowel necrosis if this collateral supply is jeopardized during revascularization.

Mesenteric Case #3
The patient is a 62-year-old female with a history of mesenteric artery disease who was treated with PTA and stent placement in the celiac artery and SMA eight years ago after presenting with symptoms of postprandial pain, weight loss, and food avoidance. Three years ago she experienced recurrence of these symptoms and was found to have in-stent restenosis of the celiac stent and stenosis distal to the SMA stent. The celiac artery in-stent restenosis was treated with sequential 4.0 × 23 and 4.0 × 13 bare metal stents (Duet, Guidant/Boston Scientific, San Jose, CA) with a good angiographic result. The SMA lesion was dilated with a 5.0 × 20 balloon with a good angiographic result. A year later she experienced another recurrence of abdominal symptoms. She underwent angiography and was found to have in-stent restenosis of the celiac artery stents with extension of the lesion into the ostia of both the hepatic and splenic arteries [Fig. 7(A)]. The patient underwent PTA of these lesions with a good angiographic

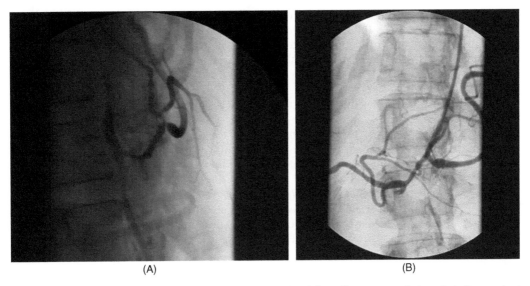

(A)   (B)

Figure 7 Before (**A**) and after (**B**) PTA for in-stent restenosis of the celiac artery and stenosis in the proximal hepatic and splenic arteries.

result [Fig. 7(B)]. One year later she again experienced recurrence of her abdominal symptoms. Angiography was performed. The patient was found to have recurrence of celiac artery in-stent restenosis and stenosis of the ostia of the hepatic and splenic arteries [Fig. 8(A)]. The SMA stent was widely patent. The patient underwent PTA of celiac, hepatic, and splenic arteries once again [Fig. 8(B)]. Fifteen months later, the patient presented with yet another recurrence of her abdominal symptoms. Ultrasound imaging demonstrated restenosis of the celiac artery stents. Repeat angiography was scheduled.

On examination, the patient's blood pressure was 140/70 mm Hg and her heart rate is 72 bpm. There was no JVD. She had a left carotid bruit and a left carotid endarterectomy (CEA) scar. Her lungs were clear. Auscultation of the heart revealed a normal S1 and S2, and an S4 gallop with no rub or heave. The patient had normal bowel sounds. Her abdomen was

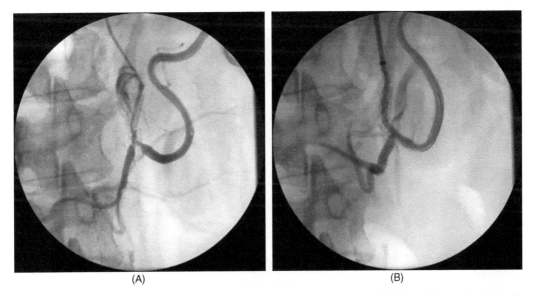

(A)   (B)

Figure 8 (**A**) Instent restenosis of the celiac artery and stenoses at the previous PTA sites in the proximal hepatic and splenic arteries. (**B**) Angiogram after PTA of the celiac, hepatic, and splenic arteries.

soft and nontender. Examination of her extremities demonstrated no clubbing nor cyanosis. Peripheral pulses were as follows: femoral pulses 1+ bilaterally, dorsalis pedis and posterior tibial pulses present only by Doppler bilaterally, brachial pulses 2+ bilaterally, and radial pulses 2+ bilaterally. Her Allen's test was normal bilaterally.

What Made the Case "Complex"?
This case was made complex by the recurrent in-stent restenosis that the patient experienced.

What Was the Clinical Indication for the Treatment of This Patient?
The clinical indication for the treatment of this patient was a history of abdominal symptoms and weight loss in the context of recurrent stenosis of the celiac, hepatic, and splenic arteries.

What Were the Potential Hazards of Treating This Patient and Anatomy?
The potential hazards associated with treating this patient and anatomy included the risk of restenosis and the risk of dissection or perforation. Additionally, there is the risk of repeated procedural radiation exposure to the patient if endovascular treatment is performed.

What Interventional Strategies Were Considered?
Surgical revascularization was considered. The patient opted for repeat endovascular treatment. Procedures that were considered included repeat PTA, brachytherapy, and drug-eluting stent (DES) placement. Repeat PTA would likely result in recurrent restenosis given the patient's history. Brachytherapy and DES placement are effective treatments for in-stent restenosis of coronary arteries (25,26). Due to the availability of DES, this option was chosen.

Which Interventional Tools Were Used to Manage This Case?
Given the patient's history of lower extremity peripheral arterial disease as well as the angle from which the celiac artery left the aorta, the right brachial artery was chosen as the point of vascular access. A 6-Fr sheath was placed in the right brachial artery. Three thousand international units of heparin were administered intravenously. A 6-Fr, 125 cm in length, multipurpose-shaped catheter was utilized to engage the celiac artery. The celiac artery was found to have critical in-stent restenosis. The hepatic and splenic arteries contained severe restenoses (Fig. 9). The celiac restenotic lesion was crossed with a 0.014-in Balance Middle Weight Universal coronary guidewire (Abbott Vascular, Abbott Park, IL). The celiac artery lesion was dilated with a 3.0 × 20 mm Quantum Maverick (Boston Scientific, San Jose, CA) coronary angioplasty balloon.

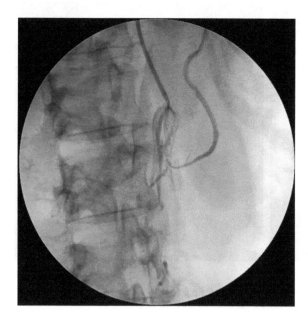

Figure 9 Angiogram demonstrating severe in-stent restenosis of the celiac artery and restenosis of the hepatic and splenic artery ostia.

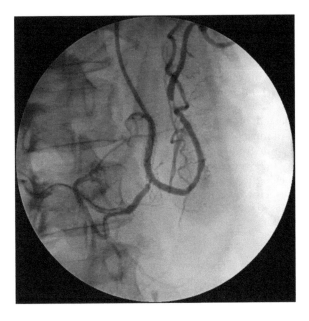

Figure 10 Final angiogram after PTA of the celiac artery followed by placement of a 3.0 × 28 Cypher DES (Cordis, Warren, NJ) in the splenic artery and a 3.5 × 23 Cypher (Cordis, Warren, NJ) in the celiac artery.

The splenic artery was stented with a 3.0 × 28 mm Cypher DES (Cordis, Warren, NJ). A second 3.5 × 23 mm Cypher DES was overlapped with the splenic artery stent and deployed extending into the celiac artery. The hepatic artery stenosis was dilated with a 3.0 × 20 mm coronary angioplasty balloon. The final angiographic result is shown in Figure 10.

Summary
Procedural and angiographic success were achieved in this case. Unfortunately within two years the patient developed recurrence of her symptoms and was found to have restenosis of the celiac artery with hepatic and splenic artery involvement. She then underwent surgical revascularization. She remained free of abdominal symptoms three years post surgery.

List of Equipment
6-French brachial artery sheath
6-French multipurpose guide catheter
0.014-in Balance Middle Weight Universal coronary guidewire (Abbott Vascular, Abbott Park, IL)
3.0 × 20 mm Quantum Maverick balloon (Boston Scientific, San Jose, CA)
3.0 × 28 and 3.5 × 23 mm Cypher stents (Cordis, Warren, NJ)

Key Learning Issues
The key learning issues in this case are to understand the high rate of restenosis after PTA or stent placement in mesenteric arteries. Potential options for the treatment of in-stent restenosis in this vascular bed include PTA, brachytherapy, and DES placement. However, no randomized clinical trials addressing in-stent restenosis in the mesenteric arteries have been published. This is in part due to the low incidence of CMI relative to coronary artery disease.

PART 3: KEY ISSUES FOR SUCCESSFUL AND SAFE TREATMENT OF COMPLEX MESENTERIC LESIONS
The key points in the management of patients with CMI are (*i*) to be as certain as possible that symptoms truly represent visceral ischemia, as the prevalence of mesenteric artery stenosis is much more common than the clinical syndrome of CMI and (*ii*) once a decision has been made to proceed with endovascular treatment, selecting the appropriate vascular access and guide catheter is necessary.

Mesenteric vascular disease is common in patients with atherosclerosis, but clinical ischemia is unusual given the redundancy of the mesenteric circulation. Patients with functional bowel complaints will not have lost weight and will not improve with mesenteric stenting. Before planning an intervention, it is important to elicit a history of significant weight loss, a history of postprandial discomfort, and anatomic evidence of occlusion or stenosis of at least two of the three mesenteric vessels. Patients who do not meet these criteria can prove to be a diagnostic challenge.

Once the patient has been carefully selected, then the next issue is to decide upon the best vascular access. The acute downward angle of most of these vessels as they arise from the aorta is often most suitable to an upper extremity, antegrade approach. Many of these lesions can be approached from the common femoral artery in retrograde fashion, but it is often a struggle and the risk of stent embolization or dislocation is high. At this time, there is no clinical trial data to support a role for DES's in mesenteric arteries. However, the restenosis rate of bare metal stents in these arteries appears to be higher than that reported in renal arteries.

REFERENCES

1. Moawad J, Gewertz BL. Chronic mesenteric ischemia. Clinical presentation and diagnosis. Surg Clin North Am 1997; 77:357–369.
2. Oldenburg WA, Lau LL, Rodenberg TJ, et al. Acute mesenteric ischemia: a clinical review. Arch Intern Med 2004; 164:1054–1062.
3. Hansen KJ, Wilson DB, Craven TE, et al. Mesenteric artery disease in the elderly. J Vasc Surg 2004; 40:45–52.
4. Thomas JH, Blake K, Pierce GE, et al. The clinical course of asymptomatic mesenteric arterial stenosis. J Vasc Surg 1998; 27:840–844.
5. Brandt LJ, Boley SJ. AGA technical review on intestinal ischemia. American Gastrointestinal Association. Gastroenterology 2000; 118:954–68.
6. Matsumoto AH, Tegtmeyer CJ, Fitzcharles EK, et al. Percutaneous transluminal angioplasty of visceral arterial stenoses: results and long-term clinical follow-up. J Vasc Interv Radiol 1995; 6:165–674.
7. Calderon M, Reul GJ, Gregoric ID, et al. Long-term results of the surgical management of symptomatic chronic intestinal ischemia. J Cardiovasc Surg (Torino) 1992; 33:723–728.
8. Christensen MG, Lorentzen JE, Schroeder TV. Revascularisation of atherosclerotic mesenteric arteries: experience in 90 consecutive patients. Eur J Vasc Surg 1994; 8:297–302.
9. Cormier JM, Fichelle JM, Vennin J, et al. Atherosclerotic occlusive disease of the superior mesenteric artery: late results of reconstructive surgery. Ann Vasc Surg 1991; 5:510–518.
10. Cunningham CG, Reilly LM, Rapp JH, et al. Chronic visceral ischemia. Three decades of progress. Ann Surg 1991; 214:276–287.
11. Gentile AT, Moneta GL, Taylor LM Jr, et al. Isolated bypass to the superior mesenteric artery for intestinal ischemia. Arch Surg 1994; 129:926–931.
12. Johnston KW, Lindsay TF, Walker PM, et al. Mesenteric arterial bypass grafts: early and late results and suggested surgical approach for chronic and acute mesenteric ischemia. Surgery 1995; 118:1–1187.
13. Kieny R, Batellier J, Kretz JG. Aortic reimplantation of the superior mesenteric artery for atherosclerotic lesions of the visceral arteries: sixty cases. Ann Vasc Surg 1990; 4:122–125.
14. Mateo RB, O'Hara PJ, Hertzer NR, et al. Elective surgical treatment of symptomatic chronic mesenteric occlusive disease: early results and late outcomes. J Vasc Surg 1999; 29:821–831.
15. McAfee MK, Cherry KJ, Jr, Naessens JM, et al. Influence of complete revascularization on chronic mesenteric ischemia. Am J Surg 1992; 164:220–224.
16. Sivamurthy N, Rhodes JM, Lee D, et al. Endovascular versus open mesenteric revascularization: immediate benefits do not equate with short-term functional outcomes. J Am Coll Surg 2006; 202:859–867.
17. Park WM, Cherry KJ Jr, Chua HK, et al. Current results of open revascularization for chronic mesenteric ischemia: a standard for comparison. J Vasc Surg 2002; 35:853–859.
18. Silva JA, White CJ, Collins TJ, et al. Endovascular therapy for chronic mesenteric ischemia. J Am Coll Cardiol 2006; 47:944–950.
19. Sharafuddin MJ, Olson CH, Sun S, et al. Endovascular treatment of celiac and mesenteric arteries stenoses: applications and results. J Vasc Surg 2003; 38:692–698.
20. Landis MS, Rajan DK, Simons ME, et al. Percutaneous management of chronic mesenteric ischemia: outcomes after intervention. J Vasc Interv Radiol 2005; 16:1319–1325.
21. Hallisey MJ, Deschaine J, Illescas FF, et al. Angioplasty for the treatment of visceral ischemia. J Vasc Interv Radiol 1995; 6:785–791.

22. Shih MC, Hagspiel KD. CTA and MRA in mesenteric ischemia: part 1, role in diagnosis and differential diagnosis. AJR Am J Roentgenol 2007; 188:452–461.
23. Agostoni P, Biondi-Zoccai GG, de Benedictis ML, et al. Radial versus femoral approach for percutaneous coronary diagnostic and interventional procedures; Systematic overview and meta-analysis of randomized trials. J Am Coll Cardiol 2004; 44:349–356.
24. Alvarez-Tostado JA, Moise MA, Bena JF, et al. The brachial artery: a critical access for endovascular procedures. J Vasc Surg 2009; 49:378–385.
25. Dibra A, Kastrati A, Alfonso F, et al. Effectiveness of drug-eluting stents in patients with bare-metal in-stent restenosis: meta-analysis of randomized trials. J Am Coll Cardiol 2007; 49:616–623.
26. Grise MA, Massullo V, Jani S, et al. Five-year clinical follow-up after intracoronary radiation: results of a randomized clinical trial. Circulation 2002; 105:2737–2740.

13 | Leriche's Disease

Hans Krankenberg, Thilo Tübler, and Michael Schlüter

Medical Care Center Prof. Mathey, Prof. Schofer, Hamburg, Germany

INTRODUCTION

The total occlusion of the infrarenal aorta by atherosclerosis or a thrombus was first described in 1814 by the physician Sir Gilbert Blane from Glasgow and almost 100 years later defined by the French surgeon René Leriche (1,2). The condition is generally diagnosed between 40 and 60 years of age; its incidence is low (3). It is located at the aortic bifurcation obliterating both common iliac arteries (4). The main symptoms are fatigue in the lower limbs, cramps in the calf area, ischemic pain of intermittent bilateral claudication, absent or diminished femoral pulse, pallor and coldness of the feet and legs, and erectile dysfunction. Symptoms related to ischemia of the lower limbs may ultimately lead to severe impairment of walking capability, resting pains, and wheelchair dependence.

To date, the predominant treatment of patients with the Leriche syndrome has been surgery with anatomical or extra-anatomical (mainly bilateral subclavian-femoral prosthetic) bypass grafting (3,5–7). The main drawback of this approach is a significant perioperative mortality, which ranges between 2.5% and 19% for anatomical bypasses (5,8–10). In patients who require repeat surgery, the mortality risk rises up to 25% (11).

In recent years, endovascular equipment and experience have developed rapidly providing a variety of tools for recanalization and enabling interventions in complex lesions and patient subsets. Iliac and superficial femoral artery occlusions as well as aortic aneurysms are nowadays treated by endovascular means with satisfying results or even—particularly in aortic aneurysms—with equal results compared to surgery (12–15). In contrast to surgery, the perioperative endovascular risk remains low and predictable in these patients with severe peripheral arterial disease (PAD).

An endovascular approach to treatment of the Leriche syndrome has only been described anecdotally (8,16–19). The complexity of the lesion encountered in Leriche's disease results from the fact that it is a chronic diffuse disease in which total vascular occlusion usually encompasses the infrarenal aorta as well as both common iliac arteries, often extending for several centimeters into the external iliac arteries. To complicate matters further, the occluded segments are frequently severely calcified.

The indication for an endovascular attempt at revascularization is the expected relief of symptoms and improvement in walking capacity in severely handicapped patients who had either been denied surgery, experienced surgical failure, or refused to undergo surgery. Thus, endovascular intervention is the only therapeutic option left to these patients.

Potential hazards of catheter-based therapy comprise target vessel rupture and perforation, aortic dissection, and visceral, in particular renal, artery occlusion, and/or dissection.

Preprocedural diagnostics include a standard treadmill test (2 mph, 12% incline), duplex ultrasonography of the abdominal aorta and iliac/infrainguinal arteries; echocardiography to evaluate left ventricular function; an assessment of the ankle brachial pressure index (ABI); and magnetic resonance angiography to estimate the occlusion lengths in the aorta and iliac arteries, as well as assess femoral, popliteal, and infrapopliteal runoff.

The interventional strategy adhered to at our institution consists of antegrade, transbrachial, recanalization of the occluded vessel segments with subsequent retrograde, transfemoral, angioplasty. The infrarenal aorta is stented electively, whereas primary nitinol stenting is the therapeutic end point for the iliac limbs.

All patients are premedicated with acetylsalicylic acid (aspirin, 100 mg/day) and clopidogrel (75 mg b.i.d.) for at least three days or receive a loading dose of 600 mg of clopidogrel immediately before the intervention.

CASE PRESENTATION

We report on a 60-year-old female patient in whom Leriche's disease was diagnosed in 1998. By the time she presented at our institution, she was wheelchair dependent and could walk no more than 5 m. Despite the presence of chronic obstructive pulmonary disease, the patient was actively smoking 20 cigarettes per day; she was hypertensive (mean daytime pressure 140 mm Hg) and hyperlipidemic (low-density lipoprotein 151 mg/dl). Left ventricular ejection fraction was 40%; left and right ABIs were 0.50 and 0.45, respectively.

Following local anesthesia, 90-cm 6-F and 7-F sheaths were placed in the left and right arm, respectively. Heparinization was begun with a bolus of 5000 units administered through the 6-F sheath; a second bolus of 5000 units of heparin was given after two hours. Throughout the procedure, the patient did not require general anesthesia.

Preprocedural magnetic resonance angiography had revealed an onset of the aortic occlusion immediately distal to the left renal artery (Fig. 1). Therefore, 0.014 in. coronary wires (Iron Man™, Abbott Vascular, Abbott Park, IL) were introduced into both renal arteries and the superior mesenteric artery by way of a 5-F angled support catheter advanced through the 7-F sheath in the right arm (Fig. 2). This protective measure would allow accessing the three arteries in case of an unexpected plaque shift or a dissection compromising their blood supply. It is not deemed necessary in patients in whom the distance between the left renal artery and the aortic occlusion is >2 cm.

Access to the target lesions was gained by means of the 6-F sheath placed in the left brachial artery. Through this sheath, diagnostic angiography was performed to verify the extent of the disease from the aorta to the iliac/femoral arteries, which was followed by the advancement of a 125-cm 5-F multipurpose catheter toward the aortic occlusion. Penetration of the occlusion by way of this catheter was attempted with a 260-cm hydrophilic, stiff, angled guidewire. Once the proximal fibrous cap of the occlusion was penetrated, the multipurpose catheter was exchanged for a 135-cm, 0.035-in. support catheter (Quick-Cross®, Spectranetics Corp., Colorado Springs, CO) that was passed through the occlusion either following the Terumo wire or "clearing the way" for it. Controlled wire passage through both the aortic and the iliac artery occlusion (Fig. 3) necessitated switching between angled and straight wires. Upon entering the femoral artery, an intraluminal position of the support catheter and wire was verified by a freely mobile

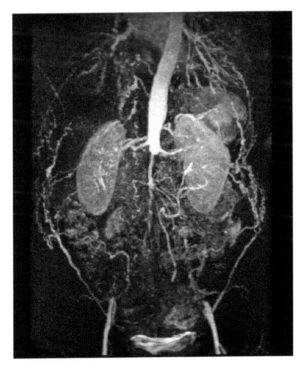

Figure 1 Preprocedural magnetic resonance angiography showing total occlusion of infrarenal aorta and both common iliac arteries.

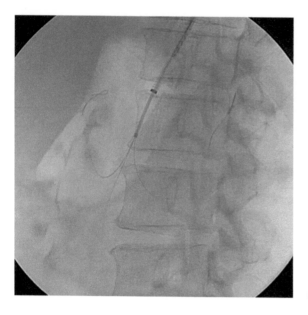

Figure 2 Coronary wires placed in superior mesenteric artery and both renal arteries.

wire tip and ultimately by an injection of contrast media through the support catheter (Fig. 4). The described recanalization technique was then repeated for the other iliac limb (Fig. 5). In cases of antegrade recanalization failure, we generally do not attempt retrograde recanalization because of the risk of an aortic dissection secondary to subintimal wire passage. Recanalization of the aorta was monitored by fluoroscopy in anteroposterior and lateral projections, whereas recanalization of the iliac arteries was preferentially monitored in the 30° contralateral anterior oblique projection.

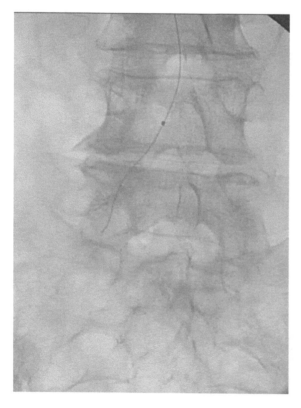

Figure 3 Wire passage of right iliac artery.

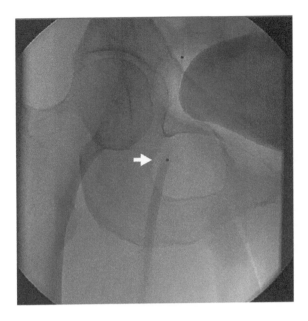

Figure 4 Angiography verifying intraluminal position of distal tip of support catheter (arrow) in right common femoral artery.

When the two wires were successfully passed into the femoral arteries, each artery was punctured under fluoroscopic guidance, targeting the endoluminal wire. By way of 8-F sheaths, the Terumo wires were snared with a 180-cm 0.035 in. looped guidewire (Fig. 6) and pulled out, resulting in single wires reaching from their entry point in the left brachial artery all the way through the aortoiliac occlusion to an exit point in either femoral artery. Both Terumo wires were then exchanged for stiffer wires over which the subsequent angioplasties were performed retrogradely from both groins.

Starting from the aortic occlusion, the entire occluded segment was predilated with a 4.0/80-mm balloon (Figs. 7–9). Balloon inflation pressure was restricted to 6 atm to minimize the risk of vessel rupture. Since the infrarenal aorta was occluded for more than 3 cm and no major thrombus burden present in this patient, the 8-F sheath on the side of the shorter (right) iliac occlusion was replaced with a 12-F sheath of 25 cm length through which a balloon expandable stent (Palmaz-Schatz™, Cordis, Warren, NJ) was placed (Fig. 10). Its correct position

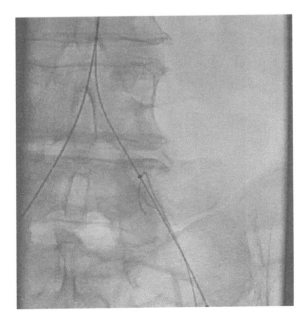

Figure 5 Wire passed through left iliac artery into left common femoral artery.

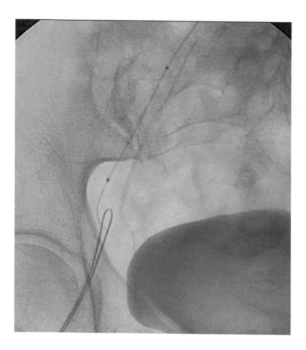

Figure 6 Snaring, with looped wire advanced retrogradely, of recanalization wire passed into right common femoral artery.

with its proximal end extending for about 1 cm beyond the aortic occlusion was verified using the roadmap technique, after which the stent was deployed at 4 to 6 atm and postdilated with two 8-mm balloons in kissing-balloon fashion (Fig. 11). In later cases, we also used the CP Stent™ (NuMED, Inc., Hopkinton, NY), which was postdilated with a 20-mm balloon-in-balloon dilatation catheter (BIB®, NuMED). In patients with an aortic occlusion of less than 2 cm in length, we prefer not to place an aortic stent.

For reconstruction of the iliac limbs, a self-expanding nitinol stent (Luminexx® 3 Vascular Stent, C.R. Bard, Inc., Murray Hill, NJ) was advanced from either groin and deployed such that

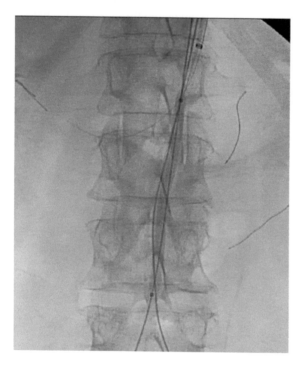

Figure 7 Predilatation of infrarenal aorta.

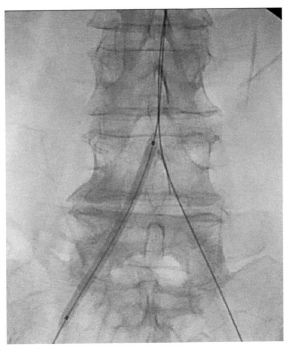

Figure 8 Predilatation of right iliac artery.

it invaded the distal end of the aortic stent by about 3 mm (Fig. 12). The nominal diameter of either iliac stent was chosen to exceed the respective iliac artery reference diameter by 1 mm. Both self-expandable stents were postdilated in kissing-balloon fashion (Fig. 13). Because the iliac occlusions could not be completely covered with 12-cm stents in this patient, one additional self-expandable nitinol stent was implanted into each iliac artery. Unimpeded blood flow through the entire reconstructed aortoiliac tract was documented by angiography (Fig. 14). In patients in whom no aortic stent is placed, the iliac artery stents are deployed such that their proximal ends extend for about 1 cm beyond the occlusion into the aorta.

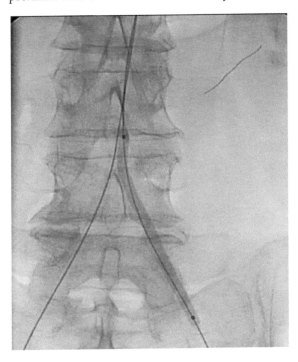

Figure 9 Predilatation of left iliac artery.

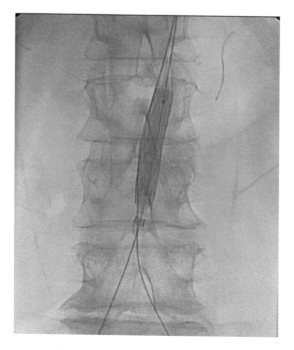

Figure 10   Placement of aortic stent.

Both groins were closed using a percutaneous suture device (Prostar XL, Abbott Vascular) to avoid vessel compression and ensure unimpeded distal runoff. Postprocedural computed tomography of the abdominal and pelvic region was performed to exclude retroperitoneal bleeding.

The patient was discharged on an oral regimen of aspirin (100 mg/day indefinitely) and clopidogrel (75 mg/day for three months). Computed tomography angiography at 12 months showed persistence of acute procedural success (Fig. 15).

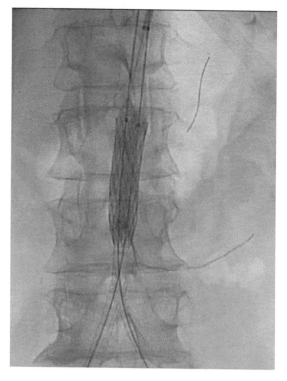

Figure 11   Kissing-balloon postdilatation of aortic stent.

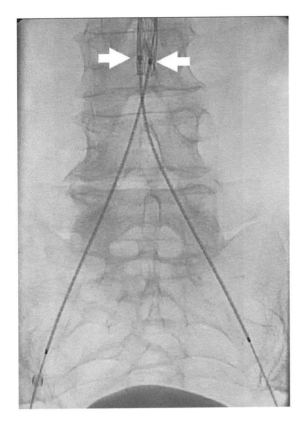

Figure 12 Placement of nitinol stents in common iliac arteries. Note proximal ends of stents extending into aortic stent (arrows).

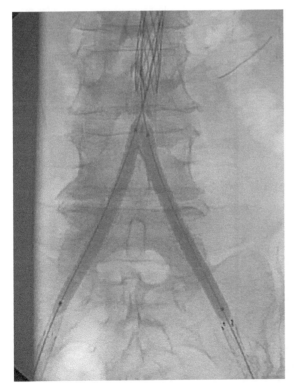

Figure 13 Simultaneous (kissing-balloon) postdilatation of iliac artery stents.

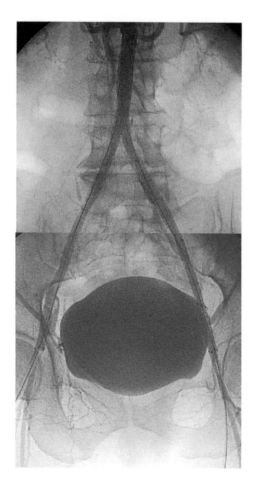

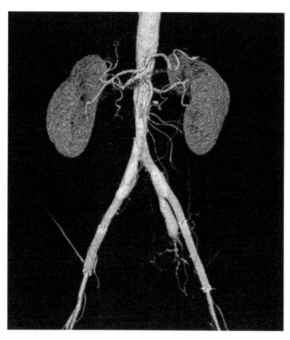

Figure 14 Composite figure of final result after placement of two stents in each iliac artery. There is unimpeded blood flow through aortic bifurcation into iliac arteries.

Figure 15 Computed tomography angiography at 12 months.

MATERIALS

	n
Sheaths	
6-F/90 cm	1
7-F/90 cm	1
8-F/25 cm	2
12-F/25 cm	1
Wires	
Iron Man^{TM}/0.014 in./300 cm	3
Terumo hydrophilic stiff angled/260 cm	1
Terumo hydrophilic stiff straight/260 cm	1
Supra Core® 35/0.035 in./260 cm	2
Catheters	
MPA2 4-F/125 cm	1
MPA 5-F/125 cm	1
IMA 5-F/100 cm	1
JR4 5-F/100 cm	1
Quick-Cross® 130 cm	1
Balloons	
4/80 mm OTW	2
6–8/80–120 mm OTW	2
8/40 mm OTW	2
20 mm BIB® OTW	1
Stents	
Palmaz-Schatz^{TM} 40/50 mm	1
CP Stent^{TM}	1
Luminexx® 3 Vascular Stent 7–9/60–120 mm	6
Vascular Closure Systems	
Prostar XL 10-F	1

RESULTS IN 11 PATIENTS

We defined "procedural success" as restored vessel patency with a residual diameter stenosis <30% and a translesion pressure gradient <20 mm Hg. In case of a residual stenosis ≥30%, postdilatation was performed using an appropriately sized balloon. Another postdilatation of the stented segments was performed if the pressure gradient exceeded 20 mm Hg.

Between 2003 and 2008, we treated 11 consecutive patients [8 men (73%), 64 ± 12 years] according to the strategy presented above. Leriche's disease had been present for a median of 3 years in these patients, ranging up to 13 years. Six patients had been denied surgery and two patients had previously undergone extra-anatomic bypass surgery with subsequent reocclusion of the grafts. The latter two patients as well as the remaining three patients all refused a surgical intervention. Bilateral endovascular success was achieved in eight patients (73%), unilateral success in the other three patients. Seven patients received aortic stents; the total stented segment length in 19 iliac arteries successfully recanalized was a median of 18 cm (range, 12–26 cm). Attesting to the safety of our treatment strategy, we encountered only one periprocedural complication, an acute thrombotic aortoiliac occlusion managed by thrombolysis. One patient with unilateral endovascular success had to undergo subsequent femorofemoral crossover bypass grafting. At a median of 14 months, significant hemodynamic improvement was observed in successfully revascularized legs (ABI, 0.79 ± 0.20 vs. 0.48 ± 0.08 at baseline; $P = 0.0004$). Walking capacity and Rutherford category of PAD had improved in all patients.

SUMMARY

The endovascular strategy for the treatment of the extended aortoiliac occlusions present in Leriche's disease appears to be safe and efficacious. It is essentially a two-step procedure.

→   In the first step, antegrade, transbrachial, wire recanalization of all occluded vascular segments usually encompassing the infrarenal aorta and both common/external iliac arteries is attempted.

○ As a protective measure, placement of coronary wires in the superior mesenteric artery and both renal arteries must precede recanalization in patients in whom inflow into these arteries may be compromised as a consequence of plaque shift or dissection.

→ Following successful antegrade recanalization, the second procedural step consists of retrograde, transfemoral, angioplasty of the previously occluded segments.

○ Predilatation of the aorta must be performed at a low pressure (≤6 atm) to avoid vessel rupture. An aortic stent is placed electively in patients with an aortic occlusion exceeding 3 cm in length and no major thrombus burden.

○ The iliac arteries are also predilated at low pressure. Nitinol stents are implanted such that their proximal ends extend into the distal aorta and that they cover the entire occluded iliac artery segments.

→ A percutaneous closure device should be used in both groins to avoid vessel compression and ensure unimpeded distal runoff. Postprocedural computed tomography of the abdominal and pelvic region should be used to exclude retroperitoneal bleeding.

REFERENCES

1. Graham R. Case of Obstructed Aorta. Communicated by Sir G. Blane. [Sir Gilbert Blane, 1747–1834]. London: Medico-Chirurgical Transactions, 1814.
2. Leriche R. Des obliterations artérielles hautes (oblitération de la terminaison de l'aorte) comme causes des insuffisances circulatoires des membres inférieurs. Bull Mem Soc Chir Paris 1923; 49:1404–1406.
3. Erskine JM, Gerbode FL, French SW III, et al. Surgical treatment of thrombotic occlusion of aorta and iliac arteries; the Leriche syndrome. AMA Arch Surg 1959; 79:85–93.
4. Leriche R. De la résection du carrefour aortico-iliaque avec double sympathectomie lombaire pour thrombose artéritique la l'aorte: le syndrome de l'oblitération termino-aortique par artérite. Presse Med 1940; 48:601–607.
5. Cooley DA, Creech O Jr, De Bakey ME. The Leriche syndrome and its surgical treatment by resection and homograft replacement. Lyon Chir 1956; 52:402–411.
6. Burgess CM. Treatment of the Leriche syndrome: a technique of endarterectomy. Arch Surg 1959; 79:487–492.
7. Sugimoto T, Ogawa K, Asada T, et al. Leriche syndrome. Surgical procedures and early and late results. Angiology 1997; 48:637–642.
8. Garcia FC, Gard PD Jr. Leriche syndrome: review of the literature and a case report. J La State Med Soc 1979; 131:263–265.
9. Stubbs DH, Kasulke RJ, Kapsch DN, et al. Populations with the Leriche syndrome. Surgery 1981; 89:612–616.
10. Genoni M, von Segesser LK, Laske A, et al. Occlusion of the distal aorta. Helv Chir Acta 1994; 60:723–728.
11. Mavioglu I, Veli Dogan O, Ozeren M, et al. Surgical management of chronic total occlusion of abdominal aorta. J Cardiovasc Surg (Torino) 2003; 44:87–93.
12. Scheinert D, Schröder M, Balzer JO, et al. Stent-supported reconstruction of the aortoiliac bifurcation with the kissing balloon technique. Circulation 1999; 100(suppl 19):II295–II300.
13. Schillinger M, Sabeti S, Loewe C, et al. Balloon angioplasty versus implantation of nitinol stents in the superficial femoral artery. N Engl J Med 2006; 354:1879–1888.
14. Krankenberg H, Schlüter M, Steinkamp HJ, et al. Nitinol stent implantation versus percutaneous transluminal angioplasty in superficial femoral artery lesions up to 10 cm in length: the femoral artery stenting trial (FAST). Circulation 2007; 116:285–292.
15. EVAR Trial Participants. Endovascular aneurysm repair versus open repair in patients with abdominal aortic aneurysm (EVAR trial 1): randomised controlled trial. Lancet 2005; 365:2179–2186.
16. Marty AT, Penkava R, Whitehead D, et al. Kissing balloon therapy for Leriche syndrome. Indiana Med 1985; 78:288–289.
17. Bean WJ, Rodan BA, Thebaut AL. Leriche syndrome: treatment with streptokinase and angioplasty. AJR Am J Roentgenol 1985; 144:1285–1286.
18. Katzenschlager R, Ahmadi A, Koppensteiner R, et al. Leriche syndrome: treatment with local lysis and subsequent percutaneous transluminal angioplasty. Vasa 1996; 25:180–183.
19. Schröder M, Friedrich K, Zipfel B, et al. Acute painless paraplegia of the legs as a manifestation of extensive acute Leriche syndrome. Clin Res Cardiol 2007; 96:240–242.

14 | Iliac Arteries

Patrick Peeters and Jürgen Verbist
Department of Cardiovascular and Thoracic Surgery, Imelda Hospital, Bonheiden, Belgium

Koen Deloose and Marc Bosiers
Department of Vascular Surgery, A.Z. Sint-Blasius, Dendermonde, Belgium

INTRODUCTION

What Makes a Lesion "Complex" in Iliac Interventions?

Although over 90% of iliac lesions can be passed with simple guidewire techniques, each endovascular attempt to treat an iliac occlusion might be compromised by failure of guidewire passage. In order to achieve optimal success when treating complex iliac lesions, the operator should know when and how ipsilateral, contralateral, and brachial access techniques should be applied. Later in section "Interventional Strategies," we will discuss the different interventional strategies that can help to treat a complex iliac case successfully.

Clinical Indications for Treatment of Complex Iliac Lesions in Iliac Interventions

The application of endovascular techniques for the treatment of short iliac stenoses and occlusion has been well accepted for several years now. A meta-analysis from 1997 by Bosch et al. (1) compared the results of six PTA studies (1300 patients) and eight stent studies (816) on iliac lesions. It revealed four-year primary patency rates of 67% after PTA and 81% after stenting. This means there is a 43% lower risk for long-term failure for stent placement over balloon angioplasty after four years. The randomized controlled Dutch Iliac Stenting trial failed in demonstrating superiority of primary stenting over PTA with additional stenting in short lesions (2–4).

A similar spirit was reflected when in 2000 the TransAtlantic Inter-Society Consensus (TASC) working group published their recommendations for the management of peripheral arterial disease. Based on the literature available and drawn up by field specialists, they are widely considered as the authoritative guidelines for use during everyday practice. One important aspect included in the TASC document is its lesion classification. It is based on response to intervention, independent of technology and techniques. The goal of this system is to indicate the best form of treatment, endovascular (TASC A) or surgical (TASC D). The lesions without strongly supportive evidence, but that are more likely to respond better to endovascular therapy (TASC B) or surgery (TASC C), need more evidence (Table 1) (5).

Owing to advancements in endovascular techniques and technology, there has been an evolution to tackle more and more complex iliac lesions and chronic iliac occlusions with minimally invasive procedures. Leville et al. (6) reported primary and secondary patency rates of 76% and 90% after three years after stenting of iliac occlusions. They concluded that endovascular treatment for iliac occlusive disease should be extended to Type C and D lesions, as stratification for the different TASC lesion classifications did not show any significant differences in outcome for primary and secondary patency rates (Fig. 1).

The TASC working group has revised and updated their recommendations, which resulted in their publication in 2007 of the Inter-Society Consensus for the Management of Peripheral Arterial Disease TASC II document (7). A concise overview of the TASC aortoiliac lesion classification and its evolution over the past few years is shown in Table 2. Lesions that are easier to be tackled by endovascular means belong to TASC A and B categories. The more complex iliac lesions are listed under TASC C and D categories.

Table 1 TASC Lesion Classification Categories

Treatment choice	TASC category
• Endovascular therapy is the treatment of choice	Type A
• Endovascular therapy is the preferred treatment after consideration of the patient's comorbidities, fully informed patient preference, and the local operator's long-term success rates	Type B
• Surgery is the preferred treatment for good-risk patients after consideration of the patient's comorbidities, fully informed patient preference, and the local operator's long-term success rates	Type C
• Surgery is the treatment of choice	Type D

Hazards and Complications

Access site complications
  – Groin hematoma
  – Retroperitoneal bleeding
  – Pseudoaneurysm
  – Arteriovenous fistula
	These complications used to be more frequent in the early years due to the need for 9-F or 10-F systems. With the current lower French sizes, groin complications are now much less common

Dissection	Hemodynamically significant dissection has been reported in 7.1% after iliac PTA. The majority of these dissections can be treated by stent implantation If a retrograde dissection into the aorta occurs, more complex endovascular repair is necessary
Perforation/rupture	This rare complication has been reported in 0.8% of the cases, especially in calcified lesion configurations. When it occurs, aggressive reversal of anticoagulants, balloon tamponade of the vessel, placement of a covered stent or surgery will have to be performed to solve the problem
Late aneurysm formation pseudoaneurysm	This complication can usually be treated with placement of a covered stent
Distal embolization	Distal embolization has been reported in 8.8–24% of the cases
Compromise/closure of internal iliac artery	

Device-related events
  – Stent thrombosis
  – Stent embolization/migration
  – Stent crush
  – Septic infection
  – Septic endarteritis
	Although these events are rare, operators should be familiar with techniques associated with snaring and retrieval of embolized stents

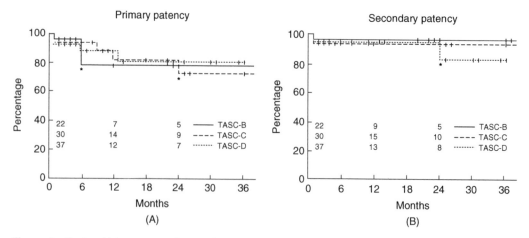

Figure 1 Kaplan–Meier curve estimates for endovascular iliac treatment stratified by TASC classification. Kaplan–Meier curve estimates for (**A**) primary and (**B**) secondary patencies in patients treated for iliac occlusion stratified by TASC. No significant difference was found between groups (6).

Table 2 TASC Classifications for Aortoiliac Lesions Evolution from 2000 to 2007

TASC 2000	TASC 2007
A lesions	**NO CHANGES**
TASC 2000 — Unilateral/bilateral single stenosis <3cm of CIA or EIA	TASC II 2007 — Unilateral/bilateral stenosis of CIA; Unilateral/bilateral single short stenosis of CIA <3cm of EIA
B lesions	**NEW**
TASC 2000 — Single stenosis 3–10cm in length; Two stenoses <5cm in the CIA and/or EIA; Unilateral CIA occlusion	TASC II 2007 — Short stenosis (<10cm) of infrarenal aorta; Unilateral CIA occlusion; Single or multiple stenosis totalling 3–10cm involving EIA; Unilateral EIA occlusion
C lesions	**NEW**
TASC 2000 — Bilateral stenosis 5–10cm of the CIA and/or EIA; Unilateral EIA occlusion; Unilateral EIA stenosis; Bilateral CIA occlusion	TASC II 2007 — Bilateral CIA occlusions; Bilateral EIA stenoses 3–10cm; Unilateral EIA stenosis; Unilateral EIA occlusion; Heavily calcified unilateral EIA occlusion
D lesions	**NO CHANGES**
TASC 2000 — Diffuse multiple stenoses involving the unilateral CIA, EIA, and CFA; Unilateral occlusions of both CIA and EIA; Bilateral EIA occlusions; Diffuse disease involving the aorta and both iliac arteries; Iliac stenoses in patient requiring aortic or iliac surgery	TASC II 2007 — Infrarenal aortoiliac occlusion; Diffuse disease involving the aorta and both iliac arteries; Diffuse multiple stenoses involving the unilateral CIA, EIA, and CFA; Unilateral occlusions of both CIA and EIA; Iliac stenoses in patients with other lesions requiring open aortic or iliac surgery

Interventional Strategies

Although the TASC stratification is an important tool to assess the extent of lesion morphology, successful endovascular treatment is not precluded for TASC C and D aortoiliac lesions. In experienced hands, endovascular treatment of complex iliac lesions is always possible, except when the common femoral artery (CFA) is occluded (for which a surgical aortobifemoral graft is indicated, preferably with profundaplasty); or when there is presence of an aortic occlusion up to the renal arteries of an aortic thrombosis. This chapter describes the different endovascular techniques and materials that can be used to successfully complete a minimally invasive intervention.

Access Techniques

Although over 90% of iliac lesions can be passed with simple guidewire techniques, each endovascular attempt to treat an iliac occlusion might be compromised by failure of guidewire passage. In order to achieve optimal success when treating complex iliac lesions, the operator should know when and how ipsilateral, contralateral, and brachial access techniques should be applied. Tables 3 and 4 give a schematic overview regarding which access technique should be followed for each type of complex iliac lesion configuration.

Since the introduction of subintimal angioplasty by Reekers and Bolia (8), it has become a common practice in many centers. However, this technique may compromise the result of the procedure, especially when an ipsilateral approach is performed, when re-entry to the true lumen is impossible or obtained at another site than the initially intended re-entry point (9). The use of re-entry catheters has recently been described by Ramjas et al. (10) as a means to successfully achieve continuity of the dissected portion with the true lumen, and to succeed in a primary stenting of the common iliac arteries. In a case report by Cho et al. (11), subintimal guidewire lesion passage in a patient who previously had aortic bypass surgery resulted in a small false lumen attached to the true aortic lumen with an intimal flap in between. A re-entry

Table 3 Total Occlusion of Common and/or External Iliac Artery

Unilateral occlusion Contralateral approach	Bilateral occlusion Brachial access

Step 1: catheterization and crossover
Access is made by puncturing the common femoral artery at the contralateral side using the Seldinger technique. A hydrophilic guidewire and a crossover catheter are advanced into the aorta. Correct positioning is confirmed by angiographic control at the iliac bifurcation
Materials
Straight sheath, 6-F, short
  – Interventional Sheath (Arrow)
  – Brite-Tip (Cordis)
  – Performer (Cook)
Crossover catheter, 6-F, 65/100 cm
  – RIM (Cook)
  – Universal Flush (Cordis)
  – Simmons 1 (Terumo)
  – Simmons 2 (Terumo)
  – Berenstein (Cordis)
Hydrophilic guidewire, 0.035″, 260 cm
  – GlideWire Flex (Terumo) (soft lesions)
  – GlideWire Stiff (Terumo) (calcified lesions)
Step 2: lesion passage
The hydrophilic guidewire and crossover catheter are advanced into the superficial femoral artery (SFA) of the contralateral limb to gain support. Then a wire exchange is done to a stiff guidewire and careful intraluminal lesion passage is performed
Materials
Stiff guidewire, 0.035″, 260 cm
  – GlideWire Stiff (Terumo)
  – Amplatz (Boston Scientific)
	Step 1: catheterization into common iliac artery
	Access is made by puncturing the brachial artery. Intraluminal lesion passage is done with a hydrophilic guidewire. The wire is installed into one of the CFA to obtain support for the catheter
	
	Materials
	Straight sheath, 6-F, long (90/100 cm) (brachial)
	  – Super-Arrow Flex (Arrow)
	  – Brite-Tip (Cordis)
	  – Flexor (Cook)
	Interventional catheter, 6-F, 150 cm
	  – Quick-Cross (Spectranetics)
	Hydrophilic guidewire, 0.035″, 260 cm
	  – GlideWire Flex (Terumo) (soft lesions)
	  – GlideWire Stiff (Terumo) (calcified lesions)
	
	Step 2: guidewire capture and securing the access site
	A short sheath is installed in the groin. Next, a snaring catheter is advanced to capture the guidewire, which is then partially pulled out of the contralateral (CFA). Next, the access site is secured by installing a 0.018″ guidewire
	Materials
	Straight sheath, 6-F, short (groin)
	  – Interventional Sheath (Arrow)
	  – Brite-Tip (Cordis)
	  – Performer (Cook)
	Guidewire, 0.018″, 260 cm
	  – GlideWire Flex (Terumo)
	  – GlideWire Stiff (Terumo)

Step 3: guidewire capture and exchange Access is made by puncturing the common femoral artery at the ipsilateral side using the Seldinger technique. Next, a snaring catheter is advanced to capture the guidewire, which is then partially pulled out of the contralateral common femoral artery (CFA). Next, the cross-over catheter can be removed Materials Straight sheath, 5-F, short Snare kit – Goose Neck (ev3)	Step 3: guidewire installment in other groin Repeat the above steps 1 and 2 for the other groin; or use the technique described under "Unilateral occlusion—Contralateral approach"

site was created by puncturing the intimal flap under intravascular ultrasound (IVUS) with a transseptal needle and the patient was successfully stented afterwards.

Interventional Tools

In order to obtain maximum and durable success, it is important to stent the entirety of the iliac segment affected by stenotic or occlusive disease. Depending on the type and location of the lesion, different devices and techniques can be applied.

Table 4 Multisegmental Stenoses of Common and/or External Iliac Arteries

Unilateral stenoses Ipsilateral approach	Bilateral stenoses Ipsilateral approach
Step 1: sheath placement and lesion crossing	Step 1: sheath placement and lesion crossing
Access is made by puncturing the ipsilateral CFA, using the Seldinger technique and under duplex guidance. Next, the lesion is crossed intraluminally with a hydrophilic guidewire	Access is made by puncturing the ipsilateral CFA, using the Seldinger technique and under duplex guidance. Next, the lesion is crossed intraluminally with a hydrophilic guidewire
Materials	Materials
— Straight sheath, 6-F, short	Straight sheath, 6-F, short
— Interventional Sheath (Arrow)	— Interventional Sheath (Arrow)
— Brite-Tip (Cordis)	— Brite-Tip (Cordis)
— Performer (Cook)	— Performer (Cook)
Hydrophilic guidewire, 0.035″, 260 cm	Hydrophilic guidewire, 0.035″, 260 cm
— GlideWire Flex (Terumo) (soft lesions)	— GlideWire Flex (Terumo) (soft lesions)
— GlideWire Stiff (Terumo) (calcified lesions)	— GlideWire Stiff (Terumo) (calcified lesions)
REMARK: If a dissection is created during ipsilateral approach, contralateral approach (as described in Table 3) is indicated	REMARK: If a dissection is created during ipsilateral approach, contralateral approach or brachial access (as described in Table 3) is indicated.

Preferably self-expanding stents are used to treat iliac arteries, they offer good trackability needed in tortuous anatomy and have an excellent radial force. It is advised to oversize any self-expanding stent with 10% to 15% in order to obtain the best result. An overview of devices for iliac lesion treatment, with their indication for use, can be found in Table 5.

Primary Stenting Versus Elective Stenting

In short iliac lesions, there is no difference in results between primary stenting and elective stenting. The randomized controlled Dutch Iliac Stenting trial failed in demonstrating superiority of primary stenting over PTA with additional stenting in short lesions (2–4). Yet, complex iliac lesions are best managed by primary stenting (Fig. 2). AbuRahma et al. (12) compared their results for primary stenting and elective stenting in short stenoses (TASC A and B) and in long stenoses (TASC C and D). In their patient cohort, there was no statistical difference in patency rates for short lesions. In long lesions, however, results for primary stenting were significantly better.

As the stent is placed without predilation, potential embolic material is trapped between the arterial wall and the stent mesh, which significantly reduces the risk of distal embolizations. Additional potential advantages of direct stenting include shorter procedural time and less radiation exposure (13).

Stent Grafting

Endovascular treatment of any lesion inherits a certain risk of vessel rupture and distal embolization. With the increasing complexity of the lesion to be treated, the risk of complications tends to follow. When arterial rupture following iliac artery PTA occurs, stenting of the artery alone results in maintenance of flow through the ruptured segment and exsanguination. Treatment with balloon occlusion alone has been reported (14), however this complication may require further revascularization (15). More recently, treatment of these complications has been performed

Table 5 Devices for Complex Iliac Lesions

Special situation	Device/example(s)
Tortuous lesion site	Self-expanding stent
Calcified lesion	Balloon expandable stent Cutting balloon
In-stent restenosis	Covered stent Cutting balloon

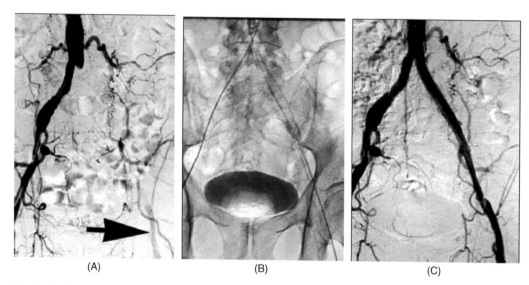

(A)   (B)   (C)

Figure 2   Example of a primary iliac stenting case (13). (**A**) Total CIA occlusion with reinjection at the level of external iliac artery (EIA) (arrow). (**B**) Direct stenting after retrograde recanalization by means of two self-expanding stents. (**C**) Good antegrade flow in the left iliac axis with preservation of the flow in the left IIA.

with covered stents (Fig. 3) with immediate exclusion obtained in 100% of patients and with primary and secondary patency rates of 87% and 100%, respectively at just under two years (16).

Distal embolization with PTA alone is not common for uncomplicated lesions, but does occur with greater frequency, as high as 24%, in the treatment of ulcerated plaques (17), with the recanalization of aortoiliac bifurcation lesions (18) or iliac occlusions (19). Stent grafts are used in our center for complex iliac lesions and have proven to effectively exclude the source of embolization (Fig. 4). In our recently published series of 91 limbs with stenotic diseased iliacs treated with the balloon expandable Atrium Advanta V12 PTFE covered stent (107 stent grafts used), we reported a successful deployment in all patients without any procedural complications including distal embolization and vessel rupture and with a primary limb patency at one year was 91.1% (20). However, even with the placement of stent grafts, embolization may remain a concern.

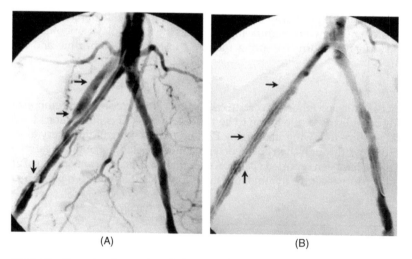

(A)   (B)

Figure 3   Example of an endograft placement (16). (**A**) Right common iliac artery (CIA) dissection (horizontal arrows) and high-grade EIA stenosis (vertical arrow). (**B**) Result after endovascular repair of the dissection with a stentgraft (8 × 60 mm) and of the stenosis with an additional Palmaz stent (7 × 30 mm).

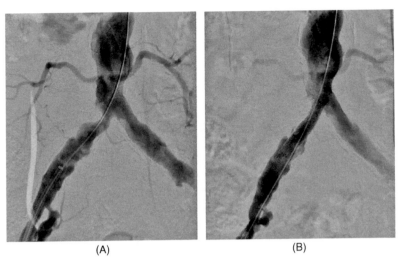

Figure 4 Example of a stentgraft placement. (**A**) Right CIA stenosis before treatment. (**B**) Result after stentgraft (8 × 38 mm) deployment.

Bifurcation Stenting

Lesions at the aortic bifurcation are traditionally treated using the "kissing balloons" technique. Simultaneous balloon dilatation at the origins of both common iliac arteries (CIAs) is advocated, even in the presence of unilateral lesion, to protect the contralateral CIA from dissection or plaque embolization. Because calcified lesions typically occurring at the aortic bifurcation are not amenable to balloon dilatation alone, "kissing stents" or "aortic reconstruction" technique is applied (Fig. 5). The aortic bifurcation reconstruction technique is technically very successful, although some have expressed fears that the proximal ends of the stents that extend into the distal aorta may serve as a nidus for thrombus formation, or cause hemolysis. Nevertheless, this fear has not been realized as has been shown by the low complication rates of this procedure. In the available study publications, different types of stent have been described, without any indication of a significant outcome. It is, however, important that both the used stents are of the same type and dimensions and they are deployed and dilated simultaneously.

Summary of Outcomes

Table 6 gives a literature overview of study results for endovascular treatment of complex iliac lesions. It shows that endovascular treatment of iliac artery occlusions can be accomplished

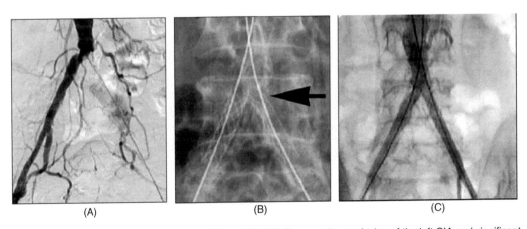

Figure 5 Example of the kissing-stent technique (16). (**A**) Preoperative occlusion of the left CIA and significant stenosis at the origin of the right CIA. (**B**) Poststenting image showing two kissing balloon expandable stents in both CIAs (arrow shows zone where kissing stents touch each other). (**C**) Postoperative good bilateral CIA flow.

Table 6 Literature Overview for Complex Iliac Lesions

References	Lesion type/device type	Technical success (%)	30-mortality (%)	PP @ 1Y (%)	PP @ 3Y (%)	PP @ 5Y (%)	PP @ 10Y (%)
1	All iliac lesions—PTA	91	1	74	68	–	–
	All iliac lesions—stent	96	0.8	86	80	–	–
23	Multisegment iliac occlusive disease	97	2	61	43	–	–
24	Kissing stents	100	0	–	86	–	–
18	Kissing stents	100	0	–	79.4	–	–
25	Kissing stents	–	–	94	–	–	–
26	Poor distal runoff—iliac stenting alone	97	–	76	66	55	–
	Poor distal runoff—iliac stenting + bypass	97	–	87	54	42	–
27	TASC C and D—surgery	96	–	85	72	64	–
	TASC C and D—endovascular	96	–	89	86	86	–
21	TASC A–D	–	–	–	87	83	49
22	TASC B–D	97.4	2.7	94	89	77	–
6	TASC C and D with concomitant infrainguinal disease	91	–	–	76	–	–
28	Kissing stents	100	–	76	63	63	–
12	All iliac lesions; primary stenting	100	–	98	87	77	–
	All iliac lesions; selective stenting	100	–	83	69	69	–
	TASC A and B primary stenting	100	–	100	98	87	–
	TASC A and B selective stenting	100	–	100	85	85	–
	TASC C and D—primary stenting	100	–	96	85	–	–
	TASC C and D—selective stenting	100	–	46	28	–	–
20	Balloon expandable covered stents	100	0	91.1	–	–	–
29	Kissing stents	–	–	–	–	–	–
30	TASC C and D—kissing stents	95.4	–	92	–	82	68
31	Cutting balloon for in-stent restenosis	92.8	–	100	–	80.7	–

via endovascular means with little morbidity and acceptable patency rates. Although evidence-based proof from controlled randomized trials is lacking, several recent publications have shown the excellent durability of iliac stenting in daily practice. Park et al. (21) described their long-term (up to 10 years) experience in their total cohort of iliac patients (TASC Type A–D lesions) and presented impressive primary patency rates of 87%, 83%, 61%, and 49% after 3, 5, 7, and 10 years of follow-up. De Roeck et al. (22) published their results after stenting of different types of iliac occlusions (TASC Type B–D) and showed primary patency rates of 94%, 89%, and 77% after one, three, and five years. They also stated that in their cohort of patients with complex aortoiliac lesions, stent failures can always be rescued endovascularly. They reported secondary patency rates of 100% after one year and 94% after three and five years. The success rate on midterm and long term is also heavily dependent on the presence of concomitant infrainguinal disease. Leville et al. (6) pointed out that surgical repair of iliac occlusions should only be referred to when all endovascular attempts are exhausted, bearing in mind the decreased perioperative morbidity and good mid-term durability.

Equipment Checklist

Contralateral approach	
Straight sheath, 6-F, short	Interventional Sheath (Arrow)
Crossover catheter, 6-F, 65/100 cm	RIM (Cook)
Snare kit	Goose Neck (ev3)
Hydrophilic guidewire, 0.035″, 260 cm	GlideWire (Terumo)
Ipsilateral approach	
Straight sheath, 6-F, short	Interventional Sheath (Arrow)
Hydrophilic guidewire, 0.035″, 260 cm	GlideWire (Terumo)
Brachial approach	
Brachial: Straight sheath, 6-F, long (90/100 cm)	Super-Arrow Flex (Arrow)
Groin: Straight sheath, 6-F, short	Interventional Sheath Flex (Arrow)
Hydrophilic guidewire, 0.035″, 260 cm	GlideWire (Terumo)
Lesion passage	
Stiff guidewire, 0.035″, 260 cm	GlideWire Stiff (Terumo) Amplatz (Boston Scientific)
Lesion treatment	
Tortuous lesion site	Self-expanding stent
Calcified lesion	Balloon expandable stent Cutting balloon
In-stent restenosis	Covered stent Cutting balloon

TEACHING CASES

Case 1: Management of an Intraprocedural Complication

What Made the Case "Complex"?
Although there was the presence of a bilateral occlusion at the level of the iliac arteries, the real difficulty with this case was the rupture after stent placement and postdilation in the right external iliac artery, which needed immediate action.

What Was the Clinical Indication for Treatment of This Patient?
A 70-year-old male patient presented in our hospital service with symptomatic PAD. He suffered from the Leriche syndrome, with intermittent claudication in the buttocks and erectile dysfunction. As clinical vascular risk factors the patient had medically controlled hypertension, hypercholesterolemia, and previous nicotine abuse (he quit smoking more than five years before). A preoperative duplex investigation showed complete absence of femoral pulses. This was confirmed by the preoperative MR Angiography, which showed a complete occlusion of the bilateral iliac arteries.

The lesion was a complete occlusion of the bilateral iliac arteries, as was confirmed by the preoperative MR Angiography (Fig. 6).

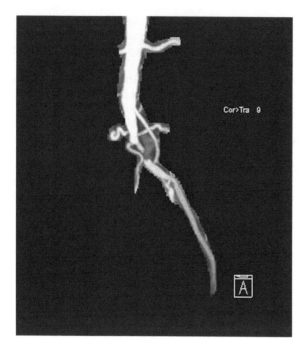

Figure 6 Complete occlusion of the bilateral iliac arteries.

What Were the Potential Hazards of Treating This Patient and Anatomy?
Ruptures need to be addressed as soon as possible as the tear in the vessel wall can lengthen. During this procedure, this was actually the case when a dilation of a covered stent, which was intended to seal the rupture, was performed.

Which Interventional Strategies Were Considered?
For the rupture, urgent complication management was necessary and the option considered was placement of a covered stent to seal the rupture.

Which Interventional Tools Were Used to Manage This Case?
− Regular PTA balloons
− Stents
   • Balloon expandable stents
   • Covered stents
− Endografts

Case Summary
Access was done via a femoral puncture on the left side with a 6-F Glidesheath (Terumo Medical Corporation, Somerset, NJ), after which intraluminal catheterization was performed into the aorta with a 0.035″ GlideWire (Terumo) guidewire. Next, an angiogram of the iliac bifurcation was done through a 6-F RIM catheter (Cook Incorporated, Bloomington, IN). Then, access was performed via a puncture in the right CFA with a short 6-F Arrow-Flex PSI sheath (Arrow International Inc.) and an X-ray-guided retrograde angiogram was taken. Subintimal antegrade catheterization and guide retrieval with an Amplatz Goose Neck® Snare catheter (ev3 Inc., Plymouth, MN) were then performed, followed by a bilateral guidewire exchange with two 0.035″ Amplatz (Boston Scientific Corporation, Natick, MA) wires.

   Due to calcifications at the bifurcation, balloon expandable stents were selected to dilate this region using the kissing-stent technique. Kissing predilation was performed with two Pheron balloons (Biotronik GmbH, Bulach, Switzerland) of 6 mm in diameter and 80 mm in length. Following was kissing stenting procedure with two balloon expandable Primus GPS stents (ev3 Inc.) of 8 mm in diameter and 57 mm long. Control angiography showed nice result with good flow. Next, the right external iliac artery was stented with a long self-expanding Protégé stent (ev3) of 8 mm in diameter and 100 mm long, which was postdilated with a Pheron balloon (Biotronik) of 7 mm in diameter and 40 mm in length. Control angiography showed blood loss due to a rupture at the external iliac artery.

At this moment the complication management to control the rupture was initiated. Blood loss was reduced by means of local control with a Pheron balloon (Biotronik) of 8 mm in diameter and 40 mm in length. Both sheaths were exchanged with an 11-F Brite Tip Interventional Sheath (Cordis Endovascular, Miami Lakes, FL) at the right side and a 9-F Arrow-Flex sheath (Arrow) at the left side, and a 33-mm aortic Equalizer balloon (Boston Scientific, Ratingen, Germany) was dilated to control the bleeding. In an attempt to seal the rupture, an Advanta V12 covered stent (Atrium Medical Corporation, Hudson, NH) of 8 mm in diameter and 38 mm in length was implanted, but angiographic control still showed a remaining small contrast flush afterwards. Therefore, another Advanta V12 covered stent (Atrium Medical) of 8 mm by 38 mm was placed immediately distal to the first, but still a residual bleeding remained. Dilation with a Pheron (Biotronik) balloon of 8 mm in diameter and 60 mm long to stop the remaining small contrast flush resulted in a new rupture. Therefore, a Viabahn (Gore & Associates, Flagstaff, AZ) endograft of 10 mm in diameter and 100 mm in length was placed. The bleeding was successfully stopped, but the graft showed to be oversized.

After this, the original procedural plan could be continued by recanalization of the left external iliac artery with primary placement of a self-expanding Protégé stent (ev3) of 8 mm in diameter and 60 mm long. After postdilation with a Star PTA balloon (Abbott Vascular, Redwood City, CA) of 7 mm in diameter and 40 mm long, final postoperative control showed a good result. The patient left the hospital two days later without any complications.

List of Equipment
- Sheaths and catheters:
  - 6-F Glidesheath (Terumo Medical Corporation, Somerset, NJ)
  - 6-F Arrow-Flex PSI sheath (Arrow International, Inc.)
  - Amplatz Goose Neck® Snare catheter (ev3 Inc., Plymouth, MN)
  - 6-F RIM Catheter (Cook Incorporated, Bloomington, IN)
  - 11-F Brite Tip Interventional Sheath (Cordis Endovascular, Miami Lakes, FL)
  - 9-F Arrow-Flex sheath (Arrow International, Inc.)
- Guidewires:
  - 0.035″ Glidewire (Terumo Medical Corporation, Somerset, NJ)
  - 0.035″ Amplatz (Boston Scientific Corporation, Natick, MA) (2×)
- Balloons:
  - 6 × 80 mm Pheron balloon (Biotronik GmbH, Bulach, Switzerland) (2×)
  - 7 × 40 mm Pheron balloon (Biotronik GmbH, Bulach, Switzerland)
  - 8 × 40 mm Pheron balloon (Biotronik GmbH, Bulach, Switzerland)
  - 33-mm aortic Equalizer balloon (Boston Scientific, Ratingen, Germany)
  - 8 × 60 mm Pheron balloon (Biotronik GmbH, Bulach, Switzerland)
  - 7 × 40 mm Star PTA balloon (Abbott Vascular, Redwood City, CA)
- Stents and endografts:
  - 8 × 57 mm Primus GPS stent (ev3 Inc., Plymouth, MN) (2×)
  - 8 × 38 mm Advanta V12 covered stent (Atrium Medical Corporation, Hudson, NH) (2×)
  - 10 × 100 Viabahn endoprosthesis (Gore & Associates, Flagstaff, AZ)
  - 8 × 60 Protégé stent (ev3 Inc., Plymouth, MN)

Key Learning Issues
In this case, the Viabahn endoprosthesis was oversized in diameter, resulting in the plicatures that can be seen on the images of the final procedure result. Despite this imperfect final result, however, it is imperative in this case to know when to quit instead of insisting too much on achieving the perfect result.

Case 2: Patient Presenting with Multisegment Lesions, Impaired Outflow, and Amputated Contralateral Leg

What Made the Case "Complex"?
This patient had a history of persisting vascular insufficiency, with several prior failed attempts of recanalization. On the left side, she had an upper leg amputation and on the right side, above-knee blood flow was provided by collaterals only. This extensive lesion configuration added significantly to this case's complexity.

What Was the Clinical Indication for Treatment of This Patient?
An 85-year-old female patient presented in our service with symptoms of mixed arterial and venous pathology. Oedemic rubor of the right big toe was reported in combination with several painful ulcerative wounds at the level of the fourth and fifth toe in the same leg. The patient had a fungal infection at the bilateral groin. Furthermore, she suffered from chronic renal insufficiency with serum creatinine levels of 2.6 mg/dl, which was treated by dialysis therapy. As further relevant clinical background, the patient did not smoke, nor had diabetes or nightly rest pain. She had had an upper leg amputation at the left side approximately two years earlier due to persisting vascular insufficiency, even after several failed attempts for recanalization.

Doppler investigation of the right leg showed a diminished flow curve at the right ankle. Due to the renal insufficiency, an nuclear magnetic resonance (NMR) angiographic investigation is done to evaluate the vascular status of the right limb. Several atheromatic vessel wall irregularities were reported at the right external iliac artery with an occlusion of the mid-third. Common and internal iliac arteries were patent. There was no opacification of the common and superficial femoral arteries, although some lateral collaterals had formed. This compromised arterial outflow increased the complexity of the case.

What Were the Potential Hazards of Treating This Patient and Anatomy?
If the endovascular intervention should fail, this patient is at high risk of another upper leg amputation.

Which Interventional Strategies Were Considered?
Considering the old age of this patient, the bad vascular circulation, the contralateral amputation, and the unfavorable overall condition of this patient, endovascular therapy was the first-line treatment considered in order to alleviate the patient from her complaints.

Which Interventional Tools Were Used to Manage This Case?
– Regular PTA balloons
– Stents
  • Balloon expandable stents
  • Covered stents

Case Summary
The patient underwent an endovascular intervention under general anesthesia. The patient was installed on the table in dorsal decubitus with the left arm on a side table. After antegrade puncture at the left brachial artery, a 5-F Glidesheath (Terumo) was brought into the left brachial artery by using the Seldinger technique under fluoroscopy.

Through a Headhunter catheter (Terumo), a 0.035″ GlideWire (Terumo) guidewire is maneuvered through the abdominal aorta up to the right common iliac artery. The guidewire is exchanged for a stiffer 0.035″ Amplatz (Boston Scientific) guidewire to gain more support, after which a 6-F Brite Tip Sheath (Cordis) of 90 cm is installed in the right common iliac. Angiographic control shows an occlusion of the right external iliac with distal reinjection of the deep femoral artery (DFA). The right superficial femoral artery (SFA) is also occluded from its origin onwards and has a heavily calcified aspect. Reinjection at the distal third of the SFA through collaterals formed from the DFA could be appreciated (Figs. 7–9).

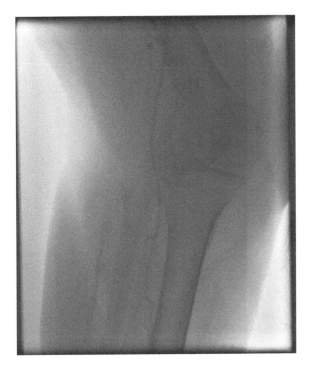

Figure 7

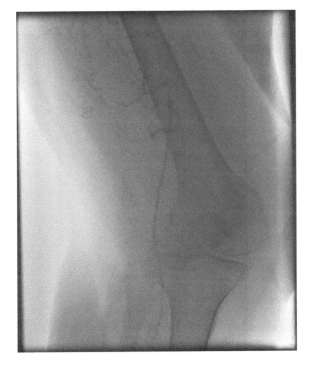

Figure 8

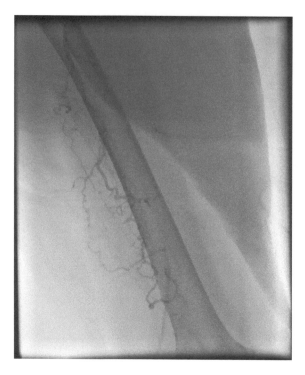

Figure 9

The Amplatz (Boston Scientific) guidewire is exchanged for a 0.018″ SV Wire (Cordis) and the common and proximal external iliac arteries are dilated with a 4 × 80 mm o.p.e.r.a. PTA catheter (Abbott Vascular), resulting in a small dissection (Fig. 10), which would be addressed later.

While the 0.018″ SV (Cordis) guidewire is left in the DFA, a 0.035″ GlideWire (Terumo) guidewire is inserted in the SFA through a long multipurpose catheter (Cook) for a selective recanalization up to popliteal level. After guidewire exchange to a 0.018″ SV Wire (Cordis), the entire femoropopliteal length is dilated with a 5 mm by 60 mm Agiltrac (Abbott Vascular)

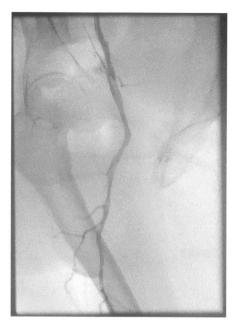

Figure 10 Dissection after dilation of the external iliac arteries.

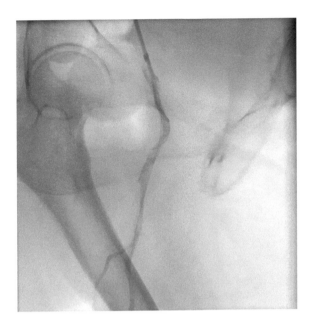

Figure 11 Dilation of the entire length of the femoropopliteal segment with a 5/60 Agiltrac balloon (Abbott Vascular).

balloon and the previously used 4 mm by 80 mm o.p.e.r.a. PTA Catheter (Abbott Vascular) balloon (Fig. 11). Control angiography showed a reasonable patency over the entire dilated tract, with the exception of a flow-limiting dissection at the segment situated in the mid-SFA and popliteal artery (Figs. 12, 13). Next, a Protégé GPS (ev3) stent of 6 mm in diameter and 150 mm long was implanted from Hunter's canal to the popliteal artery, followed by a second 6 mm by 150 mm Protégé GPS (ev3) stent at the proximal SFA (Figs. 14, 15). The gap in between these two stents was covered by an 8 mm by 100 mm Absolute (Abbott Vascular) stent, with adequate results. Postdilation was performed over the entire stented length of the SFA with a Agiltrac (Abbott Vascular) balloon of 5 mm in diameter and 60 mm in length. After checking the inflow, the second guidewire is removed from the SFA.

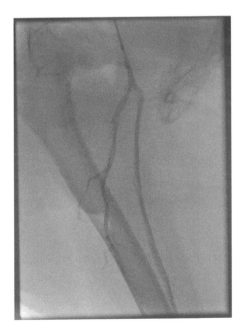

Figure 12 Flow-limiting dissection in the SFA and the popliteal artery after dilation.

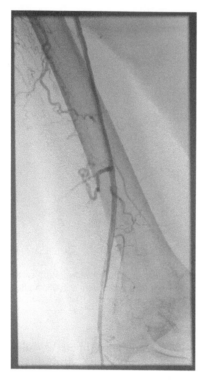

Figure 13 Flow-limiting dissection in the SFA and the popliteal artery after dilation.

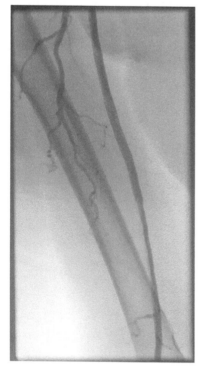

Figure 14 Stenting of the proximal SFA with a 6/150 mm Protgégé GPS stent (ev3).

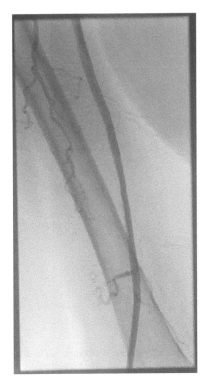

Figure 15 Stenting of the proximal SFA with a 6/150 mm Protgégé GPS stent (ev3).

Next, the Amplatz (Boston Scientific) guidewire is exchanged for a stiff 0.035″ GlideWire (Terumo) wire and, with the use of a Quick-Cross (Spectranetics, Colorado Springs, CO) catheter, the subintimal passage of the occluded segment in the DFA is achieved (Fig. 16). Next, the midportion of the DFA is treated with a self-expanding 6 mm by 40 mm Sinus-Superflex (Optimed, Ettlingen, Germany) stent and postdilation by means of the 5 mm by 60 mm Agiltrac (Abbott Vascular) balloon. Control angiography shows a good result with good flow, and without the presence of a dissection of peripheral embolization (Figs. 17, 18). Finally, a self-expanding Protégé GPS (ev3) of 6 mm in diameter and 100 mm long is placed along the length of the external iliac artery in order to improve inflow.

Final control angiography showed a good result and sheath removal was performed. The puncture site was closed by means of the Starclose closure system (Abbott Vascular).

List of Equipment
– Sheaths and catheters:
  • 5-F Glidesheath (Terumo Medical Corporation, Somerset, NJ)
  • Headhunter catheter (Terumo Medical Corporation, Somerset, NJ)
  • 6-F Brite Tip Sheath (Cordis Endovascular, Miami Lakes, FL)
  • Quick-Cross (Spectranetics, Colorado Springs, CO)
– Guidewires:
  • 0.035″ GlideWire (Terumo Medical Corporation, Somerset, NJ) (2×)
  • 0.035″ Amplatz (Boston Scientific Corporation, Natick, MA)
  • 0.018″ SV Wire (Cordis Endovascular, Miami Lakes, FL)
– Balloons:
  • 4 × 80 mm o.p.e.r.a. PTA catheter (Abbott Vascular, Redwood City, CA)
  • 5 × 60 mm Agiltrac (Abbott Vascular, Redwood City, CA)
– Stents:
  • 6 × 150 mm Protégé GPS (ev3 Inc., Plymouth, MN) (2×)
  • Sinus-Superflex (Optimed, Ettlingen, Germany)
  • 6 × 100 mm Protégé GPS (ev3 Inc., Plymouth, MN)

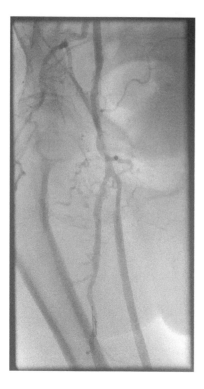

Figure 16 Subintimal passage of the occlusion located in the deep femoral artery by means of a Quick-Cross catheter (Spectranetics).

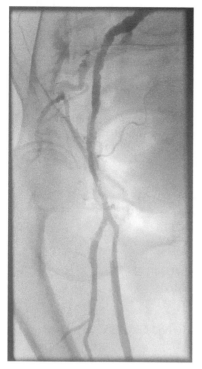

Figure 17 Control angiography shows good flow over the femoropopliteal tract.

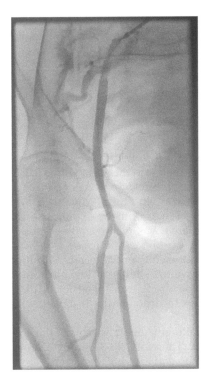

Figure 18 Control angiography shows good flow over the femoropopliteal tract.

Key Learning Issues
Recanalization of highly complex iliac disease with concomitant compromised outflow is feasible, even if a contralateral approach is impossible, through the brachial access technique. Second, treatment of all outflow lesion is a must in order to achieve the best long-term patency results.

Case 3: Patient Presenting with Multisegment Lesions Who Had a Distal Embolization During the Procedure

What Made the Case "Complex"?
Lesion passage was very difficult in this case, which is reflected in the number of catheters used to achieve the passage. Later during the procedure a distal embolization also required immediate attention.

Clinical Indication for Treatment
An 68-year-old male patient presented in our service with claudication due to a stenosis on the right and an occlusion of the left iliac arteries. As relevant clinical background, the patient is a heavy smoker with over 50 pack years, and suffers from chronic lymphatic leukemia (CLL) RAI stadium 0 and degenerative spinal pathology.

Doppler investigation of both lower limbs shows weak pulses over the entire right leg and an absence of pulses over the entire left leg. The preoperative NMR angiographic investigation shows low-grade to mid-grade stenoses from the ostium of the right common iliac artery till the external iliac artery. No relevant narrowing of the right SFA and popliteal artery was reported. There were some moderate stenoses at the below-the-knee arteries at the right side. At the left side, a postostial occlusion of the common iliac artery, with reinjection at the CFA was seen. There were no other significant arterial lesions in the left lower limb.

What Were the Potential Hazards of Treating This Patient and Anatomy?
There were no immediate hazards linked to the endovascular intervention in this patient.

Which Interventional Strategies Were Considered?

Given the bad overall health, open surgery was to be avoided. An endovascular intervention using contralateral approach immediately seemed to be the best option.

Which Interventional Tools Were Used to Manage This Case?

– Regular PTA balloons
– Stents
  • Self-expanding stents

Case Summary

Access was done via a common femoral puncture on the right side with a 6-F Glidesheath (Terumo), after which intraluminal catheterization was performed into the aorta with a 0.035″ GlideWire (Terumo) guidewire. Next, an angiogram of the iliac bifurcation was done through a 6-F RIM catheter (Cook Incorporated). Although the crossover with the RIM catheter was successful, it was impossible to obtain catheterization of the lesion in the left common iliac. Therefore, a SIM 1 catheter (Cook Incorporated) from the arch was placed and subintimal lesion passage was commenced. In order to pass the distal portion of the lesion a catheter exchange was performed to a Quick-Cross (Spectranetics) catheter. Eventually, recanalization is successful with the CFA as the re-entry site. Angiographic control shows the low bifurcation of the superficial and deep femoral arteries. Next, the guidewire is exchanged for a 0.035″ GlideWire stiff guidewire (Terumo) and a Balkin sheath (Cook Incorporated) is installed in the left common iliac artery.

   After predilation with a 7 mm by 80 mm Fox Plus balloon (Abbott Vascular), the control angiography shows a dissection and a residual stenosis. Therefore, an 8 mm by 120 mm Luminexx stent (C.R. Bard) is placed at the level of the common and external iliac arteries up to the CFA. Postdilation with a 7 mm by 80 mm Fox Plus balloon (Abbott Vascular) results in an adequate outcome of the treated segment, as confirmed by angiography.

   Due to a remaining stenosis at the postostial common iliac artery, another Luminexx stent (C.R. Bard) of 8 mm by 50 mm is implanted. After postdilation with a 4 mm by 60 mm Fox Plus balloon (Abbott Vascular), angiographic control shows a good blood flow throughout the iliac trajectory. At the middle portion of the SFA, however, blood flow interruption can be seen by angiography, which could be related to either a stenotic lesion or a distal embolization. An additional dilation with a 5 mm by 40 mm Pheron balloon (Biotronik GmbH) at the middle portion of the SFA confirms the thesis of a distal embolization. At this stage, the dilated segment in the SFA shows to be patent, but the anterior tibial artery and tibiofibular trunk are now embolized. Several laborious attempts for thrombus aspiration fail and it is chosen to first address a stenosis at the right external iliac artery. An 8 mm by 40 mm Luminexx stent (C.R. Bard) is implanted, followed by a dilation with a 7 mm by 80 mm Fox Plus balloon (Abbott Vascular) at the same treatment area.

   Next, distal embolization at the left lower leg was readdressed. This time, success was finally achieved after sheath exchange for a Destination sheath (Spectranetics) in combination with the Quick-Cross catheter (Spectranetics). The result shows a good outflow over all three below-the-knee vessels. In order to alleviate residual spasm, Cedocard is administered.

   Final control angiography showed a good result, without embolization, and sheath removal was performed. The puncture site was closed by manual compression.

List of Equipment

– Sheaths and catheters:
  • 6-F Glidesheath (Terumo Medical Corporation, Somerset, NJ)
  • 6-F RIM catheter (Cook Incorporated, Bloomington, IN)
  • SIM 1 catheter (Cook Incorporated, Bloomington, IN)
  • Quick-Cross (Spectranetics, Colorado Springs, CO)
  • Balkin sheath (Cook Incorporated, Bloomington, IN)
  • Destination sheath (Spectranetics, Colorado Springs, CO)
– Guidewires:
  • 0.035″ GlideWire (Terumo Medical Corporation, Somerset, NJ)
  • 0.035″ GlideWire stiff (Terumo Medical Corporation, Somerset, NJ)

- Balloons:
  - 7 × 80 mm Fox Plus balloon (Abbott Vascular, Redwood City, CA) (3×)
  - 4 × 60 mm Fox Plus balloon (Abbott Vascular, Redwood City, CA)
  - 5 × 40 mm Pheron balloon (Biotronik GmbH, Bulach, Switzerland)
- Stents:
  - 8 × 120 mm Luminexx stent (C.R. Bard GmbH, Karlsrühe, Germany)
  - 8 × 50 mm Luminexx stent (C.R. Bard GmbH, Karlsrühe, Germany)
  - 8 × 40 mm Luminexx stent (C.R. Bard GmbH, Karlsrühe, Germany)

Key Learning Issues

Even though endovascular iliac interventions may seem straightforward to perform, a complicated case always demands the presence of backup materials on the shelf. In this particular case, we needed the Destination sheath (Spectranetics) in combination with the Quick-Cross catheter (Spectranetics) in order to successfully treat the distal embolization.

REFERENCES

1. Bosch JL, Hunink MG. Meta-analysis of the results of percutaneous transluminal angioplasty and stent placement for aortoiliac occlusive disease. Radiology 1997; 204:87–96.
2. Tetteroo E, van der Graaf Y, Bosch JL, et al. Randomised comparison of primary stent placement versus primary angioplasty followed by selective stent placement in patients with iliac-artery occlusive disease. Dutch Iliac Stent Trial Study Group. Lancet 1998; 351:1153–1159.
3. Klein WM, van der Graaf Y, Seegers J, et al. Long-term cardiovascular morbidity, mortality, and reintervention after endovascular treatment in patients with iliac artery disease: The Dutch Iliac Stent Trial Study. Radiology 2004; 232:491–498.
4. Klein W, van der Graaf Y, Seegers J, et al. Dutch iliac stent trial: long-term results in patients randomized for primary or selective stent placement. Radiology 2006; 238:734–744.
5. Dormandy JA, Rutherford RB. Management of peripheral arterial disease (PAD). TASC Working Group. TransAtlantic Inter-Society Consensus (TASC). J Vasc Surg 2000; 31:S1–S296.
6. Leville CD, Kashyap VS, Clair DG, et al. Endovascular management of iliac artery occlusions: extending treatment to TransAtlantic Inter-Society Consensus class C and D patients. J Vasc Surg 2006; 43:32–39.
7. Norgren L, Hiatt WR, Dormandy JA, et al. Inter-Society Consensus for the Management of Peripheral Arterial Disease (TASCII). Eur J Vasc Endovasc Surg 2007; 33(suppl 1):S1–S75.
8. Reekers JA, Bolia A. Percutaneous intentional extraluminal (subintimal) recanalization: how to do it yourself. Eur J Radiol 1998; 28:192–198.
9. Lipsitz EC, Ohki T, Veith FJ, et al. Does subintimal angioplasty have a role in the treatment of severe lower extremity ischemia? J Vasc Surg 2003; 37:386–391.
10. Ramjas G, Thurley P, Habib S. The use of re-entry catheters in recanalization of chronic inflow occlusions of the common iliac artery. Cardiovasc Intervent Radiol 2008; 31(3):650–654.
11. Cho JR, Kim JS, Cho YH, et al. Subintimal angioplasty of an aortoiliac occlusion: re-entry site created using a transseptal needle under intravascular ultrasound guidance. J Endovasc Ther 2007; 14(6): 816–822.
12. AbuRahma AF, Hayes JD, Flaherty SK, et al. Primary iliac stenting versus transluminal angioplasty with selective stenting. J Vasc Surg 2007; 5:965–970.
13. Brountzos EN, Kelekis DA. Iliac artery angioplasty: technique and results. Acta Chir Belg 2004; 104:532–539.
14. Ballard JL, Sparks SR, Taylor FC, et al. Complications of iliac artery stent deployment. J Vasc Surg 1996; 24:545–553.
15. Murphy TP, Ariaratnam NS, Carney WI Jr, et al. Aortoiliac insufficiency: long-term experience with stent placement for treatment. Radiology 2004; 231:243–249.
16. Scheinert D, Ludwig J, Steinkamp HJ, et al. Treatment of catheter-induced iliac artery injuries with self-expanding endografts. J Endovasc Ther 2000; 7:213–220.
17. Vorwerk D, Gunther RW. Percutaneous interventions for treatment of iliac artery stenoses and occlusions. World J Surg 2001; 25:319–326; discussion 326–327.
18. Haulon S, Mounier-Vehier C, Gaxotte V, et al. Percutaneous reconstruction of the aortoiliac bifurcation with the 'kissing stents' technique: long-term follow-up in 106 patients. J Endovasc Ther 2002; 9: 363–368.
19. Leu AJ, Schneider E, Canova CR, et al. Long-term results after recanalisation of chronic iliac artery occlusions by combined catheter therapy without stent placement. Eur J Vasc Endovasc Surg 1999; 18:499–505.

20. Bosiers M, Iyer V, Deloose K, et al. Flemish experience using the Advanta V12 stent-graft for the treatment of iliac artery occlusive disease. J Cardiovasc Surg (Torino) 2007; 48:7–12.
21. Park KB, Do YS, Kim JH, et al. Stent placement for chronic iliac arterial occlusive disease: the results of 10 years experience in a single institution. Korean J Radiol 2005; 6:256–266.
22. De Roeck A, Hendriks J, Delrue F, et al. Long-term results of primary stenting for long and complex iliac artery occlusions. Acta Chir Belg 2006; 106:187–192.
23. Powell RJ, Fillinger M, Bettmann M, et al. The durability of endovascular treatment of multisegment iliac occlusive disease. J Vasc Surg 2000; 31(6):1178–1184.
24. d'Othée BJ, Haulon S, Mounier-Vehier C, et al. Percutaneous endovascular treatment for stenoses and occlusions of infrarenal aorta and aortoiliac bifurcation: midterm results. Eur J Vasc Endovasc Surg 2002; 24(6):516–523.
25. Mohammed F, Sarkar B, Timmons G, et al. Outcome of 'kissing stents' for aortoiliac atherosclerotic disease, including the effect on the non-diseased contralateral iliac limb. Cardiovasc Intervent Radiol 2002; 25:472–475.
26. Timaran CH, Ohki T, Gargiulo NJ III, et al. Iliac artery stenting in patients with poor distal runoff: influence of concomitant infrainguinal arterial reconstruction. J Vasc Surg 2003; 38(3):479–484.
27. Timaran CH, Prault TL, Steven SL, et al. Iliac artery stenting versus surgical reconstruction for TASC (TransAtlantic Inter-Society Consensus) type B and type C iliac lesions. J Vasc Surg 2003; 38:272–278.
28. Yilmaz S, Sindel T, Golbasi I, et al. Aortoiliac kissing stents: long-term results and analysis of risk factors affecting patency. J Endovasc Ther 2006; 13:291–301.
29. Houston BG, Bhat R, Ross R, et al. Long-term results after placement of aortic bifurcation self-expanding stents: 10 year mortality, stent restenosis, and distal disease progression. Cardiovasc Intervent Radiol 2007; 30(1):42–47.
30. Piffaretti G, Tozzi M, Lomazzi C, et al. Mid-term results of endovascular reconstruction for aortoiliac obstructive disease. Int Angiol 2007; 26:18–25.
31. Tsetis D, Belli AM, Morgan R, et al. Preliminary experience with cutting balloon angioplasty for iliac artery in-stent restenosis. J Endovasc Ther 2008; 15(2):193–202.

15 | The Femoropopliteal Segment

Andrej Schmidt and Dierk Scheinert

Parkkrankenhaus Leipzig, Medizinische Klinik I, Angiologie, Kardiologie, Herzzentrum Leipzig, Abteilung für Angiologie, Leipzig, Germany

PART 1: INTRODUCTION

What Makes a Lesion "Complex" in This Vessel Area?

During the last years, endovascular treatment of the femoropopliteal segment has been more and more accepted as a valuable treatment option. However, recanalization can be challenging in chronic total occlusions due to sever calcification, but recent development of dedicated techniques and devices has significantly increased the success rate for these lesions. Due to the high restenosis rate, long obstructions can be considered challenging as well and research to solve this problem is ongoing.

Clinical Indications for Endovascular Treatment of Complex Lesions in This Vessel Area

The decision for, whether to treat conservatively or to recanalize the vessel depends on the clinical situation and extent of the lesion.

The recent improvements in decreasing the restenosis rate of longer femoropopliteal lesions have shifted the therapeutic approach from surgery to intervention as shown in the TASC recommendations (1,2) (Table 1).

Potential Hazards of Treating Complex Lesions in This Vessel Area?

The potential risks are generally rare (Table 2). The frequency of peripheral embolization into the tibial arteries is mainly dependent on the thrombus load of the obstruction and low in chronic lesions; however, it can be high in rather acute or subacute occlusions or in stent occlusions. When embolization occurred, aspiration is the technique of choice. Local thrombolysis, dedicated thrombectomy devices [e.g., Rotarex (Straub Medical)] (3), and finally stenting of the peripheral embolus to the arterial wall is reserved in case aspiration fails. Perforation is rare and hardly ever leads to sever bleeding. The treatment options are prolonged low-pressure balloon inflation, implantation of nitinol stents, and finally covered stents. Destruction of the infrapopliteal trifurcation can occur, if the position of the tip of the guidewire is not regularly controlled during the intervention. Meticulous endovascular reconstruction and close follow-up, preferably by angiography is mandatory.

Specific Interventional Strategies and Tools for This Vessel Area

Preinterventional diagnostic workup should include duplex ultrasound. Several trials have demonstrated a good correlation between duplex ultrasound and digital subtraction angiography or magnetic resonance (MR) (8). Computed tomography (CT)- or MR-angiography plays an ancillary role for planning the intervention, for example, to rule out additional lesions in different arterial segments. Ankle brachial index (ABI) measurements are mandatory before and after recanalization to verify the interventional success.

The most frequent approach to the femoropopliteal lesion is the contralateral crossover access, mainly preferred by cardiologists, used in the retrograde femoral puncture or the ipsilateral antegrade approach, which is mainly familiar to radiologists. The contralateral approach is of advantage if the lesion involves the proximal superficial femoral artery (SFA), if an antegrade puncture is difficult as in obese patients or to avoid reduction of the inflow to the lesion by compression of the artery for hemostasis after the intervention. Antegrade ipsilateral access might be easier to perform in case of significantly kinked and calcified iliac arteries and a steep aortic bifurcation. It is clearly the access of choice in case of peripheral embolization to be able to perform embolus aspiration. A transpopliteal approach is reserved for situations, when an

Table 1 Recommendations from the TASC I and II Consensus Paper (1,2)

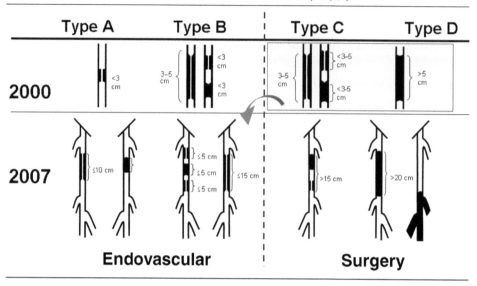

antegrade recanalization fails and a second retrograde attempt seems promising (9). A brachial approach is also possible if a femoral puncture is contraindicated as after aortobifemoral or bilateral femoropopliteal bypass surgery. The equipment for a brachial approach is however limited (Table 3). A 6-Fr sheath, either from contralateral or ipsilateral, is usually large enough for a standard procedure. For crossover, a rather stiff sheath [e.g., Balkin crossover (Cook)] is most important to avoid friction and loss of steerability and pushability of the angioplasty equipment during recanalization. Also for a popliteal approach, a 6-Fr access is safe and easy to compress manually after the intervention. However, it can be limited to 4- or 5-Fr if the guidewire is snared after retrograde wire passage and the procedure is continued via the antegrade access. Anticoagulation during the intervention usually consists of the administration of 5000 IE Heparin. If thrombotic material is visualized during the procedure, the additional administration of 5000 IE Heparin or GP IIb/IIIa inhibitors (10) should be considered.

For recanalization of total occlusions of the femoropopliteal tract, the guidewire can either be passed intraluminally through the occluded artery or via the subintimal space (11). Whether one or the other technique is more successful in terms of primary success or patency has never been proven. For an intraluminal recanalization, a hydrophilic tipped 0.018″ guidewire (e.g., V-18 Control, Boston Scientific) is the wire of choice. Other devices to intraluminally pass an occlusion are the Excimer laser (Spectranetics) or the Frontrunner CTO catheter (Cordis) (Table 4). The later device is a catheter with a jaw-like blunt tip to create a channel prior

Table 2 Potential Risks of Angioplasty of Femoropopliteal Lesion

Clinical and anatomic presentation	Potential complications	Frequency of events
Acute–subacute occlusion	Peripheral embolization of thrombus	24% (3)
Chronic total occlusion	Peripheral embolization of plaque material	Depending on embolus size Angiographically visible: <1% Filter analysis: 58% (4)
Heavily calcified lesion	Perforation	<1%
Disease involving the femoral bifurcation	Plaque shift to the profunda artery	No reports
Long segment stenting	Stent fracture	2% to >50% (5–7)
Long obstructions	Early reocclusion	<1%
Nitinol stenting	Clinical deterioration	3–5% (5)

Table 3 Recommended Devices for Complex Femoropopliteal Lesions

Special situation	Tool	Device example
Brachial access	6-F 90 cm sheath	6-F Flexor introducer sheath, 90 cm (COOK)
Balloons with sufficient shaft length for brachial access	Pacific Xtreme, 180 cm shaft length (Invatec)	
Stents with sufficient shaft length for brachial access	Sinus stents, 150 cm shaft length (Optimed)	
Femoral crossover access	6-F 40 cm sheath	6-F Balkin Up & Over Contralateral sheath, 40 cm (COOK)
Guidewire passage	Intraluminal passage	V-18 Control wire (Boston S.)
Subintimal passage	Stiff angled Terumo (Terumo)	
Inability to enter the occlusion with guidewire	Laser catheter	Excimer Turbo laser (Spectranetics)
Inability to re-enter true lumen distal to occlusion	CTO re-entry devices	Outback catheter (Cordis)
Severe perforation	Covered stents	Fluency (Bard)
Peripheral embolization	Aspiration catheter	Multipurpose 6–8-F Straight 6–8-F

to further endovascular treatment. The subintimal passage is performed using a stiff angled hydrophilic 0.035″ guidewire. A loop of the wire is used to dissect the subintimal space [Fig. 3(B)]. Re-entry from the subintimal space into the true lumen distal to the occlusion can be difficult. Dedicated re-entry catheters like the Outback (Cordis) or Pioneer catheter (Medtronic) are very successful in this regard (12,13). If the guidewire cannot be engaged into the occlusion at all, the laser can be very helpful, by creating an "entrance" for the wire into the occlusion.

After wire passage, balloon angioplasty is the standard technique. Balloons tracking over a 0.035″ guidewire can be difficult to pass through an occlusion, low-profile balloons tracking over 0.018″ or 0.014″ guidewires are therefore preferred, potentially reducing also the risk of embolization. The cutting balloon or a dedicated high-pressure balloon can be necessary in the rare case of a very rigid stenosis. Another device similar to the cutting balloon, the AngioSculpt (AngioScore/Biotronik) (Table 4) is a semicompliant balloon with an external nitinol shape-memory helical scoring edge (14) and is currently under investigation. The laser or SilverHawk atherectomy device (ev3) is used in total occlusions to facilitate balloon angioplasty or to achieve a stand-alone result (15,16); however, the success of these devices is limited in highly calcified lesions. A new laser device, the so-called "Booster laser" consisting of a catheter, which directs the laser tip into an eccentric position to increase the ablation area, is currently under investigation (17).

Stenting seems to be superior to balloon angioplasty alone in terms of patency rate only for longer lesions (6,18). Self-expanding nitinol stents are standard. More flexible stents, for example with a helical design [Everflex (ev3), LifeStent (Bard)], are preferred in the popliteal region. A disadvantage of rather flexible stents might be a lower radial force and after implantation of standard nitinol stents in highly calcified lesions recoil is not infrequent. An additional implantation of a short balloon expandable stent or nitinol stents with enhanced radial force, such as the Supera stent (IDEV-Technologies), might be a solution.

Stenting can be performed as full lesion coverage or spot stenting. In case of intentional subintimal recanalization, stenting of the proximal "entrance" to the subintimal channel and distal re-entry into the true lumen might preserve the flexibility of the artery; however, whether the patency rate is superior to long segment stenting is not proven. In fact, if the artery reoccludes, entry into the occluded distal stent can be extremely difficult and failure to reopen the artery is not infrequent.

Summary on Technical Success Rates, Acute and Long-Term Outcomes
The technical success rate in terms of possibility to pass the occlusion is, using the available tools like devices to facilitate re-entry (Pioneer, Outback catheter), very high and up to

Table 4 Specific Tools for Complex Femoropopliteal Lesions

Tool	Purpose	Figure
Frontrunner (Cordis)	Intraluminal passage of chronic total occlusions	
Outback (Cordis)	Re-entry from subintimal space to true lumen	
Pioneer (Medtronic)	Same as Outback (IVUS controlled)	
Booster laser (Spectranetics)	Atherectomy	
SilverHawk (ev3)	Atherectomy	
AngioSculpt (AngioScore/ Biotronik)	Lesions resistive to plain old balloon PTA	
Supera stent (IDEV-Technologies)	Calcified lesions	

100% (12,13). The ability to dilate the lesion with a maximally 30% residual stenosis might be lower, since highly calcified lesions have a tendency to recoil, even after implantation of self-expanding nitinol stents. Nevertheless, even if stenting is performed rather infrequent, endovascular recanalization leads to a high clinical success (15,16).

The restenosis rate after endovascular treatment of the femoropopliteal tract (Table 5) is relatively high and inversely correlated to the length of the lesion. At least for longer lesions, the systematic implantation of nitinol stents seems to improve the patency rate (6,18). A superiority of one over the other stent design has not yet been shown. Stents with a relatively high stiffness seem to show a higher frequency of stent fractures (7) compared to more flexible stents (6). Whether the use of other interventional tools and concepts such as atherectomy (Excimer-laser, SilverHawk), alternative balloon techniques (cryotherapy, cutting balloon, scoring balloon) or the implantation of covered stents (Viabahn) is superior is not proven. First results using a drug-eluting balloon are promising (19).

Table 5 Patency Rate After Femoropopliteal Recanalization

References	N pts	Lesion length (mm)	Treatment	Patency rate and follow-up period
20	121	45	Balloon angioplasty	61% (12 mo)
21	217	100	Balloon angioplasty	<30% (12 mo)
15	318	194	Excimer laser + balloon	34% (12 mo)
22	21	20	Cutting balloon	38% (6 mo)
16	45	43	SilverHawk	84% (12 mo)
20	123	45	Nitinol stent (Luminexx)	68% (12 mo)
5	116	107	Wallstent	28% (36 mo)
5	125	125	Nitinol stent (Dynalink/Absolute)	51% (36 mo)
23	47	83	Sirolimus-eluting stent (Smart)	77% (24 mo)
24	97	Up to 130	Viabahn endoprosthesis	65% (12 mo)
19	41	75	PTX-eluting balloon	83% (6 mo)

Checklist for Recommended Equipments for Complex Interventions in This Specific Vessel Area
PART 2: TEACHING CASES

Case 1: Mid-SFA Occlusion Right Side

What Made the Lesion "Complex"?
The proximal SFA leads directly to a large collateral, showing no stump, which would indicate the beginning of the occlusion [Fig. 1(A)]. Similarly, this situation is often found at the origin of the SFA as a so-called "flush" occlusion, where no stump of the occluded artery can be seen and maneuvering of the guidewire into the occlusion can be difficult.

What Was the Clinical Indication for Treatment?
The male patient suffered from claudication on both sides, but mainly right calf, maximal walking capacity 100 m, ABI at rest was 0.6 right side.

What Were the Potential Hazards of Treating This Specific Lesion?
If the beginning of the occlusion is missed and a recanalization attempt is performed within the collateral, a perforation of the collateral artery could occur.

Which Interventional Strategies Were Considered for This Lesion?
If an antegrade recanalization fails due to the missing stump, a transpopliteal access could be successful.

Which Interventional Tools Were Used to Handle the Lesion?
Due to the disease of the proximal SFA, a crossover approach was chosen. A 6-F 40 cm Balkin Up & Over sheath (Cook) was introduced. A stiff angled 0.035″ hydrophilic guidewire (Terumo) was introduced and engagement of the wire into the occlusion was attempted with the support of different 5-F diagnostic catheter with bent tips, such as a Judkins Right, Multipurpose, Vertebral, IMA catheter and angled Glide catheter (Terumo). However, all catheters did not provide enough support to hook the guidewire into the occlusion, which therefore always slipped into the collateral [Fig. 1(B)].

Summary: How Was the Case Managed?
To improve the stiffness of the support catheter, a 6-F guiding catheter could have been introduced through the 6-F sheath. In this case, a 5-F catheter with an improved stability at the tip and a sharper angle was chosen. A SOS Omni Selective catheter was modified by cutting off the recurved part of the tip giving it a 90° angled tip. Additionally, by cutting the catheters tip with the scalpel a sharper edge of the catheter tip was produced facilitating the catheter to

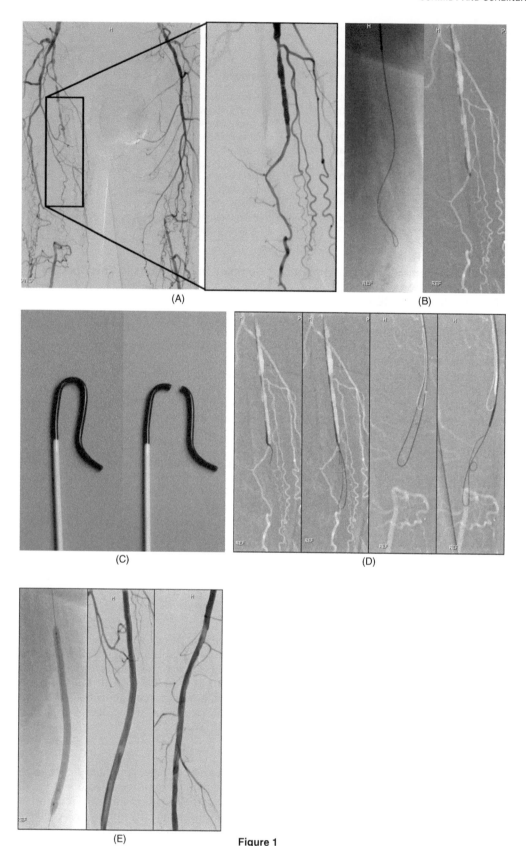

(A)

(B)

(C)

(D)

(E)

Figure 1

"hook" into the occluded artery [Fig. 1(C)]. It then was easy to engage an angled hydrophilic guidewire (Terumo) into the subintimal space, which was indicated by the loopform of the wire [Fig. 1(D)]. Also other catheters such as IMA, Judkins Right or Pigtail catheter can be modified in this manner. Re-entry of the guidewire into the distal artery was unproblematic, followed by balloon angioplasty using a 5-mm diameter balloon with a length of 120 mm. Due to the length of the lesion, primary stenting was performed using two 6/120 mm nitinol stents and postdilatation with the same balloon [Fig. 1(E)].

List of Equipment Used in This Case
- 6-F Balkin Up & Over Contralateral introducer sheath, 40 cm (COOK)
- 5-F SOS Omni Selective (Angiodynamics)
- 0.035" angled stiff guidewire, 300 cm (TERUMO)
- 5.0/120 mm Admiral Xtreme, 130 cm (Invatec)
- 6.0/120 mm Everfelx nitinol stent (ev3)

Key Learning Issues of This Specific Case
A selection of support catheters and the modification of these by cutting off the tip at different points can be helpful to engage an occlusion with the guidewire. Also, the tip of guidewires can be gradually modified in their stiffness by cutting off the tip with a sterile scissor. However, the risk of perforation might be increased.

Case 2: Heavily Calcified Popliteal Occlusion

What Made the Lesion "Complex"?
The severe calcification and not the length of an occlusion is the most important predictor of failure to recanalize CTOs of the SFA [Fig. 2(A)].

What Was the Clinical Indication for Treatment?
The male patient suffered from severe claudication of the left calf, maximal walking capacity 80 m, ABI at rest 0.55.

What Were the Potential Hazards of Treatment?
In highly calcified lesions, the risk of perforation is increased just by the mere fact that higher forces have to be applied to pass the guidewire through the lesion. Another potential hazard in calcified CTOs is the risk of dissecting the artery distal to the occlusion, thus ending up with a much longer lesion to be dilated or stented. This is, however, only a risk using a subintimal recanalization technique, where re-entry of the guidewire into the artery distal to the occlusion can be difficult due to severe calcification of the arterial wall. An intraluminal recanalization attempt is therefore preferable to avoid difficulties during re-entry; however, in case of severely calcified lesions only feasible in rather short occlusions.

Which Interventional Strategies Were Considered for This Lesion?
A crossover access can be chosen; however, pushability of the angioplasty tools is enhanced using a more direct ipsilateral antegrade approach.

Catheter-based atherectomy is considered in this case to achieve a result without the need for stenting. A laser catheter (Spectranetics) would be preferable over a SilverHawk device (ev3) in this case, because wire passage before atherectomy is not necessary using the laser and the ability of debulking severely calcified plaque is estimated to be higher for a laser using high energy (Turbo laser) compared to the SilverHawk.

If intraluminal passage of the occlusion fails, a subintimal passage could be performed. The Pioneer or the Outback catheter permits to re-enter the artery exactly distal to the occlusion to avoid ballooning and stenting further distal.

Which Interventional Tools Were Used to Handle the Lesion?
A 6-F 45-cm Arrow sheath was introduced ipsilateral, thereby having the tip of the sheath directly in front of the occlusion. After several attempts to pass the occlusion intraluminally

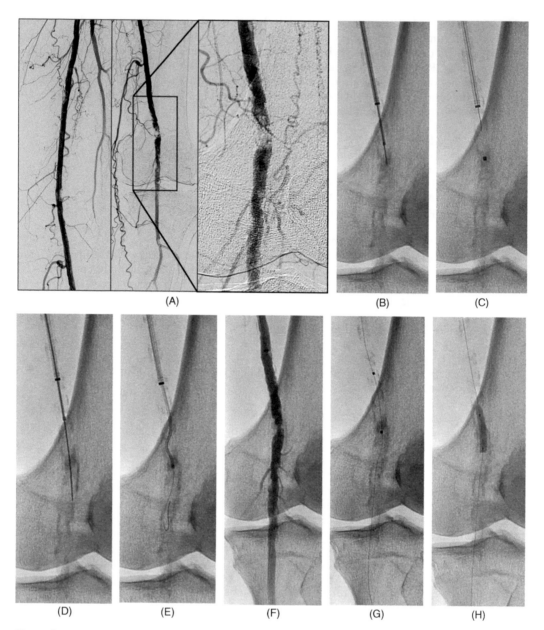

(A)   (B)   (C)

(D)   (E)   (F)   (G)   (H)

Figure 2

with a stiff straight 0.035″ hydrophilic guidewire (Terumo) supported by a 5-F multipurpose catheter, the wire was introduced in a reversed way using the very stiff end [Fig. 2(B)]; however, this was also unsuccessful in the first attempt. A 2.0-mm Turbo laser (Spectranetics) [(Fig. 2(C)] was used to pass or at least weaken the plaque. The laser catheter did not pass, although the maximal energy (60 mJ/mm^2) and a maximal pulse-repetition rate (60/sec) were used, but facilitated passage of the reversed tip of the Terumo wire [Fig. 2(D)] through the occlusion. Since leaving the wire in a reversed mode in the artery during the next interventional steps might have been hazardous in terms of potential perforation, a 5-F diagnostic catheter was positioned over the Terumo wire as far into the occlusion as possible. Thereafter, the Terumo wire was withdrawn and a 300-cm 0.014″ guidewire inserted, which easily passed the channel created by the Terumo wire [Fig. 2(E)]. Laser atherectomy was continued thereafter [Fig. 2(F)].

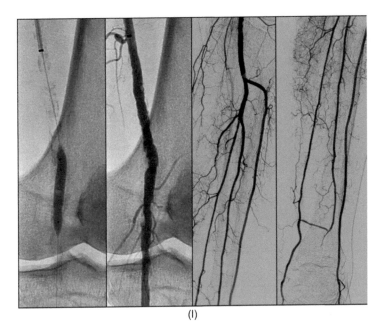

(I)

Figure 2 (*Continued*)

A high-pressure balloon, tracking over a 0.035″ guidewire, chosen due to the calcification of the lesion, did not pass the channel created by the laser [Fig. 2(G)]. A PTCA balloon with a very low crossing profile was then used for predilatation [Fig. 2(H)] followed by dilatation using a low-profile OTW balloon with a larger diameter [Fig. 2(I)].

Summary: How Was the Case Managed, Is There Anything That Could Have Been Improved?
A direct antegrade approach improved the pushability of the tools used for recanalization. A laser catheter was helpful to weaken the plaque and facilitate wire passage. If a laser device is not available, further ongoing attempts to pass the lesion with the wire might have been successful as well. The reversed tip of the wire came rather close to the arterial wall after passage of the occlusion with the risk of perforation. The reversed tip of the Terumo wire can be bent using a sterile clamp to be able to direct the wire into another position. If intraluminal wire passage would have failed, a subintimal recanalization attempt could have been attempted.

List of Equipment Used in This Case
- 6-F 45 cm Arrow sheath (Arrow)
- 0.035″ Radiofocus Terumo angled stiff guidewire, 300 cm (TERUMO)
- 3.0 OTW Elite Turbo laser catheter (Spectranetics)
- 0.014″ PT2 hydrophilic 300 cm guidewire (Boston Scientific)
- 5.0/40 mm Admiral Xtreme, 130 cm (Invatec)
- 4.0/20 Mercury PTCA catheter (Abbott)
- 5.0/40 mm Pacific Xtreme, 130 cm (Invatec)

Key Learning Issues of This Case
In case of severely calcified short CTOs, an intraluminal recanalization attempt is justified using the stiff, reversed tip of guidewires. Laser atherectomy can be helpful to facilitate guidewire passage into an occlusion.

Case 3: Severely Calcified Long SFA Occlusion

What Made the Lesion "Complex"?
The severe calcification of the occlusion clearly makes the success of an endovascular approach questionable [Fig. 3(A)].

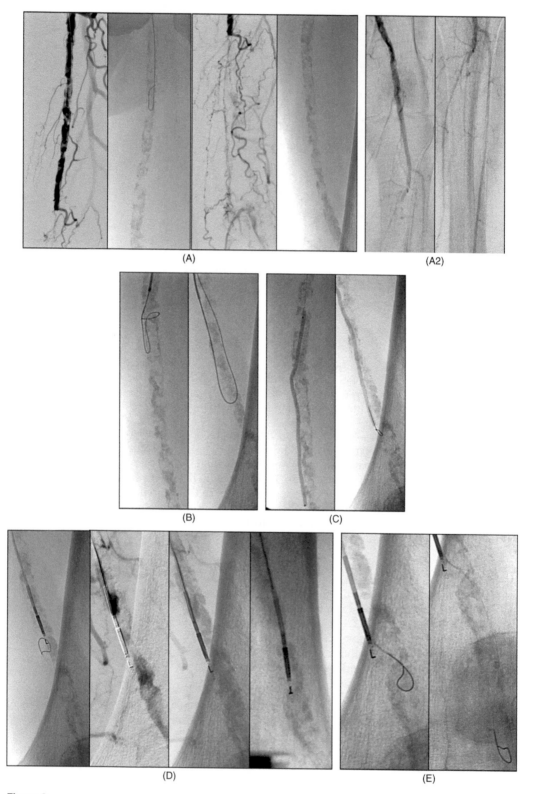

(A)

(A2)

(B)

(C)

(D)

(E)

Figure 3

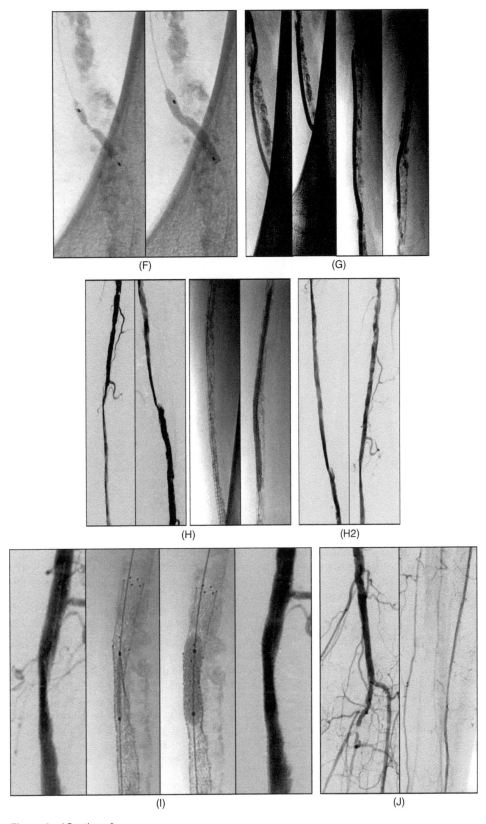

Figure 3 (*Continued*)

(*Continued on page 216*)

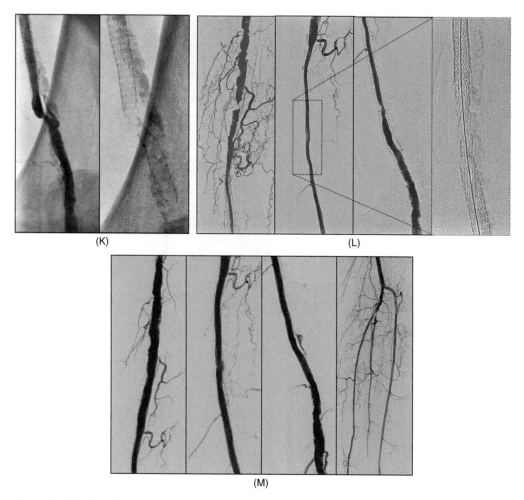

(K)   (L)

(M)

Figure 3   (*Continued*)

What Was the Clinical Indication for Treatment?

The male patient suffered from critical limb ischemia with minor gangrene of the toes. The severe calcification is typical for patients with endstage renal insufficiency. The patient was referred by a vascular surgical department for an endovascular recanalization attempt. Difficulty inserting the bypass to the highly calcified arterial wall was anticipated.

What Were the Potential Hazards of Treating This Lesion?

The risk of bleeding is clearly higher if guidewire perforation occurs right at the beginning of the occlusion, leading the blood flow from the proximal open artery directly into the surrounding tissue. In contrast, guidewire perforation within an occlusion is normally self-limiting either if the procedure is stopped at this stage or balloon angioplasty and/or stenting is performed after successful guidewire passage of the occlusion.

Dissection with the guidewire further distal of the end of the occlusion is frequent in highly calcified lesions and makes ballooning and potentially stenting further distal necessary. This scenario should be avoided not to destroy an area for a future distal bypass anastomosis.

Which Interventional Strategies Were Considered for This Lesion?

Generally two ways of endovascular recanalization can be attempted, an intraluminal or a subintimal approach. In this highly calcified artery, the subintimal way is the only chance to pass the occlusion.

Which Interventional Tools Were Used to Handle the Lesion?

After having introduced a 6-F crossover sheath, a 5-F Judkins Right catheter was used to engage the tip of the 0.035″ stiff angled hydrophilic guidewire into the subintimal space at the very beginning of the occlusion, using the so-called "percutaneous intended subintimal recanalization technique (PIER)" (11). Creating a loop with the wire a subintimal passage of the occlusion was possible [Fig. 3(B)]; however, re-entry into the patent distal artery was unsuccessful. Therefore, the Terumo wire was exchanged for a 0.014″ guidewire and predilatation was performed using a low-profile balloon (2.5/120 mm) [Fig. 3(C)] to facilitate the introduction of the Outback catheter. The marker at the tip of the catheter has to appear as a "T" in alignment with the artery and should be "L"-shaped if the position is lateral to the artery [Fig. 3(D)] to direct the curved needle from the subintimal space back into the true lumen. Thereafter, the 0.014″ guidewire is advanced through the needle into the distal SFA [Fig. 3(E)]. It can be difficult to pass a balloon through the calcified membrane, low-profile PTCA catheters are successful, if other peripheral balloon catheters fail [Fig. 3(F)]. Thereafter, gradual angioplasty using a 4.0/120 mm and 5.0/120 mm balloon was performed [Fig. 3(G)]. Due to severe recoil, nitinol stents were implanted and postdilated with the 5.0-mm balloon [Fig. 3(H)]. However, thereafter also significant residual stenoses remained due to recoil. A balloon expandable renal stent was implanted at the area of most severe recoil [Fig. 3(I)] and finally a significantly improved outflow was achieved [Fig. 3(J)].

Summary: How Was the Case Managed, Is There Anything That Could Have Been Improved, What Was the Immediate and Long-Term Outcome?

The combination of a subintimal recanalization technique and a re-entry device was successful. The Outback catheter is a very stiff device with an excellent pushability, therefore predilatation of the lesion might not have been necessary before introduction of the device. Whether a cutting or scoring balloon would have reduced the recoil after ballooning is questionable. There was a sustained improvement of the clinical situation during the next six months. Reangiography after six months showed a patent artery with severe stent fracture at the area of re-entry into the true lumen [Fig. 3(K)] and stent-in-stenting was performed. Twenty-six months later the patient suffered from recurrent claudication. A proximal subtotal de novo stenosis of the SFA and moderate restenosis in the stents with severe stent fractures not associated to restenosis were seen [Fig. 3(L)]. Figure 3(M) shows the result after additional stenting of the proximal lesion and re-PTA in the stents.

List of Equipment Used in This Case

- 6-F Balkin Up & Over Contralateral sheath, 40 cm (COOK)
- 5-F JR4 diagnostic catheter, 100 cm (Cordis)
- 0.035″ angled stiff guidewire, 300 cm (Terumo)
- 0.014″ ACS High-Torque Floppy II Extra Support, 300 cm (Abbott)
- 2.0/120 mm Amphirion Deep balloon, 120 cm (Invatec)
- Outback catheter (Cordis)
- 2.0/20 mm Mercury PTCA catheter (Abbott)
- 4.0/120 mm and 5.0/120 mm Pacific Xtreme, 130 cm (Invatec)
- 6.0/120 mm SMART nitinol stents (Cordis)
- 6.0/18 mm Genesis on Amiia renal stent (Cordis)

Key Learning Issues of This specific Case

In severely calcified SFA occlusions, only a subintimal recanalization technique is feasible. A re-entry catheter is necessary in many cases. The radial force of nitinol stents might be suboptimal in heavily calcified lesions, an additional implantation of a short balloon expandable stent might be necessary. Recanalization of heavily calcified obstructions should probably be restricted to patients with critical ischemia; in claudicants, the residual stenoses even after stenting might not yield the desired clinical result.

PART 3: KEY ISSUES FOR SUCCESSFUL AND SAFE TREATMENT OF COMPLEX FEMOROPOPLITEAL LESIONS

Success and safety of the intervention starts with the thorough consideration of the treatment options, which mainly depend on the clinical situation and morphology of the lesion. Although the complication rate of angioplasty is generally low, the equipment and knowledge of tools for treatment of complications is mandatory.

- Experience and tools for infrapopliteal interventions.
- Appropriate aspiration catheters.
- Experience in antegrade access for aspiration.
- Covered stents.

The primary success depends largely on the availability and experience with dedicated materials:

Crossover sheath that provide sufficient support.
Variety of hydrophilic-coated guidewires.
Variety of support catheters.
Re-entry device.
Nitinol stents with proven efficacy in terms of long-term patency.

Long-term success:

Close and continuous follow-up surveillance.

REFERENCES

1. Dormandy JA, Rutherford RB. Management of peripheral arterial disease (PAD). TASC Working Group TransAtlantic Inter-Society Consensus (TASC). J Vasc Surg 2000; 31(1 Pt 2):S1–S296.
2. Norgren L, Hiatt WR, Dormandy JA, et al. Inter-society consensus for the management of peripheral vascular disease (TASC II). J Vasc Surg 2007; 45(suppl S):S5–S67.
3. Duc SR, Schoch E, Pfyffer M, et al. Recanalization of acute and subacute femoropopliteal artery occlusions with the Rotarex catheter: one year follow-up, single center experience. Cardiovasc Intervent Radiol 2005; 28(5):603–610.
4. Karnabatidis D, Katsanos K, Kagadis GC, et al. Distal embolism during percutaneous revascularization of infra-aortic arterial occlusive disease: an underestimated phenomenon. J Endovasc Ther 2006; 13(3):169–180.
5. Schlager O, Dick P, Sabeti S, et al. Long-segment SFA stenting—the dark side: in-stent restenosis, clinical deterioration, and stent-fractures. J Endovasc Ther 2005; 12:676–684.
6. Schillinger M, Sabeti S, Loewe C, et al. Balloon angioplasty versus implantation of nitinol stents in the superficial femoral artery. N Engl J Med 2006; 354(18):1879–1888.
7. Scheinert D, Scheinert S, Sax J, et al. Prevalence and clinical impact of stent fractures after femoropopliteal stenting. J Am Coll Cardiol 2005; 45:312–315.
8. Schlager O, Francesconi M, Haumer M, et al. Duplex sonography versus angiography for assessment of femoropopliteal arterial disease in a "real-world" setting. J Endovasc Ther 2007; 14(4):452–459.
9. Yilmaz S, Sindel T, Lüleci E. Ultrasound-guided retrograde popliteal artery catheterization: experience in 174 consecutive patients. J Endovasc Ther 2005; 12(6):714–722.
10. Dörffler-Melly J, Mahler F, Do DD, et al. Adjunctive abciximab improves patency and functional outcomes in endovascular treatment of femoropopliteal occlusions: initial experiences. Radiology 2005; 237(3):1103–1109.
11. Laxdal E, Jenssen GL, Pedersen G, et al. Subintimal angioplasty as a treatment of femoropopliteal artery occlusions. Eur J Vasc Endovasc Surg 2003; 25:578–582.
12. Jacobs DL, Motaganahalli RL, Cox DE, et al. True lumen re-entry devices facilitate subintimal angioplasty and stenting of total chronic occlusions: initial report. J Vasc Surg 2006; 43(6):1291–1296.
13. Scheinert D, Braunlich S, Scheinert S, et al. Initial clinical experience with an IVUS-guided transmembrane puncture device to facilitate recanalization of total femoral occlusions. EuroIntervention 2005; 1:115–119.
14. Scheinert D, Peeters P, Bosiers M, et al. Results of the multicenter first-in-man study of a novel scoring balloon catheter for the treatment of infra-popliteal peripheral arterial disease. Catheter Cardiovasc Interv 2007; 70(7):1034–1039.

15. Scheinert D, Laird JR, Schroeder M, et al. Excimer laser-assisted recanalization of long chronic superficial femoral artery occlusions. J Endovasc Ther 2001; 8:156–8166.

16. Zeller T, Rastan A, Sixt S, et al. Long-term results after directional atherectomy of femoro-popliteal lesions. J Am Coll Cardiol 2006; 48(8):1573–1578.

17. Rastan A, Sixt S, Schwarzwälder U, et al. Initial experience with directed laser atherectomy using the CLiRpath photoablation atherectomy system and bias sheath in superficial femoral artery lesions. J Endovasc Ther 2007; 14(3):365–373.

18. Schillinger M, Sabeti S, Dick P, et al. Sustained benefit at 2 years of primary femoropopliteal stenting compared with balloon angioplasty with optional stenting. Circulation 2007; 115(21):2745–2749.

19. Tepe G, Zeller T, Albrecht T, et al. Local delivery of paclitaxel to inhibit restenosis during angioplasty of the leg. N Engl J Med 2008; 358(7):689–699.

20. Krankenberg H, Schlüter M, Steinkamp HJ, et al. Nitinol stent implantation versus percutaneous transluminal angioplasty in superficial femoral artery lesions up to 10 cm in length: the femoral artery stenting trial (FAST). Circulation 2007; 116(3):285–292.

21. Capek P, McLean GK, Berkowitz HD. Femoropopliteal angioplasty. Factors influencing long-term success. Circulation 1991; 83:170–180.

22. Amighi J, Schillinger M, Dick P, et al. De novo superficial femoropopliteal artery lesions: peripheral cutting balloon angioplasty and restenosis rates-randomized controlled trial. Radiology 2008; 247(1):267–272.

23. Duda SH, Bosiers M, Lammer J, et al. Drug-eluting and bare nitinol stents for the treatment of atherosclerotic lesions in the superficial femoral artery: long-term results from the SIROCCO trial. J Endovasc Ther 2006; 13(6):701–710.

24. Saxon RR, Dake MD, Volgelzang RL, et al. Randomized, multicenter study comparing expanded polytetrafluoroethylene-covered endoprosthesis placement with percutaneous transluminal angioplasty in the treatment of superficial femoral artery occlusive disease. J Vasc Interv Radiol 2008; 19(6):823–832.

16 | The Tibioperoneal Segment

Lanfroi Graziani

Invasive Cardiology Unit, Istituto Clinico Città di Brescia, Brescia, Italy

Hubert Wallner

Kardinal Schwarzenberg´sches Krankenhaus, Schwarzach, Salzburg, Austria

PART 1: INTRODUCTION

Ischemic diabetic foot ulcer is the main cause of nontraumatic amputations in western countries (1).

For patients aged 65 to 74 years, diabetes heightens the risk of amputation more than 20-fold, putting these patients at great risk of limb loss; 20% of subjects with diabetes develop a foot ulcer in the course of life, and 33% of them, if untreated, frequently undergo amputation (2–5).

The most common indication for intervention in the tibial–peroneal segment (Table 1) is represented by the condition of critical limb ischemia (CLI) (6).

Diagnosis of CLI is possible in the presence of pain at rest or ulceration or gangrene with or without ankle pressure less than 50 to 70 mm Hg or transcutaneous oxygen tension ($TcPO_2$) values lesser than 30 to 50 mm Hg (7).

In general, the development of CLI condition strictly depends on the efficiency of collateral circulation but, it has been fully demonstrated that in diabetics, the development and formation of collateral circulation is significantly reduced or absent and thus the majority of patients with CLI are diabetic (8–10).

As a consequence, it is also possible in a limited percentage of cases that diabetics may develop a condition of CLI, even in the presence of isolated obstruction of only one of their tibial arteries.

This condition rarely recognized if not foreseen, makes it quite impossible in some cases to identify the CLI presence, simply for the mere existence of at least one valid tibial pulse.

Only in 1984, thanks to a group of American vascular surgeons, was it possible to establish that the best treatment in diabetics with ischemic foot lesions was to provide direct flow to the foot arteries (11), but even now peripheral ischemia remains frequently undiagnosed.

The frequent false negative result of the ankle brachial index (ABI) measurement complicates even more the possibility of recognizing the condition of CLI particularly in diabetics, due to the poor compression of leg arteries for the presence of diffuse calcifications along their course.

It has been noticed, in fact, that an increase of the ABI index greater than 1.3 must be considered as a suspected false negative value in subjects with CLI.

Poorly diffused and utilized only in the area of diabetic foot centers is the $TcPO_2$ measurement that, however, represents one of the most important diagnostic tests in the demonstration of the CLI condition.

From a procedural point of view, the condition that complicates the treatment further, is the need to use the femoral approach for the endovascular recanalization of most tibial artery occlusions.

The antegrade approach, which offers conditions of absolute advantage with respect to the traditional crossover aortailiac technique, has not been sufficiently popularized over the last few years and limits the feasibility of extreme interventions, even today.

Moreover, the management of hemostasis subsequent to the antegrade approach is considered by some as difficult and a possible cause of complications (Table 2).

Table 1 Clinical Indications for the Treatment of Complex Lesions in Tibial–Peroneal Interventions

1. The avoidance of limb amputation or reducing the level of amputation when this proves to be unavoidable
2. The presence of pain at rest in patients with CLI, with or without ulceration. Due to the frequent coexistence of diabetic neuropathy, the presence of pain can vary consistently (12)
3. The presence of ischemic ulcerations that often represent the initial manifestation of a CLI condition
4. Further indication is represented by the presence of a healed ischemic ulceration in a persistent CLI condition to prevent ulcer recurrence
5. Symptomatic claudication, often absent due to the associated neuropathy (13), does not represent a possible indication in the absence of a CLI condition

CLI represents the most common indication for tibioperoneal interventions.

In reality, a correct antegrade puncture and catheterization technique and an appropriate learning curve determine a rate of complications absolutely comparable to that of the classic femoral retrograde approach.

Due to the reduced diameter of tibial vessels, often diffusely occluded and calcified, regular techniques in use for the femoral and popliteal recanalization segment do not have the same applications, leaving ample possibility in the utilization of techniques derived from angioplasty of coronary vessels.

Moreover, the requirement of sufficient experience in the use of coronary-type devices represents a further element of complexity in the tibial–peroneal interventions (Table 3).

Finally, the frequent coexistence of necrosis and infection requires the competence of a diabetic foot center for appropriate surgical treatment promoting wound healing and limb salvage.

Usually the revascularization precedes surgical foot care.

Along with normal risk conditions of endovascular procedures, such as renal failure, hematoma, bleeding, hemorrhage, dissection, and thrombosis at the puncture site, interventions in the tibial and peroneal segment present additional risks of accidental vessel perforation and rupture.

The risk of significant hemorrhage due to perforation is very low, as well as the possibility of partial vessel laceration or rupture even in case the dilatation is performed with a balloon of a diameter slightly bigger than the regular size of the vessel.

These conditions can be easily managed and treated with the application of a tourniquet around the trauma site, maintaining a pressure value greater than the systolic one and proceeding with reversed heparin therapy using protamine sulfate (14).

During the procedure, it is preferable to keep or maintain the guide inside the artery for an eventual continuation and completion of the treatment with balloon dilatation and stenting.

Other possible complications are embolization and thrombosis of the tibial–peroneal and foot vessels.

The formation of emboli could be relatively frequent in the presence of a fresh thrombus in a femoral or popliteal site.

Its treatment could be selective transcatheter lysis by urokinase infusion, or more commonly thrombus aspiration using a 5 to 6-F coronary guiding catheter.

In resistant cases, a stent implantation in the thrombus occluded site is advisable, for a quick re-establishment of the arterial flow.

Table 2 Hazards and Complications in Extreme Interventions

Complication	Cause	Incidence (%)	Treatment
Perforation	Guidewire	5	Tamponade (tourniquet)
Rupture	Balloon oversize	3	Tamponade (tourniquet)
Thrombosis	Insufficient heparinization	2	Full dose of heparin, frequent ACT assessment
Embolization	Wire catheter manipulation	2	Lysis, catheter aspiration
Spasm	Balloon inflation, guidewire	20	Selective nitroglycerin

Table 3 Interventional Tools

Special procedure	Device/s
Long tibial stenosis/occlusion crossing (regular)	Boston Sci. PT Graphic Super Support™.014 G.W., Invatec Ampirion Deep™ balloon
Long tibial stenosis/occlusion crossing (difficult)	Terumo 3 mm J tipped 0.035 G.W., Cordis 4 Fr Berenstein™ cath.
Long tibial stenosis/occlusion crossing (difficult)	Boston Sci. 0.035 straight G.W., Cordis 4 Fr Berenstein cath.
Stenting of long lesions (self-expandable nitinol stents)	Invatec Maris Deep™, Abbott Vascular Xpert™, Biotronic Astron Pulsar™
Stenting of proximal lesions (balloon expandable coronary stents)	Medtronic Driver™, Boston Sci. Taxus™
Kissing-balloon dilatation of bifurcation lesions	Medtronic Sprinter Legend™ coronary balloon
Atherectomy of bifurcation/ostial lesions	Ev3 Fox Hollow™
Focal hard lesions dilatation	Boston Sci. Cutting Balloon™ and Cordis 4 Fr Berenstein cath.
Re-entry maneuver after CTO subintimal crossing	Boston Sci. V18™ G.W.
Extremely hard lesions dilatation	Boston Sci. Quantum™ coronary balloon
Extremely tight lesion dilatation	Boston Sci. Maverick™ coronary balloon

Thrombosis of the tibial arterial vessels during the procedure is usually due to an insufficient heparinization. Prevention of such a condition can be obtained by the frequent monitoring of the activated coagulation time (ACT) during the procedure.

Our data on procedural complications (15,16) (L.G., unpublished data) referred to 1500 consecutive interventions in diabetics with CLI between 1998 and 2000 are:

Minor complications (no surgery or transfusion required): 6%
Major complications: 2%
Mortality: 0.2%

Preinterventional Diagnostic Workup

Only in less than 28% of cases the condition of CLI is sustained by an exclusive involvement of the tibial–peroneal arteries (17).

CLI conditions, particularly in the presence of ischemic ulcerations, are usually caused by multilevel involvement of the femoral, popliteal, and tibial–peroneal segments.

The approach to the endovascular treatment of tibial vessel obstruction must be chosen in order to allow for easy manoeuvrability of catheters, guides, and other devices. The antegrade femoral approach is the best solution for this purpose.

MRI and TC angiography and Doppler ultrasound examinations are useful preliminary tests to detect the anatomical complexity of a planned procedure.

In the absence of iliac arteries lesions, since 1998 in our centers, the procedure has always begun with the performance of a direct antegrade femoral angiography using a 19 G single-wall needle to establish the best entry site for intervention.

Then we proceed with the advancement of a short angled 0.035 Teflon-coated guidewire along the first segment of the superficial femoral artery and then with the positioning of a 5 to 6-F vascular introducer.

Interventional Strategies

In the presence of multilevel lesions, the initial procedure is to cross the proximal lesions as far as reaching the dorsalis pedis artery, or plantar artery, or in cases where this is not possible, the peroneal artery (PA).

During the procedure, 5000 UI of sodium heparin is injected.

Crossing the tibial vessel obstructions is usually performed by a 0.014 coronary-type guidewire and low-profile over-the-wire (OTW) balloon catheters with the diameter of the balloon selected on the basis of the diameter of the most distal segment to be dilated (Fig. 1).

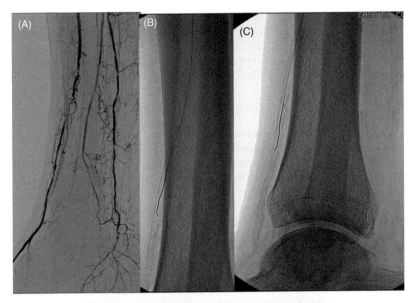

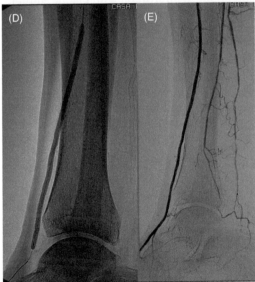

Figure 1 (A) Anterior tibial artery (AT) occlusion in a diabetic with ischemic foot ulcer. (B–D) The occlusion was crossed with a 0.014 coronary wire followed by balloon angioplasty dilatation using a 3.0 × 120 mm Amphirion Deep balloon. (E) Optimal final result. The ulcer healed after some weeks.

The broad selections of .014-inch dedicated wire systems for chronic total occlusions in coronary systems offer versatile solutions in below the knee lesions and are utilized in following techniques:

Controlled drilling: the guide wire is advanced using gentle movements.

Sliding technique with controlled drilling: very lubricious polymer covered guide wires are used to slide through narrow lesions or functional occlusions.

Penetration technique: penetrating the obstruction aiming at the target. The direction of the guide wire is more precisely controlled. Tapered tip guide wires permit higher penetrating forces but the following balloon advancement could be very difficult due to increased friction under calcified plaques.

Alternative techniques are the use of the 4-F diagnostic Berenstein catheter and a straight 0.035 Teflon-coated guidewire, replaced by a 3 mm J tipped 0.035 Terumo wire if a subintimal recanalization is required.

In all patients with multilevel lesions, the first vessel to be treated must be the most distal, which is usually represented by one of the two tibial vessels, to get direct flow to the foot at the completion of the procedure.

Ideally direct flow should be assured along the tibial and foot artery that supplies the ischemic lesion, when present.

Alternative techniques such as plantar arch crossing, collateral dilatation (Fig. 2) or retrograde tibial artery recanalization, can represent possible options (18,19).

Whenever possible, the goal of the procedure is to get direct flow to the dorsalis pedis artery in case of toe lesions or to the plantar artery in case of calcanear lesions.

The most common and effective technique for below-the-knee (BTK) revascularization is transluminal angioplasty using the new generation of OTW low-profile long balloons.

These very low profile and tapered to 0.014 balloons could be used over the several specialized coronary-type guidewires available, with a 70% of successful recanalization of chronically occluded tibial–peroneal arteries.

Elective or provisional stenting is used in case of:

1. complex lesions that involve the bifurcation of the popliteal artery (Fig. 3);
2. lesions of tibial arteries ostium and popliteal bifurcation with plaque shifting (Fig. 4);
3. persistent recoiling of proximal tibial arteries lesions;
4. short embolus not amenable to selective thrombolysis or aspiration thrombectomy;
5. extensive flow-limiting dissection;
6. elective stenting in stenosis of bypass graft anastomosis and ostial lesions (Fig. 5).

The new generation of self-expandable nitinol stents designed for use in tibial vessels has expanded the indications in obstructions of considerable lengths, and particularly in the case of lesion recurrence after balloon angioplasty, but their long-term result is under evaluation.

Normally, balloon expandable stent implantation is avoided in foot arteries and medium distal tibial vessels due to the concrete risk of stent crushing after ABI measurement or physical examination with pulse palpation.

A possible alternative to stenting in proximal bifurcation lesion is the kissing-balloon dilatation (Fig. 6)

Direct atherectomy using the Fox Hollow™ device (20) can be considered appropriate in the case of eccentric plaques, complex lesions of popliteal bifurcation involving the origin of tibial branches, and in-stent restenosis in BTK arteries (Fig. 7).

In these lesions, encouraging results have been achieved using drug-eluting coronary-type stent (DES) implantation (21). The frequently diffuse tibial artery obstructive involvement in a typically multilevel disease limits the use of DES to short lesions in proximal segments, without the privilege of ascribing the clinical result to this otherwise crucial device as in the coronary tree.

The most effective technique in tibial–peroneal segments is balloon angioplasty dilatation.

General rules for its performance are well established (22–31) and are represented by the following:

1. Prolonged dilatations, greater than three minutes.
2. Gradual high-pressure balloon inflation.
3. The balloon diameter at the maximum inflation pressure must be similar or slightly exceed the normal vessel size.
4. The length of the balloon must approach or slightly exceed the length of the lesion.

Cutting balloon dilatation (Fig. 8), laser recanalization, and cryoplasty balloon dilatation are alternative techniques that have to be tested in large series of CLI patients (32–34).

The common multilevel disease of CLI also means that, in case of endovascular treatment, different techniques and devices are used during the same procedure.

Therefore, studies specifically addressing a single technique and/or device in subjects with CLI could depend on the concomitant treatment of other vascular segments with different

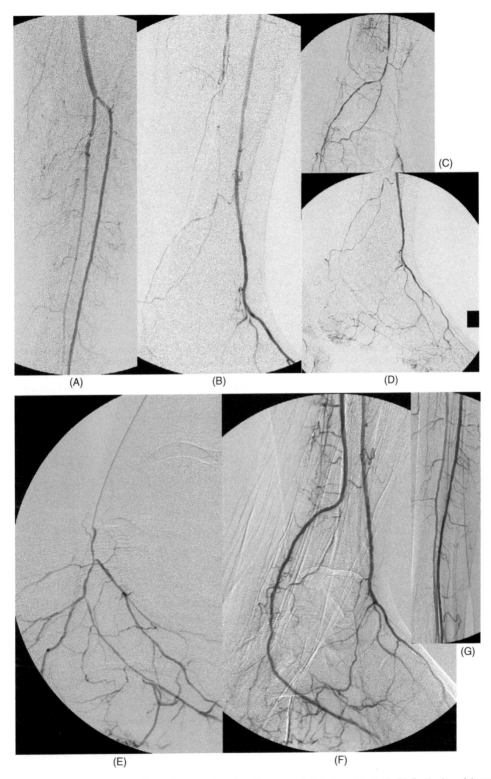

Figure 2 Ischemic nonhealing calcanear ulcer in a 60-year-old diabetic patient. (**A–D**) Occlusion of the posterior tibial (PT) artery and stenosis of the peroneal artery (PA). Typical appearance of lack of collaterals formation in posterior aspect of the foot. (**E–G**) A 0.014-coronary support wire was advanced along the PA and its posterior perforating branch to reach the plantar artery. Final balloon dilatation using the 3.0 × 120 mm Amphirion Deep balloon with direct flow to the plantar artery. The lesion healed after ulcerectomy.

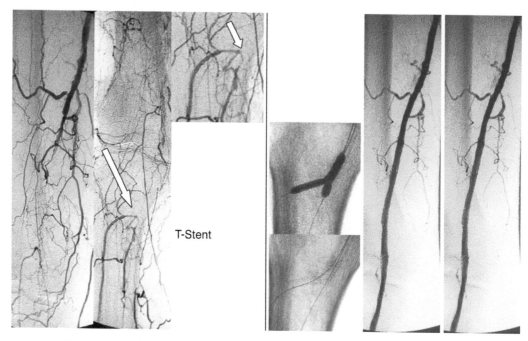

T-Stent

Figure 3 Complex femoral popliteal and ostial tibial recanalization in a 76-year-old man; diabetes, ischemic ulcer, and dry gangrene of the right forefoot. To maintain the patency of both AT and PA ostium (arrow), a T-stent implantation was performed using two Medtronic chromium–cobalt 3.5-mm coronary stents. The stent for the AT was implanted first followed by the second with final kissing-balloon inflation. A 12-cm long nitinol stent was implanted in the fem–pop segment. CLI was relieved and the patient underwent a transmetatarsal amputation with limb salvage.

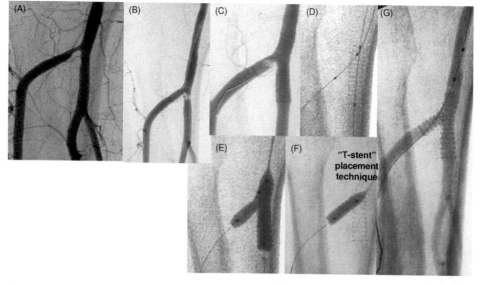

Figure 4 (**A–G**) A 49-year-old woman patient with diabetes, with smoking background, who had ischemic nonhealing ulcer of the great toe. Ostial, noncalcified soft stenosis of the AT, prone to prolapse into the tibioperoneal (TP) trunk. This was the case after 3.5 mm balloon dilatation, with plaque shifting into the trunk. This kind of bifurcation lesion required a 4.0- and 3.5-mm Medtronic chromium–cobalt coronary stent in TP trunk and AT, respectively, with final kissing-balloon dilatation. The lesion healed in two weeks.

STENTING

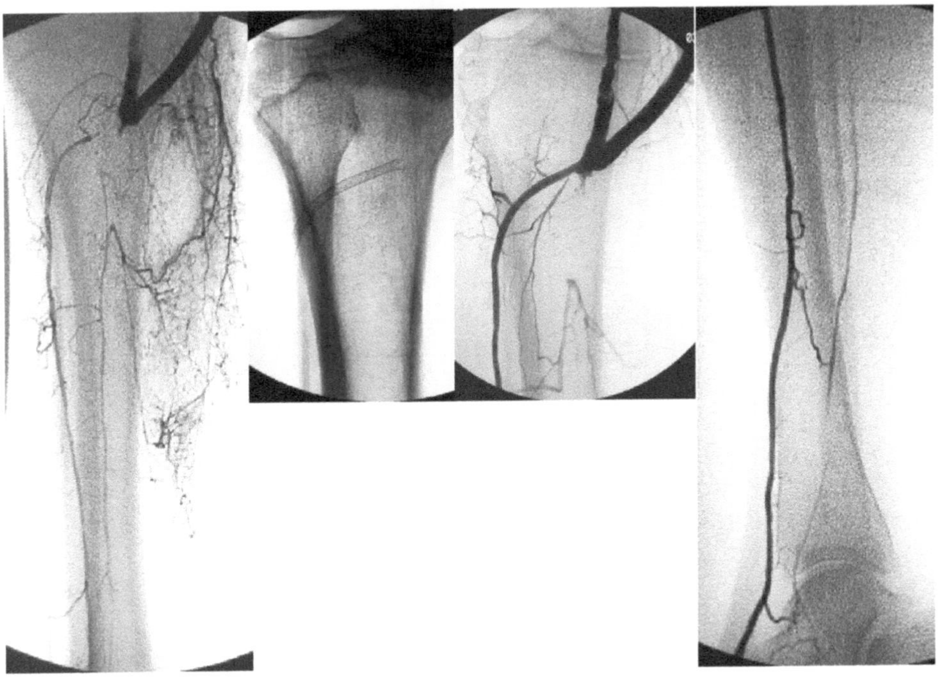

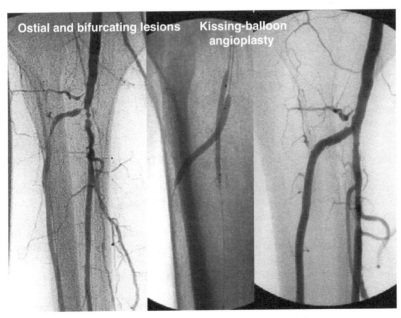

Figure 5 Persistent CLI and foot lesion in a 69-year-old diabetic patient with a normally patent fem–pop bypass graft. Occlusion of the distal anastomosis. Procedure: antegrade approach, AT occlusion was crossed with an extra support hydrophilic coronary wire and 3.5 mm coronary balloon, Magic Wallstent® deployment. Final balloon dilatation. The lesion healed after one month.

Ostial and bifurcating lesions   Kissing-balloon angioplasty

Figure 6 Kissing-balloon dilatation of a true bifurcate lesion of the TP trunk using two 3.0 × 40 mm Amphirion Deep balloons inflated at 14 atm. Perfect final angiographic result.

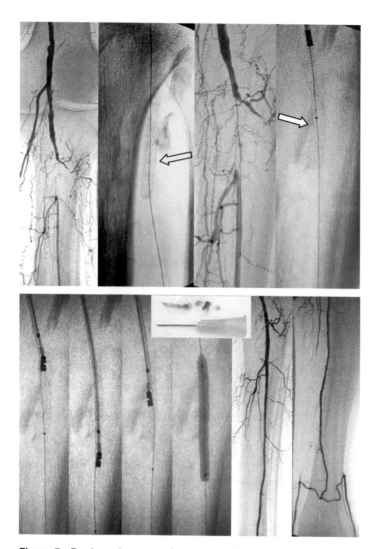

Figure 7 Previous placement of a bare metal stent in the TP trunk of a 62-year-old claudicant, nondiabetic, smoker. The stent (arrows) occluded after three months. The sequence shows a 0.014 wire crossing the occlusion followed by intimal hyperplasia removal using the Fox Hollow atherotome (fragments in a box). Final 4.0 mm Amphirion Deep balloon dilatation.

techniques. This has to be considered when judging the real impact of a single technique/device on outcome.

The interest in testing new endovascular solutions to be used in the tibioperoneal territory makes urgent the need of appropriate evaluation criteria to assess the benefit on clinical outcome and the long-term patency of the treated vessels.

The new criteria should consider new morphologic classifications (17) to stratify the patients in classes of homogeneous vascular involvement and appropriate clinical and instrumental measurement of the result.

The goal of extreme intervention in patients with CLI is in fact not long-term patency, but rather the avoidance of a major amputation.

Even in subjects with end-stage renal disease (ESRD) and chronic dialysis, extreme interventions showed to be feasible and effective (Table 4), with a limb salvage rate similar to the highest reported in literature for surgical series (35). These patients have an increased risk of CLI and limb loss and are accompanied by diffuse vascular calcifications and involvement of distal infrapopliteal and foot arteries that makes extreme interventions challenging.

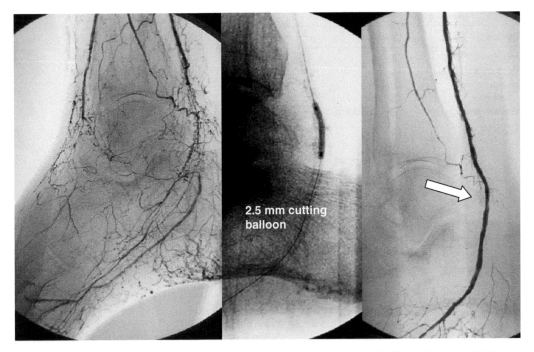

Figure 8 ESRD, 61-year-old dialyzed male. CLI and dry gangrene of the foot. Multilevel disease with tibial and foot arteries calcified stenoses and occlusions. Initial attempt of complete PT and plantar artery recanalization using the Amphirion Deep balloon and a high-pressure coronary balloon at 20 atm was ineffective, due to the presence of an extremely hard focal lesion. A 2.5-mm cutting balloon was then inflated at 18 atm with good result. The patient underwent only a transmetatarsal amputation with limb salvage.

A strict cooperation with a specialized foot center is crucial in obtaining the best results.

Although restenosis rates of 40% to 50% can be expected in these patients, due to lesion diffusion in a typical multilevel disease, limb salvage can be achieved in more than 90% of cases, primarily dependent on restoration of straight-line flow to the foot.

Furthermore, as in surgical practice, clinical and instrumental follow-up surveillance and subsequent early reintervention in case of restenosis can prolong long-term patency and the clinical benefit.

Repeat intervention, much less invasive if compared to surgical options, performed to enhance secondary patency is probably underused, even if well tolerated and often done on an outpatient basis. A list of recommended devices for complex cases is reported in Table 5.

Table 4 Results of Endovascular Treatment of Combined Tibio-peroneal and Femoropopliteal Lesions in Subjects with CLI

Author	Patients/ lesions	Technical success %	Mortality %	Limb salvage %	Primary patency
Faglia 2005	993 (1,191)	83	0.1	88 (5 yrs)	—
Dorros 2001	270	91	0.4	91 (5 yrs)	—
Lofberg 1996	94	88	2.4	72 (3 yrs)	—
Soder 2000	72	74	—	80 (18 mo)	48%, (18 mo)
Brillu 2001	37	94.5	—	87 (2 yrs)	—
Rand 2006	37/57	—	2.0	98 (6 mo)	61-83%, (6 mo)
Staffa 2003	18	—	—	—	78%, (6 mo)
Matsagas 2003	67	88	4.0	98 (3 yrs)	52%, (2 yrs)
Balmer 2002	66	—	—	94 (12 mo)	44%, (1 yr)
Ferraresi 2009	107	98	—	93 (3 yrs)	42%, (1 yr)

Source: Modified from Ref. 6.

Table 5 Recommended Devices for Complex Tibioperoneal Interventions

Device	Company	Type	Code
Needle	Cordis	19 G	502–654
Vascular introducer	Terumo	Regular	RS B50K10MQ
Multipurpose catheter	Cordis	Berenstein 4-F	451–415 HO
Guidewire	Boston Scientific	Coronary stiff	14905-01
		Coronary intermediate	14902-01
		Short 0.035	49–209
		0.035 support exchange	46–592
		0.035 straight	49–150
		0.018 V18™	46–852
	Medtronic	Couguar™	CGRXT190HS
		Zinger™	ZNGRS180HS
		Persuader™	9PSDR180HS
	Terumo	0.035 angled	RFGA35153M
		0.035 angled stiff	RFHR35183M
		0.035 3 mm J	RFPA35183M
Guiding catheter	Medtronic	6-F	LA6SR60
Angioplasty balloons	Invatec	OTW long balloons	Amphirion Deep™ series
	Boston Scientific	RX coronary, regular and high pressure	Maverick™ series, Quantum™ series
		Cutting Balloon™	BPM125015B
	Medtronic	RX coronary, regular	Sprinter Legend™ series
	Abbott	OTW small vessels 0.018	82156-54-01
Stent	Invatec	Small vessels	Maris Deep™ series
	Abbott	Small vessels	X-Pert™ series
	Biotronic	Small vessels	Astron Pulsar™ series
	Boston Scientific	RX coronary DES	Taxus™ coronary stent series
	Medtronic	RX coronary	Driver™ series
Atherotome	Ev3	Small vessels	Fox Hollow™ series

PART 2: TEACHING CASES

Case 1: Retrograde Recanalization of the Plantar and Distal Posterior Tibial Artery Through the Plantar Arch (18) [Fig. 9(A)–9(K)]. Case Description in the Text.

a. What made the lesion "complex" in this specific case? The calcanear ischemic ulcer is a well-established possible cause of limb loss in diabetics. The AT was occluded proximally, the dorsalis pedis artery was normal, and the PA was very thin and diffusely stenosed/occluded with the absence of well-developed collaterals to be used in order to reach the plantar artery with alternative techniques. The posterior tibial (PT) was diffusely occluded, but the plantar branch was patent [Fig. 9(A)–9(C)]. It was impossible to reopen the PT by the classic retrograde technique. In this case, there was a typical lack of sufficient collateral formation (8–10) toward the posterior aspect of the foot so that it was urged PT and plantar arteries revascularization. The possibility of a femoral-distal saphenous bypass graft using the distal PT was also considered, but due to the presence of a large calcanear infected wound this hypothesis was excluded by vascular surgeons.

b. What was the clinical indication for treatment of this specific case? The clinical indication was the presence of a large ischemic infected calcanear ulcer in a diabetic subject. TcPO$_2$ was 20 at the dorsum of the foot but probably did not reflect the ischemia in the posterior aspect of the foot. There was a high risk of major amputation in eventual failure of intervention.

c. What were the potential hazards of treating this specific patient and this lesion? There is a potential risk of dissection during the plantar arch crossing using the coronary-type support

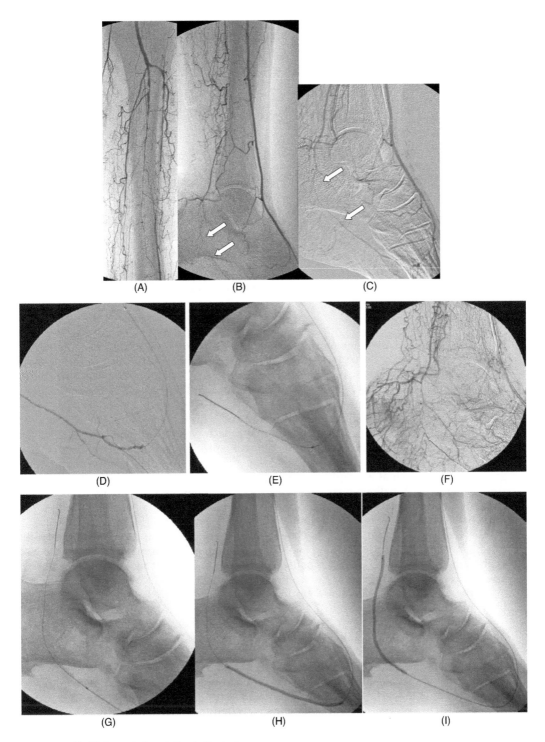

Figure 9 (**A–K**) Case 1, description in the text.

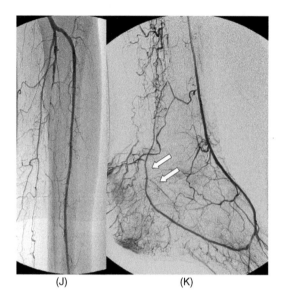

(J)   (K)   **Figure 9**   *(Continued)*

wire. Crossing the plantar arch requires a complete angiographic study of the segment and careful manipulation of the 0.014 wire in order to promptly reach the plantar artery without inducing spasm or dissection. Intra-arterial nitroglycerine injection could prevent the spasm. During the balloon inflation, there is a risk of rupture of the plantar artery with possible plantar hematoma formation.

d.   Which interventional strategies were considered and which interventional tools were used to handle this lesion? The antegrade femoral approach was the only one considered. The contralateral crossover technique does not allow the precise manipulation maneuvers necessary to cross tibial arteries occlusions. A 5-F regular introducer sheath was placed at the groin. The intraluminal attempt to reopen the PT was done using both the 2.0 × 80 mm Amphirion Deep™ balloon over a 0.014 PT Graphic Super Support™ wire and the 0.035 straight wire inside a 4-F Berenstein catheter. The procedure was unsuccessful due to the unfavorable anatomy. Subintimal technique was not taken into consideration in this case for the risk of arterial rupture. The same balloon was then directed to the AT ostium and the 0.014 wire carefully advanced along the AT occlusion in an intraluminal fashion. Followed by the balloon, the wire crossed part of the plantar arch and a direct angiogram of the plantar artery was taken injecting 50% dilute contrast through the balloon catheter [Fig. 9(D)].

The wire was then advanced up to the distal third of the PT and a dilatation was performed at 14 atm [Fig. 9(E)–9(I)]. Proximal TP was dilated using an Amphirion Deep™ 3 × 120 mm inflated at 14 atm. The control angiogram showed a good result with direct flow to the distal PT and plantar artery and clear evidence of the inflammatory hyperemia around the wound [Fig. 9(J) and 9(K)].

e.   Summary: How was the case managed, is there anything that could have been improved, what was the immediate and long-term outcome? Antiplatelet thyenopiridine therapy was maintained indefinitely. The pain at rest immediately ceased and two days after the patient was admitted to a specialized foot center for ulcerectomy and conservative cares. The wound completely healed after three months.

f.   List of contemporary equipments that should be used in this case:
   ○   Selective catheter (4-F Berenstein type)
   ○   Guidewire 0.035 (regular, teflon coated)
   ○   Guidewire 0.014 (PT Graphic Super Support™)
   ○   Long balloon (Amphirion Deep™ OTW)

g.   Key learning issues of this specific case: Retrograde recanalization of the plantar artery is a well-established technique in case of failure of the antegrade PT recanalization.

Case 2: Retrograde Pedal Access (38) for Anterior Tibial Artery Recanalization [Fig. 10(A)–10(M)]. Case Description in the Text.

a. What made the lesion "complex" in this specific case? In this case of ischemic diabetic left great toe ulcer, the PT was diffusely occluded with no visible stump to attempt an antegrade recanalization. The AT was occluded near its origin, showing a truly unfavorable anatomy due to the presence of a well-developed collateral branch running along the occlusion. There was diffuse disease of AT downward but a normally patent dorsalis pedis artery [Fig. 10(A)–10(C)]. Alternative technique using transluminal angioplasty of PA branches was not considered in this case for the poor development of the anterior perforating branch of the PA (19). Several attempts made to cross the AT occlusion intraluminally had failed. No subintimal attempt was done for the risk of collateral branch rupture requiring therapeutic AT embolization and/or the procedure abortion.

b. What was the clinical indication for treatment of this specific case? In case of CLI and foot lesions in diabetics, a normally perfused PA cannot improve the TcPO$_2$ values significantly, due to the frequent lack of efficient collateral formation (8–10). In this case, TcPO$_2$ was 28. Direct flow to one of the foot arteries is often necessary for limb salvage in diabetics (11), therefore every effort should be made to provide direct flow to foot arteries.

As an alternative, a possible femoral dorsalis pedis bypass graft surgery was not considered due to the previous utilization of the saphena veins in a prior coronary bypass surgery.

c. What were the potential hazards of treating this specific patient and this lesion? During the dorsalis pedis artery puncture attempt, the vessel could be damaged with possible dissection or thrombosis, compromising any further interventions and/or possible bypass surgery alternatives.

d. Which interventional strategies were considered and which interventional tools were used to handle this lesion? The antegrade femoral approach was the only strategy considered. The contralateral crossover technique does not allow for the precise manipulation maneuvers necessary to cross tibial arteries occlusions. A 5-F regular introducer sheath was placed at the groin and an OTW 2 × 40 mm Amphirion Deep™ balloon was advanced in the proximal AT over a PT Graphic Super Support™ wire and several attempts were made to cross the occlusion unsuccessfully. Considering the complete patency and the good size of the dorsalis pedis artery, the dorsum of the foot was scrubbed for a retrograde pedal access using regular 19 G single-wall needle and a short customized angled tip 0.035 Boston Scientific wire. A smaller needle was not selected in this case of slowly perfused distal artery, for the possible scarce evidence of backflow and the difficult maneuverability of the necessary 0.021 wire in tortuous segments. Under fluoro guidance during contrast injection from the groin, the dorsalis pedis artery was punctured and a 4-F Pediatric introducer (Terumo) was placed [Fig. 10(D) and 10(E)]. The 0.014 PT Graphic SS™ wire was then advanced to cross the AT occlusion [Fig. 10(F) and 10 (G)]. The procedure was accomplished but with difficulty. A complete AT dilatation was performed from below, using a 3 × 120 mm Amphirion Deep™ balloon inflated at 12 atm with good final result [Fig. 10 (H)–10(K)]. Both sheaths were then removed with final moderate compression on the pedal entry site.

e. Summary: How was the case managed, is there anything that could have been improved, what was the immediate and long-term outcome? A residual focal moderate stenosis remained proximally, even with prolonged dilatation [Fig. 10(H) and 10(I)]. Stent placement was not taken into consideration as the stenosis did not limit the flow significantly and because no definite dates are available on stent use in the tibial territory. Antiplatelet thyenopiridine therapy was maintained indefinitely. The pain at rest immediately ceased and the lesion healed after three weeks of conservative care. A month later at the time of the right leg intervention, an antegrade angiogram through the 19 G needle was performed showing a persistent good result [Fig. 10(L) and 10(M)]. The dorsalis pedis pulse was normal on physical examination.

f. List of contemporary equipments that should be used in this case:
   ○ Guidewire 0.014 (PT Graphic Super Support™)
   ○ Long balloon (Amphirion Deep™ OTW)
   ○ Vascular introducer (Terumo, pediatric type 4-F)

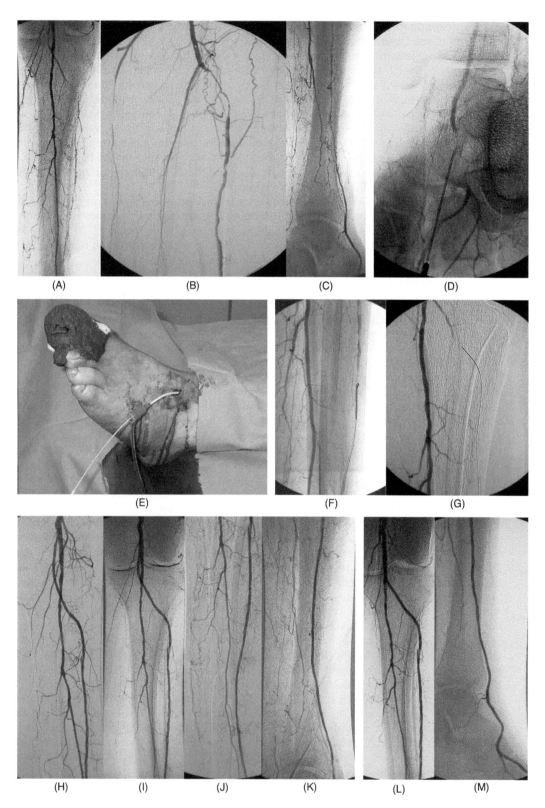

Figure 10 (**A–M**) Case 2, description in the text.

g. Key learning issues of this specific case: According to our experience, classic antegrade recanalization of chronically occluded tibioperoneal arteries could be successfully performed in more than 70% of cases. Only in few selected cases with good-size pedal arteries and good distal run-off, a retrograde approach through the dorsalis pedis or distal PT arteries should be considered. The retrograde pedal access could not represent a regular alternative in case of frequent failure in crossing the occlusions from above, due to lack of operator's skill and experience. Careful procedure performance and meticulous arterial puncture is usually required. The placement of a 4-F pediatric introducer is always advisable, in order to prevent complications at the entry site, to allow easy insertion of most devices, thus avoiding the requirement of complicate maneuvers in converting the retrograde into the antegrade approach, from above.

Case 3: Antegrade Recanalization of a Chronically Occluded Anterior Tibial and Dorsalis Pedis Arteries [Fig. 11(A)–11(F)]. Case Description in the Text.

a. What made the lesion "complex" in this specific case? Complete occlusion of most AT and complete occlusion of the entire dorsalis pedis artery are conditions that usually prevent the attempt of endovascular treatment even in the presence of an experienced operator. In addition, the PT and the origin of the plantar artery were occluded [Fig. 11(A)–11(C)]. The presence of ischemic changes, mostly in the forefoot area, could be normally approached even with a PT and plantar artery recanalization, but several attempts made with different techniques had failed. As in most diabetics, providing direct flow to the PA is rarely sufficient in the presence of CLI and initial foot lesions. In this case, the absence of well evident medial calcifications along the occluded segments represented an adjunctive drawback during intervention performance.

b. What was the clinical indication for treatment of this specific case? CLI, pain at rest, border-line forefoot lesion, and TcPO$_2$ of 15 in a diabetic patient with the absence of tibial pulses at Duplex scanning represented the indications for intervention. No surgical alternatives were considered due to the absence of recipient vessel in the foot. Novel alternative techniques such as balloon angioplasty PA collaterals recanalization (19) were also considered due to the apparent favorable anatomy of the posterior perforating branch. After a brief discussion, the first option remained the antegrade recanalization of the AT and dorsalis pedis arteries, as most plausible.

c. What were the potential hazards of treating this specific patient and this lesion? The most important risk to consider was the failure of the endovascular procedure in association with the worsening of symptoms and thus possible indication of leg amputation.

d. Which interventional strategies were considered and which interventional tools were used to handle this lesion? The antegrade femoral approach was the only one considered. The contralateral crossover technique does not allow the precise manipulation maneuvers necessary to cross tibial arteries occlusions. A 5-F regular introducer sheath was placed at the groin and an OTW 2 × 80 mm Amphirion Deep™ balloon was advanced in the proximal AT over a PT Graphic Super Support™ wire. Careful advancement of the catheter wire system using alternate oblique views was made, in order to keep the wire aligned to the expected course of the AT and dorsalis pedis arteries. Finally but surprisingly the wire tip slides into the plantar arch and its position was confirmed by contrast injection from the introducer. A balloon dilatation of the distal segment was performed at 15 atm. A 2.5 × 120 mm Amphirion Deep™ balloon inflated at 14 atm was used for the AT. A good final angiographic result was achieved with the complete revascularization, and direct flow to the plantar arch was acquired [Fig. 11(D)–11(F)].

e. Summary: How was the case managed, is there anything that could have been improved, what was the immediate and long-term outcome? Antiplatelet thyenopiridine therapy was maintained indefinitely. There was an immediate improvement in foot vascularization with cessation of ischemic symptoms. The clinical result was maintained during six months follow-up.

f. List of contemporary equipments that should be used in this case:
   o Guidewire 0.014 (PT Graphic Super Support™)
   o Long balloon (Amphirion Deep™ OTW)
   o Vascular introducer (Terumo, pediatric type 4-F)

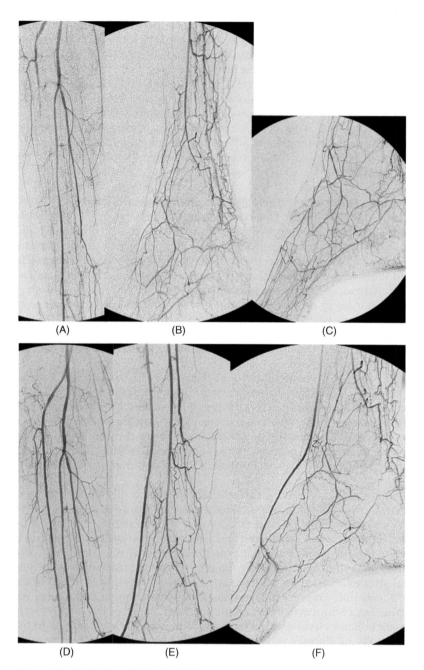

(A)   (B)   (C)

(D)   (E)   (F)

Figure 11   (**A–F**) Case 3, description in the text.

g. Key learning issues of this specific case: Chronically hypoperfused arteries may reduce their lumen completely to favor the flow redistribution along the residual patent conduits, as the PA circulation in this particular case. In this case, the phenomena could have lead to the evidence of the false complete dorsalis pedis artery occlusion that was in fact easily reopened after intervention. Preliminary angiography can fail in assessing the real status of peripheral circulation, giving an excessive pessimistic picture that can influence the final operators' decision.

REFERENCES

1. International Diabetes Federation. Diabetes Atlas, 2000. Economist 2000; 8196:132.
2. Diabetes-related amputations of lower extremities in the Medicare population of Minnesota, 1993–1995. MMWR Morb Mortal Wkly Rep 1998; 47:649–652.
3. Levin ME. Preventing amputation in the patient with diabetes. Diabetes Care 1995; 18:1383–1394.
4. Apelqvist J, Bakker K, van Houtum WH, et al. International consensus and practical guidelines on the management and the prevention of the diabetic foot. International Working Group on the Diabetic Foot. Diabetes Metab Res Rev 2000; 16(suppl 1):S84–S92.
5. Dormandy JA, Rutherford RB. Management of peripheral arterial disease. TASC Working Group. J Vasc Surg 2000; 31(suppl):S1–S296.
6. Graziani L, Piaggesi A. Indications and clinical outcomes for below knee endovascular therapy. Catheter Cardiovasc Interv 2010; 75:433–443.
7. Norgren L, Hiatt WR, Dormandy JA, et al; on behalf of the TASC II Working Group. Inter-society consensus for the management of peripheral arterial disease (TASC II). Eur J Vasc Endovasc Surg 2007; 33:S1–S75.
8. Abaci A, Kahraman S, Eryol NK, et al. Effect of diabetes mellitus on formation of coronary collateral vessels. Circulation 1999; 99:2239–2242.
9. Waltenberger J. Impaired collateral vessel development in diabetes: potential cellular mechanisms and therapeutic implications. Cardiovasc Res 2001; 49(3):554–560.
10. Weihrauch D, Lohr NL, Mraovic B, et al. Chronic hyperglycaemia attenuates coronary collateral development and impairs proliferative properties of myocardial interstitial fluid by production of angiostatin. Circulation 2004; 109:2343–2348.
11. LoGerfo FW, Coffman JD. Vascular and microvascular disease in the diabetic foot: Implications for foot care. N Engl J Med 1984; 311:1615–1619.
12. Faglia E, Favales F, Aldeghi A, et al. Change in major amputation rate in a center dedicated to diabetic foot care during the 1980s: prognostic determinants for major amputation. J Diabet Complications 1998; 12:96–102.
13. Faglia E, Favales F, Morabito A. New ulceration, new major amputation, and survival rates in diabetic subjects hospitalized for foot ulceration from 1990 to 1993. Diabetes Care 2001; 24:78–83.
14. Minar E, Graziani L. Complications in tibioperoneal interventions. In: Shillinger M, Minar E, eds. Complications in Peripheral Vascular Interventions. London: Informa UK Ltd, 2007:201–207.
15. Faglia E, Dalla Paola L, Clerici G, et al. Peripheral angioplasty as the first-choice revascularization procedure in diabetic patients with critical limb ischemia: prospective study of 993 consecutive patients hospitalized and followed between 1999 and 2003. Eur J Vasc Endovasc Surg 2005; 29: 620–627.
16. Graziani L. Unpublished data.
17. Graziani L, Silvestro A, Bertone V, et al. Vascular involvement in diabetic subjects with ischemic foot ulcer: a new morphologic categorization of disease severity. Eur J Vasc Endovasc Surg 2007; 33: 453–460.
18. Graziani L, Silvestro A. Clinical vision. 17:2-7, Gosling ed. UK, April 2006.
19. Graziani L, Silvestro A, Monge L, et al. Transluminal angioplasty of peroneal artery branches in diabetics: initial technical experience. Cardiovasc Interv Radiol 2008; 31(1):49–55.
20. Kandzari DE, Kiesz RS, Allie D, et al. Procedural and clinical outcomes with catheter-based plaque excision in critical limb ischemia. J Endovasc Ther 2006; 13:12–22.
21. Rosales OR, Mathewkutty S, Gnaim C. Drug eluting stents for below the knee lesions in patients with critical limb ischemia: long-term follow-up [published online ahead of print April 15, 2008]. Catheter Cardiovasc Interv.
22. Sarembock IJ, LaVeau PJ, Sigal SL, et al. Influence of inflation pressure and balloon size on the development of intimal hyperplasia after balloon angioplasty. A study in the atherosclerotic rabbit. Circulation 1989; 80:1029–1040.
23. Nichols AB, Smith R, Berke AD, et al. Importance of balloon size in coronary angioplasty. J Am Coll Cardiol 1989; 13(5):1094–1100.
24. Ilia R, Cabin H, McConnell S, et al. Coronary angioplasty with gradual versus rapid balloon inflation: initial results and complications. Cathet Cardiovasc Diagn 1993; 29(3):199–202.
25. Ohman EM, Marquis JF, Ricci DR, et al. A randomized comparison of the effects of gradual prolonged versus standard primary balloon inflation on early and late outcome. Results of a multicenter clinical trial. Perfusion Balloon Catheter Study Group. Circulation 1994; 89:1118–1125.
26. Eltchaninoff H, Cribier A, Koning R, et al. Effects of prolonged sequential balloon inflations on results of coronary angioplasty. Am J Cardiol 1996; 77(12):1062–1066.
27. Hering D, Haude M, Caspari G, et al. Effect of high insufflation pressures on elastic recoil forces and vascular resistance after balloon dilatation. Z Kardiol 1996; 85(4):273–280.

28. Schmitz HJ, Erbel R, Meyer J, et al. Influence of vessel dilatation on restenosis after successful percu-taneous transluminal coronary angioplasty. Am Heart J 1996; 131(5):884–891.
29. Manninen HI, Soder HK, Matsi PJ, et al. Prolonged dilation improves an unsatisfactory primary result of femoropopliteal artery angioplasty: usefulness of a perfusion balloon catheter. J Vasc Interv Radiol 1997; 8(4):627–632.
30. Miketic S, Carlsson J, Tebbe U. Influence of gradually increased slow balloon inflation on restenosis after coronary angioplasty. Am Heart J 1998; 135(4):709–713.
31. Soder HK, Manninen HI, Rasanen HT, et al. Failure of prolonged dilation to improve long-term patency of femoropopliteal artery angioplasty: results of a prospective trial. J Vasc Interv Radiol 2002; 13(4):361–369.
32. Ansel GM, Sample NS, Botti CF, et al. Cutting balloon angioplasty of the popliteal and infrapopliteal vessels for symptomatic limb ischemia. Cathet Cardiovasc Interv 2004; 61:1–4.
33. Laird JR, Zeller T, Gray BH, et al. Limb salvage following laser-assisted angioplasty for critical limb ischemia: results of the LACI multicenter trial. J Endovasc Ther 2006; 13:1–11.
34. Zvonimir K. CryoPlasty for treatment of popliteal and tibioperoneal disease. Endovasc Today 2006; 12(suppl):S13–S15.
35. Graziani L, Silvestro A, Bertone V, et al. Percutaneous transluminal angioplasty is feasible and effective in patients on chronic dialysis with severe peripheral artery disease. Nephrol Dial Transplant 2007; 22(4):1144–1149.
36. Dorros G, Jaff MR, Dorros AM, et al. Tibioperoneal (outflow lesion) angioplasty can be used as a primary treatment in 235 patients with critical limb ischemia: five-year follow-up. Circulation 2001; 104:2057–2062.
37. Lofberg AM, Lorelius LE, Karacagil S, et al. The use of below-knee percutaneous transluminal angio-plasty in arterial occlusive disease casing chronic critical limb ischemia. Cardiovasc Interv Radiol 1996; 19:317–322.
38. Soder HK, Manninen HI, Jaakkola P, et al. Prospective trial of infrapopliteal artery balloon angioplasty for critical limb ischemia: angiographic and clinical results. J Vasc Interv Radiol 2000; 11:1021–1031.
39. Brillu C, Picquet J, Villapdierna F, et al. Percutaneous transluminal angioplasty for management of critical limb ischemia in arteries below the knee. Ann Vasc Surg 2001; 15:175–181.
40. Botti CF, Ansel GM, Silver MJ, et al. Percutaneous retrograde tibial access in limb salvage. J Endovasc Ther 2003; 10(3):614–618.

17 | Dialysis Fistulas

Patrick Haage

Department of Diagnostic and Interventional Radiology, HELIOS Klinikum Wuppertal, University Hospital Witten/Herdecke, Wuppertal, Germany

Dierk Vorwerk

Department of Diagnostic and Interventional Radiology, Klinikum Ingolstadt, Ingolstadt, Germany

PART 1: INTRODUCTION

Dysfunction of arteriovenous (AV) fistulae is a problem frequently encountered in the hemodialysis patient. Since the number of patients with end-stage renal disease treated by hemodialysis is rising gradually (1), the selection of an adequate treatment technique to maintain vascular access is of utmost importance for patient and physician. Today, the interventional procedure is considered a valid and sometimes superior alternative to surgical revision, being safe, easy to perform, and clinically successful. Literature does not show a significant discrepancy pertaining to technical outcome, complication rate, and follow-up patency rates when surgery and intervention are evaluated (2–4).

WHAT MAKES A LESION "COMPLEX" WHEN TREATING DIALYSIS FISTULAS?

There are typical situations that render the percutaneous intervention complex, for example, long-segment thromboses, older occlusions, and manifold operated patients with a confusing vascular anatomy. Often it is not until the diagnostic angiography that the interventionalist can realize the complexity of the case at hand.

CLINICAL INDICATIONS FOR TREATMENT OF COMPLEX LESIONS IN DIALYSIS FISTULAS

Indications (5) for the percutaneous treatment of a dysfunctional, possibly complex AV access lesion are outlined in Table 1.

HAZARDS AND COMPLICATIONS

Table 2 defines the possible complications resulting from an intervention, which seem to be more frequent in thrombosed rather than stenosed fistulae (6). Beathard et al. (7) reported from a large collection of data from over 14,000 cases treated in different situations including both access thromboses and stenoses. They found an overall rate of 3.54% for complications on the whole; 3.26% were graded as minor whereas 0.28% was graded as major. Technical problems like venous rupture are highest in upper arm AV fistula interventions (8). Complication rates vary greatly depending on stenosis type (e.g., calcified, eccentric, recoil prone), severity, location, and number, extent of thrombosis if present, type and age of occlusion as well as on operator experience and the clinical situation.

INTERVENTIONAL STRATEGIES AND INTERVENTIONAL TOOLS

Preinterventional Diagnostic Workup of Patients with AV Fistula Problems

Clinical examination still is the most important method for the diagnosis of obstructions in AV fistulae. Nevertheless, the decision on whether clinical examination alone is sufficient or additional imaging examination must be performed before treatment depends on local customs, experience, and practice. In cases of percutaneous treatment of stenoses, pre, intra, and postoperative angiography must be conducted. Angiography entirely for diagnostic purposes without concomitant treatment should be avoided.

Whenever an obstruction is suspected, duplex ultrasonography can be performed to locate and to quantify the degree of diameter reduction due to the stenosis and can be helpful in defining thrombus extent. Complete access should be depicted by Digital Subtraction Angiography

Table 1   Indications for AV Fistula Interventions

Reduction of vessel diameter >50% plus reduction in access flow, measured dialysis dose or previous
  thrombosis
Access thrombosis
Small aneurysms distant to the anastomosis
Severe central venous obstructions that lead to inadequate hemodialysis or with impairing upper extremity
  swelling and persistent pain

(DSA) with diluted iodine to detect all significant stenoses eligible for intervention. If an arterial inflow stenosis is suspected, a 4-F diagnostic catheter can be introduced through the access via the anastomosis up into the arterial tree (9). Due to the recent reports of Nephrogenic Systemic Fibrosis, magnetic resonance angiography (MRA) should be if at all considered only in selected cases.

Access Routes and Peri-interventional Imaging

The preferred access route for complete anatomy depiction is the brachial artery. Firstly, the brachial artery should be palpated in the cubital fossa beneath the aponeurosis of the biceps muscle. After application of very little local anesthesia, the brachial artery can be retrogradely punctured in one-wall technique with a 22-gauge cannula with Teflon sheath (e.g., Abbott, Sligo, Ireland). To evade dislodgement, the sheath should be completely inserted into the artery in Seldinger technique with the use of a short 0.018″ guidewire. Access pathology can then be visualized and monitored throughout the complete intervention. When the dysfunction is clinically or sonographically evident, definitely due to an outflow problem distal to the AV anastomosis, direct antegrade puncture of the postanastomotic vein is an option and brachial puncture may be abstained from.

A tourniquet is applied for vein congestion to select a venous puncture site by palpation. Puncturing an occluded or stenosed segment can accordingly be avoided. In selected cases, additional Doppler ultrasound may be necessary. Depending on the obstruction location, the outflow vein is punctured in a retrograde fashion against the flow direction or antegradely with the flow with the use of local anesthesia and a 16-gauge sheath needle (e.g., Abbott), which is then exchanged for a 5–7-F (size dependent on balloon/device size) introducer sheath (e.g., Terumo, Tokyo, Japan). Sometimes dilation of the puncture site may be necessary. To overcome tortuous vessel segments, the obstructed segment is passed preferably with a 4–5-F multipurpose (hydrophilic) catheter (e.g., Cook, Bjaeverskov, Denmark) and a hydrophilic-coated and steerable 0.035-in. guidewire (e.g., Terumo). As mentioned before, antegrade distal venous puncture may be required for treatment of an upstream venous problem. In patients with a brachiocephalic upper arm fistula, an antegrade puncture close to the anastomosis is recommended. In long-segment thromboses, a combined retrograde and antegrade approach may be necessary to access and remove all clots.

Table 2   Potential Complications from AV Fistula Interventions

Potential complication	Frequency
Venous rupture	~8%
Formation of pseudoaneurysms at puncture or dilatation site requiring surgery	<0.5%
Infection and bacteremia	<0.5%
Severe hematoma requiring surgical evacuation	<0.2%
Mesenteric infarction, significant blood loss, iododermitis, metabolic acidosis, pulmonary edema	Each <0.1%
Symptomatic pulmonary embolism	<<1%
Arterial embolism	Very rare, but in 2–6% of thrombosed upper arm brachiocephalic fistulae
Major complications such as uncontrollable rupture with access loss	0.3–2%

Complex Stenoses

After visualization of the stenoses, selection of the access route, sheath placement, and negotiation of the obstruction, balloon dilation is indicated.

In radiocephalic AV fistulas, up to 75% of stenoses are to be found close to the AV anastomosis and ~25% in the venous outflow tract (8,10). In brachiocephalic and/or basilic AV fistulas, the characteristic location is at the intersection of the cephalic with the subclavian vein and the basilic with the axillary vein (8). PTA is indicated as the treatment of choice in stenoses of the anastomotic area in the upper forearm, the upper arm, and at the junction of the superficial vein with the deep venous system. PTA is also feasible in stenoses of the anastomotic area located in the lower forearm as an alternative to surgical treatment. After the stenoses have been passed with the hydrophilic guidewire and diagnostic catheter, a balloon catheter is advanced over the guidewire after diagnostic catheter removal. The balloon (recommended diameter: 3–5 mm close to the anastomosis, 5–8 mm in the upper arm; up to 14 mm in the central vasculature; length 20–40 mm) is appropriately positioned across the target lesion. Careful, slow inflation and dilatation with preferably high-pressure (20 atm) and ultra high-pressure (30 atm) angioplasty balloons for up to one to two minutes is recommended, which may be repeated. An inflation device with a pressure gauge with a 1:1 mixture of contrast medium and saline solution is obligatory.

If the stenoses cannot be dilated sufficiently by conventional PTA, they can be treated with a peripheral cutting balloon (PCB, Boston Scientific, Ratingen, Germany) (11). The PCB due to its atherotomes is supposed to disrupt the elastic and fibrotic continuity of the vessel wall that causes elastic recoil. The incisions alleviate dilatation of the stenosis and make the procedure less painful for the patient. Despite the complete expansion of the PTA balloon (without a waist) of sufficient diameter, the dilated vessel wall may still collapse immediately or shortly after removal of the balloon. This can be treated with stent implantation. However, stent placement in the needling areas of fistulas should rather be reserved for acute PTA-induced ruptures not controllable by prolonged balloon inflation. To our experience even stenoses longer than 5 cm can be approached radiologically. A restenosis can be treated radiologically (with or without a stent) in the same fashion. For interventions of stenoses we regularly administer 2000 to 5000 IU Heparin periprocedurally.

Complex Thromboses

AV fistula thrombosis should be treated as soon as possible or within 48 hours. The duration and site of AV fistula thrombosis as well as the type of access are important determinants of treatment outcome. Literature (12,13) suggests that thrombosed AV fistulae should, preferably, be treated by interventional radiology. The solitary exception may be forearm AV fistulae, thrombosed due to anastomotic stenosis. It is likely that in such cases, proximal reanastomosis will also grant good results. Interventional thrombolysis can be performed mechanically, pharmacomechanically or pharmacologically (Tables 3 and 4) (14).

Table 3 Thrombolysis Techniques in Occluded AV Fistulae

Technique	Dosage
Two crossed infusion catheters, one directed toward the arterial and one toward the venous side	Starting bolus 250,000 U urokinase mixed with heparin; additional dosing on a need-be basis for residual thrombus, PTA afterwards
Lyse and wait: crossed-catheter technique in the interventional preoperative area	Urokinase (e.g., 250,000 IU) + Heparin (e.g., 5000 IU) via small needle (20/22G) injected over 60 sec (volume ~10 mL)—angiographic intervention to dilate stenoses 30–120 min after
Lyse and go: crossed-catheter technique	Urokinase (e.g., 250,000 IU) + Heparin (e.g., 5000 IU) via small catheter (20/22G) injected over 60 sec (volume ~10 mL) and immediate percutaneous intervention with mechanical support
Pulse spray thrombolysis: two crossed catheters with multiple side holes = greater surface area coverage	Vigorous and fast injections of urokinase or rtPA every 30 sec—volume of each injection ~0.3 mL

Table 4 Examples of Percutaneous Thrombectomy Devices

Device type	Trade name
Rotating basket	Arrow-Trerotola Over-the-wire PTD
Rotating screw	Straub Rotarex
Laser	Spectranetics Excimer
Brush	Cragg thrombolytic brush catheter
Pigtail	Cook rotating pigtail catheters
Hydrodynamic	Possis AngioJet DVX Thrombectomy catheter

Various types of exclusively mechanical percutaneous thrombectomy have been proposed in the last decade that may be used as a single means to remove clotted material. However, the diversity and multiplicity of different mechanical native fistula thrombectomy techniques and interventions are far too numerous to re-evaluate herein. In general, after sheath placement the following modus operandi can be applied.

In cases of a very *short plug-like thrombus* selectively obstructing the AV anastomosis, maceration of the thrombus can be attempted by balloon angioplasty alone. In most instances, this thrombus located close to the anastomosis. Retrograde cannulation of the outflow vein is appropriate. The AV anastomosis is then cautiously passed by a 4–5-F multipurpose catheter and a hydrophilic guidewire, which is advanced into the inflow artery. There is only a nominal risk of arterial thrombus dislodgement during this maneuver. Next, the 4–5-F catheter is exchanged for a balloon catheter (3–5 mm diameter), which is inflated at the area of thrombosis. Treatment should be ended when an optimal opening of the underlying stenosis has been achieved.

Treatment of *complex long-segment thromboses* of the AV fistula can be performed with a wide array of different thrombectomy devices (Table 4). A combination of these devices with drug thrombolysis [urokinase, recombinant tissue plasminogen activator (rtPA)] is possible; it may accelerate and improve the result. It is advised only to use systems that are over-the-wire devices (OTD) to circumvent avoidable vessel wall injury.

We prefer to advance the thrombectomy catheter OTD as close to the anastomotic region as possible, or to cross it and then to retrieve the system while activated. Several passes of the system commonly have to be performed until no residual thrombus can be detected. No special technique is needed to prevent potential central embolization; the introducer sheath usually adequately blocks the venous outflow for larger emboli. During the active mechanical thrombectomy maneuver, the AV anastomosis should be digitally compressed to avoid retrograde thrombus dislodgment.

In some cases, the most distal thrombus close to the anastomosis needs to be dilated with a 5- to 6-mm balloon to permit some inflow into the proximal fistula before use of the thrombectomy catheter system.

Balloon dilatation should be regularly performed either to treat the underlying stenosis or to compress residual thrombus material. Balloon catheter size is usually 5–7 × 20 or 40 mm, 3–5 × 20 mm balloons are chosen for angioplasty close to the AV anastomosis. Cutting balloons and self-expanding stents may be necessary in cases of complex, angioplasty-resistant stenoses.

Concerning the device choice, either type of method for fistula recanalization is appropriate and should be based on the experience of the interventional radiologist with the respective therapeutic modality. It is improbable that the declotting method in dialysis shunts, whether pharmacomechanical or purely mechanical, has a considerable effect on short- or long-term patency (15).

Periprocedural parenteral anticoagulation should be administered regularly at the beginning of the intervention (5000 IU heparin). After procedure termination, continued heparinization with 1000 IU/hr for at least 24 hours in inpatients and three subcutaneous 7500 IU injections per day for 24 hours in outpatients is suitable. Antibiotics need not be routinely used.

Stent Placement/Complex Central Venous Obstruction

Central venous stenoses or occlusions in hemodialysis patients are considered to be due to high flow states in contrast to the low flow normally seen in veins and occur at sites of turbulence, such as valves or kinked vessels (16,17). Treatment of central venous obstruction should be performed percutaneously by PTA with/without stent (5).

After preimplantation angiography to study the vessel pathology and following antegrade venous puncture of a shunt-leading vein by a 20-gauge sheath needle (e.g., Abbocath, Abbott), intervention is done via an antegrade approach in Seldinger technique. Recanalization is usually tried using a hydrophilic-coated and steerable 0.035-in. guidewire (e.g., Terumo) for vessel stenosis and a straight guidewire with movable core (e.g., Cook) for occlusion. After safe passage of the obstructed segment, a balloon catheter of adequate size, usually 8 to 12 mm is to be advanced into the segment and subsequently dilated. If stent placement is considered necessary, a self-expanding stent, which is flexible enough to allow implantation even in kinked vessels, is positioned. Stent dilatation with a balloon of suitable size after deployment must be regularly employed to ensure as close contact to the venous wall as possible.

Traversing the lesion and recanalization should primarily be attempted with a brachial approach, except when the outflow vein is severely kinked or the obstruction cannot be negotiated; then a transfemoral access may be chosen. PTA can then be performed transfemorally, followed by stent placement transbrachially. "Through and through" access as described by Ingram (18), where the guidewire placed transbrachially is pulled out through the femoral access may be necessary in patients with extremely rigid and sharply angulated right-sided stenosis of the proximal subclavian vein.

Periprocedural anticoagulation is mandatory and is administered intravenously at the beginning of the intervention (5000 IU heparin). Outpatient treatment consists of three subcutaneous 7500 IU injections per day for 24 hours. Intravenous administration of 1000 IU per hour for 24 hours is the protocol of choice for inpatients. One hundred milligrams of acetylsalicylic acid a day as a chronic oral medication is recommended. In general, there is no need for perioperative medication. If restenosis within the stent with or without the demonstration of collateral veins or stenosis anywhere along the venous outflow tract is found on follow-up, reintervention is indicated (19).

Overall, looking at the results that can be achieved in trained hands, the primary patency rate of the treated thrombosed forearm AV fistula at 12 months is much higher than in grafts (49% vs. 14%). One-year secondary patency rates are 80% in forearm and 50% in upper arm AV fistulae (20). In dialysis fistulas, the combination of a thrombolytic agent (urokinase, rtPA) with PTA demonstrates immediate success rate of 94%. One study reported a success rate of 93% and a primary patency rate at one year of 70% (21). In another survey, 81 percutaneous treatments of thrombosed AV fistulae were performed (13). Flow restoration was achieved in almost 90% of the AV fistulae. The primary one-year patency rate was 26% and the secondary one-year patency rate 51%.

Patency rates are more favorable in the central venous lesions (22). Table 5 depicts the outcome data for this patient group.

SUMMARY OF OUTCOMES

In conclusion, all interventions in the dysfunctional AV fistula may be elaborate in the first place or may appear to be more complex than expected during the course of the intervention. Treatment must be adjusted to each individual case. Nevertheless, certain courses of action are uniform. In Table 6, devices for the percutaneous approach are listed.

EQUIPMENTS CHECKLIST
PART 2: TEACHING CASES

Case 1

Cryoplasty: This case shows a standard as well as high-pressure balloon angioplasty-resistant lesion (Figs. 1–4).

a. What made the lesion "complex" in this specific case? The difficulty of the case is attributable to the often and regularly observed resistance or recoil of stenoses in the venous outflow tract of the hemodialysis access. Even after repeated PTA, first with a standard PTA balloon

Table 5 Treatment Outcomes After Endovascular Central AV Fistula Treatment

References	Stent type	n pts	Primary patency (%)			Secondary patency (%)		
			6 mo	12 mo	24 mo	6 mo	12 mo	24 mo
PTA + stent								
23	Wallst.	26	54	21	32	55	46	29
24	Wallst.	18	73	49		83	85	
25	Mix	23		76	61			
26	Mix	35		22	9		72	79
19	Wallst.	50	84	56	28	97	89	81
27	Wallst.	14		70	50	100	84	84
28	Wallst.	27	72	45	30	100	100	100
29	Gianturco	8	11	11		89	78	
30	Mix	19		68			93	
31	Mix	13	71	71			100	
Sole PTA								
23			62	29	38	77	73	59
32		32	38	20				
33		62						
34		35		43	0		80	64
35		40				70		
29		10	23	12		100	100	

(12 atm) and afterwards with a high-pressure balloon (> 20 atm) a sufficient lumen could not be accomplished (Figs. 1 and 2).

b. What was the clinical indication for treatment of this specific case? The indication for the treatment was native fistula dysfunction with access flow measurements of less than 300 mL/min.

c. What were the potential hazards of treating this specific patient and this lesion? Hematoma, pain, restenosis of the dilated vessel, access infection, thrombus formation, complete vessel occlusion, dissection or perforation.

d. Which interventional strategies were considered and which interventional tools were used to handle this lesion? PTA with the PCB or cryoplasty. Cryotherapy combines the

Table 6 Checklist with Recommended Devices for Complex AV Fistula Interventions

Situation	Tool	Device example(s)
Brachial access (Diagnostic)	• 22-gauge cannula with Teflon sheath	
Pass the lesion	• Guidewire	Hydrophilic 0.035 in. (stenosis) Straight guidewire with movable core (occlusion)
	• Diagnostic catheter (4/5-F)	Multipurpose, straight
Stenosis (PTA)	• Balloon catheter	High-pressure (20 atm)/ultra high-pressure (30 atm) angioplasty balloons
Resistant lesion/recoil	• Alternative device	Cutting balloon Cryoplasty balloon
Femoral access (Venous)	• Diagnostic (4/5-F) • Guiding catheter (6-F)	Multipurpose, Aachen 1, straight
Thrombosis	• PTA balloon (short) • Thrombectomy device (long) • Drugs (long)	Angioplasty balloon Table 4 Table 3
Reobstruction	• Balloon catheter	High-pressure (20 atm)/ultra high-pressure (30 atm) angioplasty balloons
Vessel rupture	• Balloon catheter • Stent (if prolonged PTA fails)	Angioplasty balloon (Covered) stent

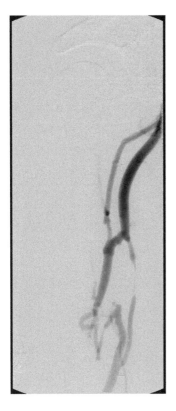

Figure 1   Venous outflow high grade stenosis before treatment.

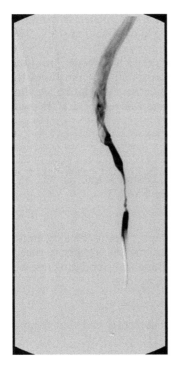

Figure 2   Unchanged morphology of stenosis after repeated PTA.

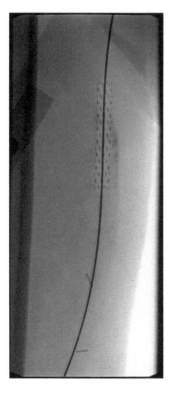

Figure 3 Inflated cryoballoon.

application of cold therapy with angioplasty using a peripheral dilatation system, a coaxial, dual balloon design (Boston Scientific). Gas is contained in the inner balloon. Radiopaque markers increase balloon visibility during the fluoroscopically guided intervention. The balloon is placed over the stenosis in an over-the-wire procedure and is inflated with nitrous oxide gas (Fig. 3). The vessel wall is then cooled with a 20-second treatment at -10°C. Two inflations were carried out.

e.   Summary: How was the case managed, is there anything that could have been improved, what was the immediate and long-term outcome? The demonstrated case illustrates the standard approach and escalation scheme to vascular access stenoses: standard PTA, then high-pressure PTA, finally use of PCB or cryoballoons. The access was patent straight away and could be used for immediate, unproblematic dialysis (Fig. 4).

f.   List of contemporary equipments that should be used in this case:
  ○   Guidewire 0.035″ hydrophilic coated
  ○   Diagnostic catheter 4–5-F (Straight or MP)
  ○   Balloon Dilatation Catheter 5–6 × 20/40 mm (e.g., SMASH, Boston Scientific)
  ○   High-pressure PTA Balloon 5–6 × 20/40 mm (e.g., Conquest, Bard)
  ○   PCB device or
  ○   PolarCath peripheral dilatation system

g.   Key learning issues of this specific case: If conventional and high-pressure balloon angioplasty is unsuccessful, an alternative to cutting balloon treatment may be cryoplasty, potentially not only improving access blood circulation but also simultaneously inhibiting restenosis through an altered plaque response, less elastic recoil, and apoptosis.

Case 2

Access combination technique: This case shows a combined transbrachial and transfemoral approach due to an unattainable antegrade recanalization (Figs. 5–11).

a.   What made the lesion "complex" in this specific case? The complexity of the case results from the failure to transbrachially cross the occluded segment with the straight guidewire with movable core together with a multipurpose catheter.

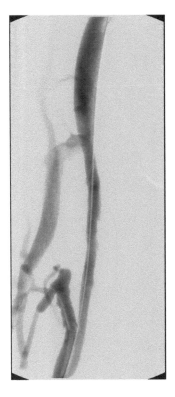

Figure 4 Result after PolarCath treatment.

b. What was the clinical indication for treatment of this specific case? The indication for treatment was chronic swelling of the access arm with disabling pain and paresthesia.
c. What were the potential hazards of treating this specific patient and this lesion? Local bleeding at both catheter insertion sites, venous perforation and disruption, early rethrombosis, embolism, stent misplacement, immediate or delayed central migration of the endoprosthesis.
d. Which interventional strategies were considered and which interventional tools were used to handle this lesion? Usually the intervention is performed via an antegrade approach through the venous outflow tract in Seldinger technique. Recanalization is attempted with a hydrophilic 0.035-in. guidewire (Terumo, Leuven, Belgium) for vessel stenosis or a straight guidewire with a movable core (Cook, Bjaeverskov, Denmark) for occlusion. Since the obstruction could not be negotiated with the brachial approach (Fig. 5), recanalization was tried transfemorally with a hydrophilic guidewire and a straight 5-F catheter (Fig. 6). After safe retrograde passage of the obstructed segment (Fig. 7), a 6-mm and subsequently 7-mm

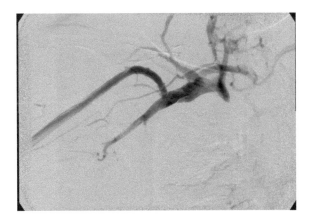

Figure 5 DSA shows occlusion of the right brachiocephalic vein with pronounced collateral flow.

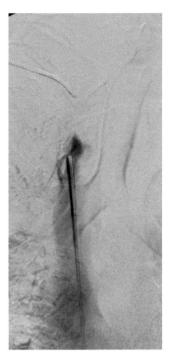

Figure 6 Transfemoral occlusion negotiation.

balloon catheter was advanced into the segment via a long sheath and dilated by hand, without pressure monitoring (Figs. 8 and 9). Inflation time each was >30 seconds. Then, a flexible, self-expanding 14/40 mm SMART Control stent (Cordis, Langenfeld, Germany) was deployed transbrachially. The stent was dilated with a 10/40 mm and 12/40 mm XXL balloon after deployment to ensure as close contact to the venous wall as possible (Fig. 10). Restoration of flow and vanishing of collateral vessels after placement was achieved (Fig. 11).

e. Summary: How was the case managed, is there anything that could have been improved, what was the immediate and long-term outcome? The introduced case illustrates the standard approach to central venous obstruction and reaction to failure of

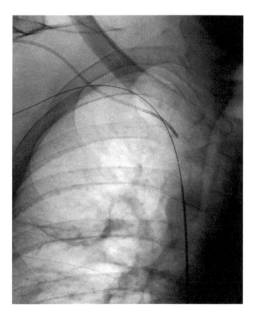

Figure 7 After transfemoral occlusion passing.

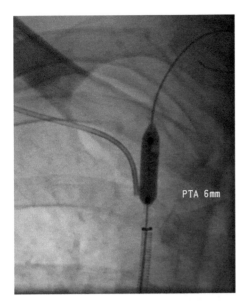

Figure 8 Transfemoral PTA.

this method. If by antegrade approach the lesion cannot be overcome, then the only reasonable alternative is to access transfemorally. In the discussed patient, pain and paresthesia were reduced to a minimum and the access patent with normal dialysis protocols during an observation period of 16 months.

f. List of contemporary equipments that should be used in this case:
    - Guidewire 0.035″ hydrophilic coated (e.g., Terumo) or straight with movable core
    - Diagnostic catheter 5-F (Straight or MP)
    - Guiding catheter 6-F (Straight, e.g., COOK, Denmark)
    - High-pressure PTA Balloon 6–7 × 40 mm (e.g., POWERFLEX EXTREME, Cordis)
    - 14/40 mm self-expanding Nitinol stent system (e.g., S.M.A.R.T. CONTROL, Cordis)
    - Balloon dilatation catheter 10–12 × 40 mm (e.g., Fox, Abbott; XXL, Boston Scientific)
g. Key learning issues of this specific case: In upper torso occlusion, to achieve exact stent placement a transbrachial approach by antegradely puncturing the outflow vein in Seldinger

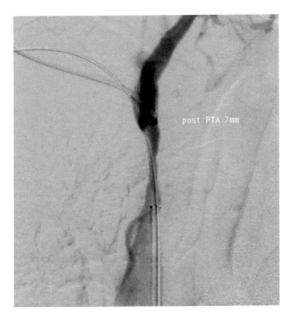

Figure 9 Result after transfemoral PTA.

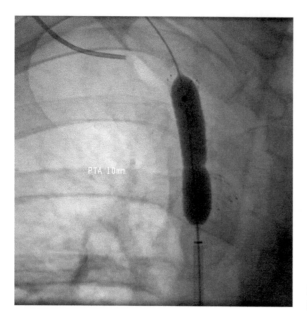

Figure 10   In-stent PTA immediately after stent placement.

technique should be used. If the outflow vein is severely kinked or too small and the obstruction cannot be negotiated with a brachial approach, a transfemoral approach is a possible alternative. In this case, primary stent placement is recommended.

Case 3

Mechanical thrombectomy and near-anastomosis stent placement: This case shows the rather exceptional mechanical treatment of partly thrombosed venous aneurysms with additional outflow endoprosthesis deployment (Figs. 12–17).

a. What made the lesion "complex" in this specific case? The patient was primarily planned for treatment of an outflow stenosis (Fig. 12). After diagnostic angiography and ineffective

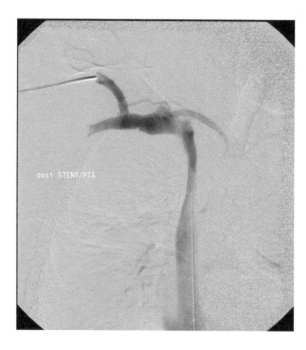

Figure 11   Final result shows that unobstructed patency has been re-established.

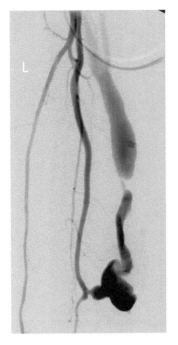

Figure 12 Arterial DSA demonstrates partly thrombosed aneurysm and stenosis in the outflow vein.

    PTA due to stenosis recoil, flow enhancement had to be attempted by central thrombus dislocation and additionally flow redirection with stent placement.

b. What was the clinical indication for treatment of this specific case? The initial indication for the treatment was a malfunctioning AV shunt with declining access flow.

c. What were the potential hazards of treating this specific patient and this lesion? Procedure-related access site bleeding, soaring thrombus formation, complete venous vessel occlusion, dissection or perforation, distal arterial or pulmonary embolism, access infection.

d. Which interventional strategies were considered and which interventional tools were used to handle this lesion? Typically, the percutaneous intervention is performed via a retrograde approach in Seldinger technique for postanastomotic obstructions. Passage is done with a hydrophilic, 0.035-in. guidewire and a diagnostic catheter (Fig. 13), followed by PTA. In this setting, angioplasty with 4-mm and 6-mm regular and high-pressure PTA balloons was ineffective and thrombus volume increased (Fig. 14), requiring immediate thrombus maceration and dislocation with a rotating 5-F pigtail catheter (Figs. 15 and 16). To circumvent the access abandonment due to complete vessel occlusion, a lineup of four overlapping self-expanding SMART Control stent (Cordis, Langenfeld, Germany) with diameters of 8 and 9 mm, respectively, were placed. Ultimately, adequate and unobstructed blood flow was attained (Fig. 17).

e. Summary: How was the case managed, is there anything that could have been improved, what was the immediate and long-term outcome? The presented case shows the difficulties the interventionist may encounter during a supposedly standard PTA. In retrospect, a primary surgical approach with aneurysm resection would have been a viable alternative. In case of stent placement, however, it became necessary to pave the complete distance from the AV anastomosis beyond the venous stenosis. The postinterventional short- and long-term (15 months restenosis free interval) result was excellent without development of early or late complications.

f. List of contemporary equipments that should be used in this case:
   ○ Guidewire 0.035″ hydrophilic coated
   ○ Diagnostic catheter 4–5-F (Straight, Aachen 1)
   ○ Balloon dilatation catheter 4 + 6 × 20 mm (e.g., SMASH, Boston Scientific)
   ○ High-pressure PTA balloon 4 + 6 × 20 mm (e.g., Conquest, Bard)
   ○ 5-F pigtail rotating catheter

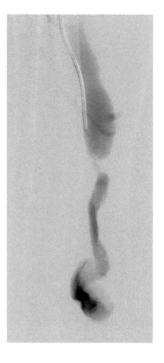

Figure 13 Retrograde approach and canalization with straight catheter and guidewire.

    ○ Self-expanding Nitinol stent system 8 + 9/30 + 60 mm (e. g. S.M.A.R.T. CONTROL, Cordis)

g. Key learning issues of this specific case: In case of conventional and high-pressure balloon angioplasty failure, with peri-interventional progressive thrombus formation proximal to the stenosis, a combination procedure of manual mechanical thrombectomy and endoprosthesis placement may become necessary to avoid complete occlusion, permit and ensure access patency while avoiding additional open surgery.

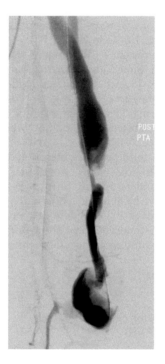

Figure 14 After futile retrograde PTA attempt.

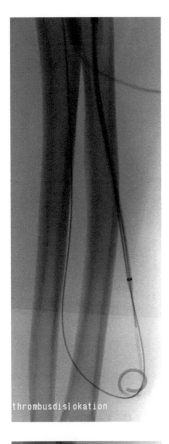

Figure 15 Manual mechanical thrombus dislocation with rotating pigtail catheter.

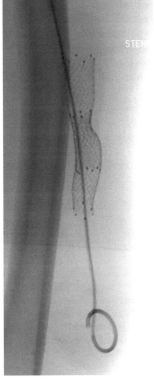

Figure 16 Stent placement covering the PTA-resistant stenosis.

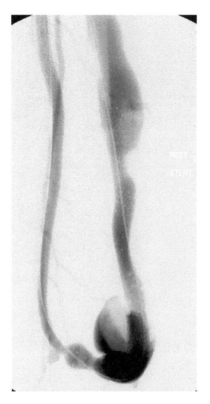

Figure 17 Unrestricted flow after placement of four overlapping self-expanding stents.

PART 3: KEY ISSUES FOR SUCCESSFUL AND SAFE TREATMENT OF COMPLEX AV FISTULA LESIONS

- High-quality treatment of AV fistula dysfunction is a complex undertaking in which the interventional radiologist, vascular surgeon, and nephrologist should collaborate closely.
- The primary percutaneous treatment approach is a very viable alternative to more invasive procedures. As long as less-invasive equivalent therapeutic alternatives to preserve the AV access are feasible, the existing vascular access should be sustained.
- In stenoses and short-segment thromboses, percutaneous transluminal angioplasty is the first treatment option.
- In access thrombosis percutaneous thrombectomy, whether pharmacomechanical or purely mechanical, has no major effect on patency. Each type of method for access recanalization is suitable and should be based on the experience of the interventionist with the therapeutic modality.
- In case of central venous obstruction, treatment should be performed percutaneously by PTA with additional stent implantation, if necessary.

REFERENCES

1. U.S. Renal Data System. USRDS 2007 Annual Data Report: Atlas of Chronic Kidney Disease and End-Stage Renal Disease in the United States. Bethesda, MD: National Institutes of Health, National Institute of Diabetes and Digestive and Kidney Diseases, 2007.
2. Dapunt O, Feurstein M, Rendl KH, et al. Transluminal angioplasty versus conventional operation in the treatment of haemodialysis fistula stenosis: results from a 5-year study. Br J Surg 1987; 74:1004–1005.
3. McCutcheon B, Weatherford D, Maxwell G, et al. A preliminary investigation of balloon angioplasty versus surgical treatment of thrombosed dialysis access grafts. Am Surg 2003; 69:663–667.
4. Uflacker R, Rajagopalan PR, Selby JB, et al; Investigators of the Clinical Trial Sponsored by Microvena Corporation. Thrombosed dialysis access grafts: randomized comparison of the Amplatz thrombectomy device and surgical thromboembolectomy. Eur Radiol 2004; 14:2009–2014.
5. Tordoir J, Canaud B, Haage P, et al. EBPG on vascular access. Nephrol Dial Transplant 2007; 22(suppl 2):88–117.

6. Miyayama S, Matsui O, Taki K, et al. Occluded Brescia-cimino hemodialysis fistulas: endovascular treatment with both brachial arterial and venous access using the pull-through technique. Cardiovasc Intervent Radiol 2005; 28:806–812.
7. Beathard GA, Litchfield T; Physician Operators Forum of RMS Lifeline, Inc. Effectiveness and safety of dialysis vascular access procedures performed by interventional nephrologists. Kidney Int 2004; 66:1622–1232.
8. Turmel-Rodrigues L, Pengloan J, Baudin S, et al. Treatment of stenosis and thrombosis in haemodialysis fistulas and grafts by interventional radiology. Nephrol Dial Transplant 2000; 15:2029–2036.
9. Duijm LE, Liem YS, van der Rijt RH, et al. Inflow stenoses in dysfunctional hemodialysis access fistulae and grafts. Am J Kidney Dis 2006; 48:98–105.
10. Turmel-Rodrigues L, Pengloan J, Blanchier D, et al. Insufficient dialysis shunts: improved long-term patency rates with close hemodynamic monitoring, repeated percutaneous balloon angioplasty, and stent placement. Radiology 1993; 187:273–278.
11. Vorwerk D, Adam G, Müller-Leisse C, et al. Hemodialysis fistulas and grafts: use of cutting balloons to dilate venous stenoses. Radiology 1996; 201:864–867.
12. Vorwerk D. Non-traumatic vascular emergencies: management of occluded hemodialysis shunts and venous access. Eur Radiol 2002; 12:2644–2650.
13. Haage P, Vorwerk D, Wildberger JE, et al. Percutaneous treatment of thrombosed primary arteriovenous hemodialysis access fistulae. Kidney Int 2000; 57:1169–1175.
14. Bush RL, Lin PH, Lumsden AB. Management of thrombosed dialysis access: thrombectomy versus thrombolysis. Semin Vasc Surg 2004; 17:32–39.
15. Gray RJ. Percutaneous intervention for permanent hemodialysis access: a review. J Vasc Interv Radiol 1997; 8:313–327.
16. Glanz S, Gordon DH, Butt K, et al. The role of percutaneous angioplasty in the management of chronic hemodialysis fistulas. Ann Surg 1987; 206:777–781.
17. Schwab SJ, Quarles LD, Middleton JP, et al. Hemodialysis-associated subclavian vein stenosis. Kidney Int 1988; 33:1156–1159.
18. Ingram TL, Reid SH, Tisnado J, et al. Percutaneous transluminal angioplasty of brachiocephalic vein stenoses in patients with dialysis shunts. Radiology 1988; 166:45–47.
19. Haage P, Vorwerk D, Piroth W, et al. Treatment of hemodialysis-related central venous stenosis or occlusion: results of primary wallstent placement and follow-up in 50 patients. Radiology 1999; 212:175–180.
20. Hingorani A, Ascher E, Kallakuri S, et al. Impact of reintervention for failing upper-extremity arteriovenous autogenous access for hemodialysis. J Vasc Surg 2001; 34:1004–1009.
21. Liang HL, Pan HB, Chung HM, et al. Restoration of thrombosed Brescia-Cimino dialysis fistulas by using percutaneous transluminal angioplasty. Radiology 2002; 223:339–344.
22. Mansour M, Kamper L, Altenburg A, et al. Radiological central vein treatment in vascular access. J Vasc Access 2008; 9:85–101.
23. Bakken AM, Protack CD, Saad WE, et al. Long-term outcomes of primary angioplasty and primary stenting of central venous stenosis in hemodialysis patients. J Vasc Surg 2007; 45:776–783.
24. Chen CY, LiangG HL, Pan HB, et al. Metallic stenting for treatment of central venous obstruction in hemodialysis patients. J Chin Med Assoc 2003; 66:166–172.
25. Mickley V. Stent or bypass? Treatment results in benign central venous obstruction. Zentralbl Chir 2001; 126:445–449.
26. Oderich GS, Treiman GS, Schneider P, et al. Stent placement for treatment of central and peripheral venous obstruction: a long-term multi-institutional experience. J Vasc Surg 2000; 32:760–769.
27. Mickley V, Görich J, Rilinger N, et al. Stenting of central venous stenoses in hemodialysis patients: long-term results. Kidney Int 1997; 51:277–280.
28. Vorwerk D, Guenther RW, Mann H, et al. Venous stenoses and occlusions in hemodialysis shunts: follow-up results of stent placement in 65 patients. Radiology 1995; 195;140–146.
29. Quinn SF, Schuman ES, Demlow TA, et al. Percutaneous transluminal angioplasty versus endovascular stent placement in the treatment of venous stenoses in patients undergoing hemodialysis: intermediate results. J Vasc Interv Radiol 1995; 6:851–855.
30. Shoenfeld R, Hermans H, Novick A, et al. Stenting of proximal venous obstructions to maintain hemodialysis access. J Vasc Surg 1994; 19:532–538.
31. Bhatia DS, Money SR, Ochsner JL, et al. Comparison of surgical bypass and percutaneous balloon dilatation with primary stent placement in the treatment of central venous obstruction in the dialysis patient: one-year follow-up. Ann Vasc Surg 1996; 10:452–455.
32. Maya ID, Saddekni S, Allon M. Treatment of refractory central vein stenosis in hemodialysis patients with stents. Semin Dial 2007; 20:78–82.

33. Levit RD, Cohen RM, Kwak A, et al. Asymptomatic central venous stenosis in hemodialysis patients. Radiology 2006; 238:1051–1056.
34. Surowiec SM, Fegley AJ, Tanski WJ, et al. Endovascular management of central venous stenoses in the hemodialysis patient: results of percutaneous therapy. Vasc Endovasc Surg 2004; 38: 349–354.
35. Kalman PG, Lindsay TF, Clarke K, et al. Management of upper extremity central venous obstruction using interventional radiology. Ann Vasc Surg 1998; 12;202–206.

18 | Venous Interventions for Iliofemoral DVT

Anthony J. Comerota and Marilyn H. Gravett

Jobst Vascular Center, Toledo, Ohio, U.S.A.

PART 1: INTRODUCTION

Acute deep venous thrombosis (DVT) represents a disease spectrum ranging from asymptomatic calf vein thrombosis to the painful swollen limb of phlegmasia cerulea dolens resulting from extensive multisegment DVT. Although patient presentation and extent of venous thrombosis vary considerably, national and international guidelines for the treatment of acute DVT had, until recently, demonstrated a "one-size-fits-all" approach by recommending a single treatment—anticoagulation alone—for all variants of DVT. The latest published guidelines of the American College of Chest Physicians (ACCP) Consensus Conference on Antithrombotic and Thrombolytic Therapy include recommendations that depart significantly from previous versions (1). In the guideline, authors recognized the link between extensive venous thrombosis and severe long-term postthrombotic morbidity and acknowledged the existing evidence supporting a strategy of thrombus removal using treatment techniques that include contemporary venous thrombectomy, catheter-directed thrombolysis, and pharmacomechanical thrombolysis.

What Makes a Lesion Complex in Venous Interventions?

The departure from anticoagulation alone to adopt a strategy of thrombus removal is what makes this approach complex. It is basically the physician's misunderstanding of the pathophysiology of postthrombotic venous disease that leads to its severe morbidity. Physicians often fail to recognize that luminal venous obstruction resulting from persistent residual thrombus is the major contributor to ambulatory venous hypertension, and hence the clinical morbidity of chronic venous disease. This obstruction can be efficiently eliminated early during the phase of acute DVT; however, recanalization of the chronically occluded venous system is not associated with the same ease of treatment or the same degree of success.

Key factors contributing to the revision of the ACCP guidelines were studies demonstrating that patients with postthrombotic syndrome suffer significant reduction in their quality of life (QOL) and that the severity of their initial DVT is predictive of postthrombotic morbidity (2,3). Nowhere are these outcomes more evident than in patients with iliofemoral DVT, a clinically relevant subset of patients with acute DVT who suffer the most severe postthrombotic sequelae (4–6). If iliofemoral DVT patients are treated with anticoagulation alone, 90% will have ambulatory venous hypertension resulting in venous insufficiency, 40% will experience venous claudication, and up to 15% will develop venous ulceration within five years (5,6). All of these patients will have reduced QOL (7). The body of evidence demonstrates that a strategy of thrombus removal offers patients with iliofemoral DVT the best long-term outcome and is therefore the preferred management for their disease.

Unfortunately, many physicians fail to discern the difference in pathophysiology between primary and postthrombotic venous insufficiency and consequently underestimate the value of thrombus removal in preventing postthrombotic morbidity, especially in patients with iliofemoral disease. The pathophysiology of postthrombotic venous insufficiency is ambulatory venous hypertension, which is defined as an elevated venous pressure during exercise (8,9). Key anatomical components that contribute to ambulatory venous hypertension are *venous obstruction* and *venous valvular incompetence*. Studies demonstrate that patients with chronic venous obstruction, particularly those with multisegment and/or iliofemoral venous obstruction, have the most severe postthrombotic sequelae (8,10). Although ultrasonography can assess valvular function by quantifying valve closure times, obstruction adversely affects venous hemodynamics long before imaging techniques can detect it. The inability to quantitate obstruction has contributed to widespread underappreciation of its contribution to postthrombotic pathophysiology.

Management of Iliofemoral DVT

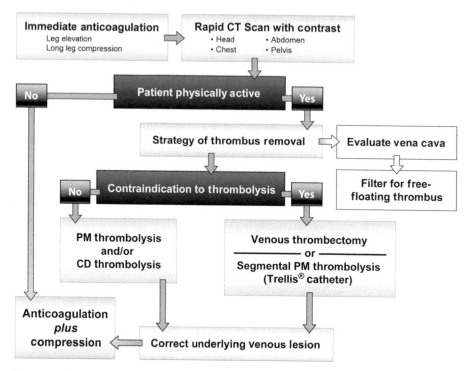

Figure 1   Algorithm illustrating our current treatment protocol for patients with iliofemoral DVT.

Experimental canine studies of acute DVT have shown that successful thrombolysis preserves endothelial function and valve competence (11,12). Natural history studies of acute DVT have shown that patients with persistent venous obstruction treated with anticoagulation alone developed distal valve incompetence, even when distal veins were not involved at onset with thrombus (13–15). Moreover, if spontaneous lysis occurred early (clot lysis within 90 days), valve function was frequently preserved (15). It is intuitive that successfully removing acute thrombus eliminates luminal obstruction and, if thrombus is eliminated early (within days/weeks), preserves valve function.

Advances in all methods of eliminating thrombus from the deep venous system have occurred in the last 10 to 15 years, and this chapter will review three key strategies: (*i*) contemporary venous thrombectomy, (*ii*) intrathrombus catheter-directed thrombolysis, and (*iii*) pharmacomechanical thrombolysis.

Clinical Indications for Treatment of Complex Lesions in Venous Interventions

All patients with iliofemoral DVT should be evaluated and considered for a strategy of thrombus removal. Assuming the patient is ambulatory, contraindications to either surgical or catheter-based treatment should be carefully assessed. The algorithm shown in Figure 1 illustrates our current management strategy for patients with iliofemoral DVT and provides a decision matrix for selecting the appropriate treatment strategy.

Patients who have occlusive thrombus of the common femoral vein have essentially obliterated venous drainage from their lower extremity, which leads to severe postthrombotic morbidity. Although most individuals diagnosed with acute DVT can be treated as outpatients, these patients should be admitted and considered for a treatment strategy that includes thrombus removal. Another subset of patients likely to suffer severe postthrombotic morbidity are those with thrombotic obliteration of their popliteal vein and adjoining proximal tibial veins. Because adequate collaterals do not develop, these patients incur severe distal venous hypertension.

Table 1   Evidence-Based Recommendations for the Treatment of Patients with Iliofemoral DVT (1)

Recommendation	Grade
In patients with extensive (iliofemoral) DVT, operative venous thrombectomy may be used to reduce acute symptoms and postthrombotic morbidity	2B
Following venous thrombectomy, the same duration and intensity of anticoagulation should be used as in those who do not undergo thrombectomy	1C
In patients with extensive proximal DVT and low risk for bleeding, catheter-directed thrombolysis (CDT) can be used to reduce acute symptoms and postthrombotic morbidity	2B
Pharmacomechanical thrombolysis should be considered in preference to CDT alone	2C
Following CDT, underlying venous lesions should be corrected	2C
Following CDT, the same intensity and duration of anticoagulation should be used for those who are not treated with CDT	1C
Patients with acute DVT should be treated with a 30–40 mm Hg compression stocking to reduce postthrombotic morbidity	1A

The 8th ACCP guidelines on antithrombotic therapy recommend catheter-directed thrombolysis for patients with acute iliofemoral DVT who are appropriate risk candidates (Table 1). The writing committee emphasized the importance of correcting underlying venous lesions following successful thrombus removal and noted that, when using catheter-directed thrombolysis, pharmacomechanical techniques may be useful to shorten treatment time. They further emphasized that the same intensity and duration of anticoagulant therapy be given to patients treated with thrombolysis and venous thrombectomy as those treated with anticoagulation alone, underscoring the value of ongoing therapeutic anticoagulation to reduce the risk of rethrombosis.

Contemporary venous thrombectomy is recommended as an option for those patients who have contraindications to thrombolysis or in medical communities where catheter-based techniques are not available. There are few contraindications to operative thrombectomy, old thrombus ($\geq$10 days) that adheres to the vein wall being the most important.

Patients with spontaneous and extensive venous thrombosis often have a clinically obvious etiology, such as trauma, an underlying thrombophilia, or an occult cancer. Earlier in our experience we routinely performed a complete thrombophilia evaluation; however, today we believe it is less important and not necessary for proper treatment of the patient during both acute and follow-up phases. The implications of a thrombophilia evaluation should be carefully considered, as some patients may face health insurance restrictions, increased premiums, and perhaps employment restrictions. However, young patients who intend to have children may benefit from such an evaluation, as the results may be relevant for family planning as well as future care. Similarly, a family history of venous thromboembolic disease suggests the need for a thrombophilia evaluation.

Both the proximal and distal extent of thrombus should be clearly defined in all patients, including imaging of the vena cava. If a patient has nonocclusive vena caval thrombus, we recommend a vena caval filter for those undergoing catheter-based techniques. If operating, either proximal balloon occlusion or filtration of the cava is warranted.

For patients with normal renal function, we strongly recommend a computed tomographic (CT) scan of the head, chest, abdomen, and pelvis with contrast. In at least 50% of patients with acute iliofemoral DVT, an asymptomatic pulmonary embolism (PE) will be found. This may not require immediate therapy but the diagnosis of PE will be appreciated in the subsequent three- to five-day period, when up to 25% of these patients develop pleuritic chest pain (16). Awareness of the presence of an asymptomatic PE when the patient presents permits the physician to confidently treat the patient, knowing that delayed symptoms of pleuritic irritation were neither a complication of the strategy of thrombus removal nor a failure of anticoagulation.

Hazards and Complications

Many physicians are understandably concerned about the risk of procedure-related PE. Patients with nonobstructive thrombus in their vena cava have the highest risk of procedure-related PE (*Case #1*), so it is vital to determine both proximal and distal extent of thrombus, with particular attention paid to the amount and level of vena caval involvement. Knowing this will assist in deciding whether or not vena caval filtration or another form of embolic protection should be used. Nonocclusive thrombus in the vena cava is a clear indication for a vena caval filter before catheter-directed thrombolysis and proximal caval protection during venous thrombectomy.

Traditional concerns about bleeding risk with thrombolytic agents are reduced by the use of intrathrombus infusion as well as adjunctive pharmacomechanical techniques. Reducing the dose of lytic agent as well as the duration of treatment lessens the systemic response to the infused plasminogen activator (17).

Interventional Strategies

Contemporary venous thrombectomy has the potential of offering patients with acute iliofemoral DVT an opportunity for rapid removal of thrombus and restoration of normal venous drainage, resulting in a significant reduction in postthrombotic morbidity. The long-term benefits of venous thrombectomy relate to its ability to restore venous patency, especially of the iliofemoral segment, and maintain distal valve competence. Both are influenced by initial technical success and avoiding recurrent thrombosis. Initial success in achieving patency is, in turn, influenced by timely intervention and attention to technical detail.

Intrathrombus catheter-directed thrombolysis evolved from earlier attempts to use systemic thrombolysis as treatment for acute DVT. Although systemic thrombolysis removed thrombus more effectively than anticoagulation alone, results were less than optimal (18), and high rates of bleeding complications occurred. Because plasminogen activators were administered intravenously, they failed to adequately penetrate thrombus, leading to higher rates of lytic failure (19).

The essential mechanism of thrombolysis is the activation of fibrin-bound plasminogen to form the active enzyme plasmin, which dissolves thrombus (20). During thrombosis, circulating Glu-plasminogen binds to fibrin and is converted to Lys-plasminogen within the thrombus, which has greater affinity for plasminogen activators. The intrathrombus delivery of plasminogen activators activates Lys-plasminogen to form plasmin. Moreover, intrathrombus techniques protect the plasminogen activators from neutralization by circulating plasminogen activator inhibitor (PAI-1) and protect the generated plasmin from immediate neutralization by circulating antiplasmins. Finally, infusing plasminogen activators directly into thrombus reduces both the dose and duration necessary to achieve lytic success, thereby reducing the likelihood of complications.

Pharmacomechanical thrombolysis, one of the newer strategies for thrombus removal, involves adding pharmacomechanical techniques to catheter-directed thrombolysis. Pharmacomechanical therapies have the potential to significantly shorten treatment times and reduce the amount of lytic agent required to achieve lysis, thereby making treatment both more cost-effective and safer for patients.

Interventional Tools

Mechanical techniques used alone or in conjunction with thrombolysis to clear the venous system more rapidly have demonstrated varying results. Vedantham et al. (21) reviewed the effectiveness of several mechanical devices in combination with thrombolysis in 28 patients. Devices used included the Amplatz (ev3, Inc, Plymouth, MN), AngioJet® (Possis Medical, Minneapolis, MN), Trerotolo (Arrow International, Reading, PA), and Oasis (Boston Scientific/Medi-tech, Natick, MA) catheter systems. Venographic scoring was performed throughout the procedures. When mechanical thrombectomy was used as the sole treatment, only 26% of thrombus was removed, whereas 82% of thrombus was removed when a plasminogen activator solution was added (including nonresponding patients with chronic occlusions). Mechanical thrombectomy alone was successful when used to eliminate intraprocedural thrombus, which is typically gelatinous and not crosslinked with fibrin. Overall infusion time averaged approximately 17 hours and major bleeding complications occurred in 14% of patients.

An eight-year experience using pharmacomechanical thrombolysis in 98 patients was reported by Lin et al. (22) Forty-six patients received catheter-directed thrombolysis while 52 received pharmacomechanical thrombolysis using the AngioJet rheolytic thrombectomy catheter. Those undergoing pharmacomechanical treatment had significantly fewer

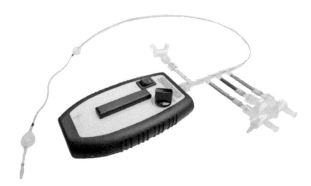

Figure 2 The Trellis-8 peripheral infusion system (Bacchus Vascular, Santa Clara, CA) delivers the lytic agent into the thrombus segmented between two occluding balloons. A dispersion wire inserted into the center of the catheter assumes a spiral configuration, dispenses the lytic agent, and mechanically macerates the thrombus. The resulting liquefied and small particulate thrombus is aspirated to minimize or avoid a systemic lytic effect.

phlebograms, reduced ICU and hospital stays, and fewer blood transfusions. Kasirajan et al. (23) treated a small patient group with rheolytic thrombectomy and demonstrated that mechanical thrombectomy was less effective when used alone than when combined with a plasminogen activator solution.

An interesting new pharmacomechanical catheter, the EKOS® EndoWave™ system (Bothell, WA), uses ultrasound-accelerated thrombolysis to remove acute thrombus. Parikh et al. (24) recently reported their initial clinical experience in 52 patients with both upper and lower extremity acute DVT. Using a variety of lytic agents, they reported that complete lysis (≥90%) was observed in 70% of patients, with overall lysis (complete plus partial) in 91%. Only 4% of patients had major complications (puncture site hematomas) and median infusion time was 22 hours.

One of the more promising pharmacomechanical techniques is isolated, segmental pharmacomechanical thrombolysis (ISPMT), which is achieved using the Trellis® catheter (Bacchus Vascular, Santa Clara, CA). This double-balloon catheter (Fig. 2) is guided into the thrombosed venous segment, with the proximal balloon positioned at the upper edge of the thrombus. Once the balloons are inflated, a plasminogen activator is infused into the thrombosed segment that has been isolated by the balloons. The intervening catheter assumes a spiral configuration and rotates at 1500 rpms for approximately 15 to 20 minutes, followed by aspiration of the liquefied and fragmented thrombus. If successful, the catheter is repositioned to treat additional segments. However, if residual thrombus persists, repeat treatment or adjunctive interventions (rheolytic thrombectomy, ultrasound-accelerated thrombolysis, balloon angioplasty, or stenting) are performed.

Summary of Outcomes
The pooled data shown in Table 2 (25–31) illustrate patency rates achieved with venous thrombectomy. Recent improvements to the technique include the use of the venous thrombectomy catheter (large balloon), fluoroscopic guidance, completion intraoperative phlebography, correction of an underlying venous stenosis, construction of an arteriovenous fistula (AVF), and immediate and prolonged therapeutic anticoagulation. These additions should substantially improve acute and long-term results.

Table 2 Venous Thrombectomy with Arteriovenous Fistula: Long-Term Valve Competence of Femoropopliteal Venous Segment

References	No.	Follow-up (mo)	Femoral-popliteal valve competence
25	31	6	52
26	53	10	42
27	17	91	82
28	37	24	56
29	37	55	80
30	150	60	80
31	27	60	30
Total	352	45 mo (mean)	63% (mean)

Table 3 Efficacy and Complications of Catheter-Directed Thrombolysis in Three Series

	Bjarnason et al. (33) (*n* = 77) (%)	Mewissen et al. (34) (*n* = 287) (%)	Comerota and Kagan (35) (*n* = 58) (%)
Initial success	79	83	84
Iliac	63	64	78
Femoral	40	47	—
Primary patency at 1 yr			
Iliac	63	64	78
Femoral	40	47	—
Iliac stent: patency at 1 yr			
+ stent	54	74	89
− stent	75	53	71
Complications			
Major bleed	5	11	9
Intracranial bleeding	0	<1	0
Pulmonary embolism	1	1	0
Fatal pulmonary embolism	0	0.2	0
Death secondary to lysis	0	0.4	0% (?2%)[a]

[a]Death due to multiorgan system failure 30 days post lysis, thought not related to lytic therapy.

Many investigators have reported good outcomes of catheter-directed thrombolysis for acute DVT; these have been previously discussed in detail (32). Three large reports (422 patients) demonstrated success rates of approximately 80% [Table 3 (33–35)], rates that likely would have been higher had the studies treated only patients with acute iliofemoral DVT. As investigators developed confidence with the technique, more patients were referred with severe symptoms longer after their acute presentation; the less than optimal results are included as a reflection of treating older (>1 month) thrombus. Bleeding complications occurred in 5% to 10%, most commonly at the venous access site. Intracranial bleeding and fatal PE were rare, occurring in only four patients in these three series.

Early studies using ISPMT demonstrate reduced treatment times and dose of lytic agents. Martinez et al. (17) reported on 52 consecutive limbs treated for iliofemoral DVT, 27 of which were treated with catheter-directed thrombolysis and 25 with ISPMT plus catheter-directed thrombolysis when necessary. Treatment outcomes and thrombus burden were quantified. Most (93%) were treated with recombinant tissue plasminogen activator (rt-PA), and all underwent venoplasty and stenting to correct underlying stenoses. All were treated with long-term therapeutic anticoagulation. Of the 27 legs treated with catheter-directed thrombolysis, 16 required adjunctive mechanical treatment to clear the thrombus; of the 25 limbs treated with ISPMT, only 7 required additional techniques. Moreover, a larger percentage of thrombus was removed with ISPMT. Complete lysis ($\geq$ 90%) was achieved in 11% of limbs receiving catheter-directed thrombolysis compared with 28% in ISPMT-treated limbs (P = 0.077). Treatment duration was decreased (23.4 vs. 55.4 hours, P < 0.001) and rt-PA dose reduced (33.4 vs. 59.3 mg, P = 0.009) with ISPMT. Bleeding complications occurred in 5% of both groups.

PART 2: TEACHING CASES

Case 1: Contemporary Venous Thrombectomy

What Made the Case Complex?

A 24-year-old woman who was 32 weeks pregnant presented to the emergency department in the evening with a swollen, painful left lower extremity and right-sided pleuritic chest pain. Her left leg had become progressively more symptomatic during the past three days and she had begun to feel lethargic, short of breath, and was experiencing right chest discomfort with deep breathing. She was a nonsmoker with no family or personal history of venous thromboembolic disease. Upon physical examination, the patient had a swollen, cyanotic left leg that was tender

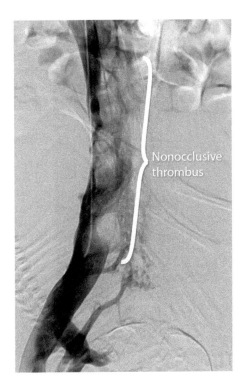

Nonocclusive
thrombus

Figure 3   An iliocavagram performed to evaluate the proximal
extent of thrombus shows clot extending from the common iliac
vein into the vena cava and up to the level of the renal veins.

to palpation, especially palpating the common femoral vein. Her left thigh and calf measured
73 cm and 45 cm, compared to 64 cm and 40 cm on the right.

What Was the Clinical Indication for Treatment of This Patient?
This patient's presentation was clinically consistent with iliofemoral DVT associated with a PE.
The adventitia of the femoral vein is innervated with sensory nerves; therefore, pain to palpation
of the femoral vein as a result of its distension is a frequent physical finding. The femoral vein
distends as a result of the associated venous hypertension and thrombosis.

The patient was started on intravenous heparin. A venous duplex scan revealed thrombosis of the left external iliac, common femoral, femoral, popliteal, posterior tibial, and proximal
great saphenous veins. A subsequent iliocavagram was performed to evaluate the proximal
extent of thrombus and potential vena caval involvement. It confirmed thrombosis of the left
common iliac vein and extensive clot in the vena cava extending to the level of the renal
veins (Fig. 3).

What Were the Potential Hazards of Treating This Patient and Anatomy?
Patients presenting during off hours to the emergency department who are at high clinical risk
of a venous thromboembolic condition should be anticoagulated until a definitive diagnosis is
made. A CT scan of the chest or ventilation/perfusion (V/Q) lung scan was not performed in
this patient because she was pregnant and the clinical probability of a PE was high. Since this
patient is being managed for acute DVT, her treatment would not be altered by the V/Q scan
findings. There is also reluctance to expose the pregnant patient to the excessive radiation of CT
scans or a radioisotope.

Which Interventional Strategies Were Considered?
Standard ascending phlebography was not necessary, since the clinical presentation and venous
duplex established the diagnosis with a high degree of accuracy. Once anticoagulation was
started and therapeutic, it was not necessary and actually counterproductive to maintain the
patient at bed rest. An echocardiogram is advisable in all patients who have the diagnosis of PE
to evaluate its impact on right ventricular function; however, it was not necessary in this patient

to perform an "off hours" echocardiogram since the patient had no evidence of hemodynamic compromise and could wait to be properly treated until the next business day.

A retrievable Gunther Tulip filter (William Cook, Europe) was placed in the suprarenal inferior vena cava (IVC) under fluoroscopic guidance. Post procedure, a discussion was held with the patient and family to review alternative treatment to eliminate thrombus, including catheter-directed thrombolysis, pharmacomechanical thrombolysis, and operative venous thrombectomy. The decision was made to proceed with venous thrombectomy.

Summary

The patient was taken to the operating room for a venous thrombectomy under fluoroscopic guidance with fetal monitoring. A cut-down was performed on the left common femoral and femoral veins, with exposure of the saphenofemoral junction. A longitudinal venotomy was performed at the level of the saphenofemoral junction, followed by protrusion of a large amount of acute thrombus (Fig. 4). The leg was raised and a tight rubber bandage applied with minimal extrusion of the infrainguinal thrombus. Attempts to pass a catheter from the inguinal ligament distally into the femoral vein and attempts to pass a guidewire distally were unsuccessful.

A cut-down on the posterior tibial vein in the lower leg was performed. Following a posterior tibial venotomy, a #3 Fogarty catheter was passed upwards through the thrombosed venous system, exiting the common femoral venotomy. This catheter was used to guide a #4 Fogarty catheter distally through the venous valves by placing both catheter tips within a 14-gauge silastic IV catheter sheath after the hub was amputated. Following a mechanical balloon catheter thrombectomy, the leg was flushed with a heparin saline solution using a bulb syringe, which flushed additional thrombus from the common femoral venotomy. After clamping the femoral vein, the deep venous system was then filled with 300 cc of a dilute recombinant tissue plasminogen solution (6 mg rt-PA in 300 cc).

The iliofemoral and vena caval thrombectomy was performed under fluoroscopic guidance, filling the balloon with contrast to ensure that the suprarenal caval filter was not dislodged. After completing the thrombectomy, an operative iliocavagram was performed to assess the adequacy of thrombectomy and to ensure unobstructed venous drainage into the vena cava. An iliac vein stenosis was observed.

A balloon angioplasty catheter was placed into the lesion and an angioplasty performed. The iliac vein was dilated to 14 mm without evidence of recoil.

An AVF using the proximal saphenous vein anastomosed to the superficial femoral artery increases flow velocity through the iliofemoral venous system, reducing the risk of rethrombosis.

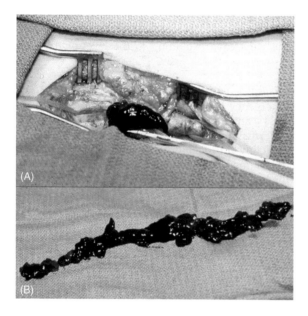

Figure 4 (A) A venotomy performed at the level of the saphenofemoral junction is followed by protrusion of a large amount of acute thrombus. (B) Thrombus removed from iliofemoral venous system during thrombectomy.

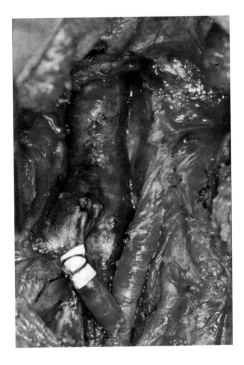

Figure 5 Following venous thrombectomy, an AVF was constructed to increase the flow velocity through the iliofemoral venous system, reducing the risk of rethrombosis. A small piece of PTFE wrapped around the saphenous AVF and looped with O-Prolene served as a guide should the AVF require closure in the future.

A thrombectomy of the proximal great saphenous vein was required in this patient, as is often the case. Since the goal of the AVF is to increase venous blood flow velocity but not venous pressure, the size of the anastomosis is limited to 3.5 to 4 mm, in order to avoid a steal and avoid venous hypertension. A small piece of polytetrafluoroethylene (PTFE) is wrapped around the saphenous AVF and looped with a 2-cm piece of O-Prolene, which is left in the subcutaneous tissue (Fig. 5). This will serve as a guide should the AVF require operative closure in the future. However, since the AVF is small, it is considered permanent and closure is not anticipated and rarely required. Common femoral venous pressure is recorded before and after the AVF is opened. It should show no change. If the AVF increases femoral venous pressure, an iliac vein stenosis should be suspected, or the AVF is too large.

To further reduce the risk of rethrombosis, a heparin infusion catheter (pediatric feeding tube) is placed into the proximal posterior tibial vein and brought out through a separate stab wound adjacent to the lower leg incision. Infusing unfractionated heparin through this catheter to achieve a therapeutic PTT ensures a high concentration of heparin in the target vein, a concentration much higher than would be achieved if the patient was treated with standard IV anticoagulation through an arm vein. A monofilament suture is looped around the posterior tibial vein cephalad to catheter entry and brought out through the skin and secured with a sterile button. This is used to occlude the vein after five to six days when the catheter is removed following full oral anticoagulation with warfarin.

In the case of this pregnant patient, IV anticoagulation through the leg veins was maintained for four days, after which she was converted to subcutaneous enoxaparin at 1 mg/kg q12 hours. The catheter was removed and the patient discharged. The patient was maintained on S.Q. enoxaparin 1 mg/kg BID until she delivered a healthy baby six weeks later.

Case 2: Catheter-Directed Thrombolysis

What Made the Case Complex?
A 37-year-old gentleman was referred for left lower extremity phlegmasia cerulea dolens eight days after undergoing an uneventful elective total colectomy for ulcerative colitis.

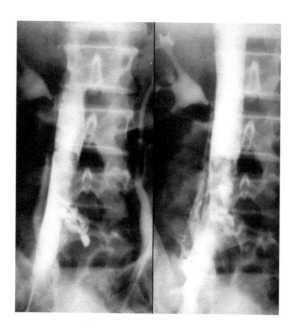

Figure 6 Contralateral iliocavagrams demonstrated nonocclusive thrombus in the vena cava,
illustrating importance of identifying the proximal
extent of thrombus.

What Was the Clinical Indication for Treatment of This Patient?

An ascending phlebogram showed thrombus in the femoral vein, common femoral vein, and iliofemoral venous system of his left leg. A contralateral iliocavagram illustrated nonocclusive thrombus of his vena cava (Fig. 6)

What Were the Potential Hazards of Treating This Patient and Anatomy?

Patients at highest risk of procedure-related PE are those with nonocclusive thrombus in their vena cava, as was revealed by this patient's iliocavagrams. It is important to image the proximal and distal extent of thrombus, and particularly the amount and level of vena caval involvement. A vena caval filter (Fig. 7) was placed in this patient to prevent a large PE from occurring during catheter-directed thrombolysis.

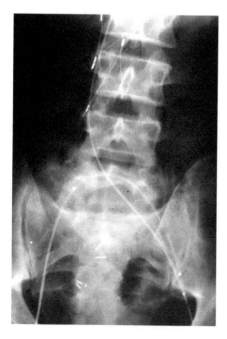

Figure 7 A Bird's nest filter was placed in the IVC to prevent a large PE from occurring during catheter-directed thrombolysis.

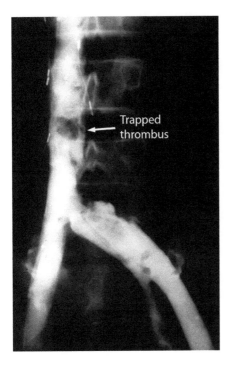

Figure 8 Completion cavagram revealed trapped thrombus inside the IVC filter, preventing a pulmonary embolus.

Which Interventional Tools Were Used to Manage This Case?
Catheter-directed thrombolysis was begun by accessing the left popliteal vein via an ultrasound-guided popliteal vein puncture. Long-segment side-hole infusion catheters were placed into the acute thrombus in the femoral vein and iliofemoral venous system.

Summary
Lytic therapy was successful; however, it demonstrated that there was compression of the left common iliac vein as it is crossed by the right common iliac artery, representing a typical May–Thurner picture. Venoplasty and stenting were performed to restore unobstructed venous drainage into the vena cava.

A completion cavagram demonstrated that the IVC filter indeed trapped an embolus in transit (Fig. 8).

The patient was subsequently treated with therapeutic anticoagulation using unfractionated heparin converted to oral anticoagulation with Coumadin targeting an international normalized ratio (INR) of 2.5. The patient was placed in a 30 to 40 mm Hg ankle gradient compression stocking and discharged.

On follow-up, the patient had minimal if any swelling, even when not wearing his compression stockings. The lower extremity venous system remained patent with valve function in the borderline normal range [venous valve closure times of 0.5–0.7 seconds and a venous filling index on air plethysmography (APG) of 2.2].

Case 3: Pharmacomechanical Thrombolysis

What Made the Case Complex?
A sixty-eight-year-old male was referred with phlegmasia cerulea dolens one day after a major abdominal operation.

What Was the Clinical Indication for Treatment of This Patient?
Venous ultrasound demonstrated extensive venous thrombosis extending from the calf veins to the vena cava, which was confirmed with ascending phlebography (Fig. 9).

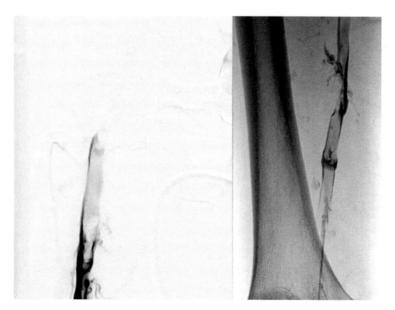

Figure 9   Phlebography illustrated extensive venous thrombosis that extended from the calf to the vena cava.

What Were the Potential Hazards of Treating This Patient and Anatomy?

A CT scan showed PE and extensive mediastinal and retroperitoneal lymphadenopathy. CT scans of the abdomen and pelvis also demonstrated retroperitoneal lymphadenopathy consistent with lymphoma.

Which Interventional Tools Were Used to Manage This Case?

The iliofemoral thrombosis was treated expediently with the Trellis catheter (Fig. 10), using ISPMT with 15-minute runs, aspirating liquified thrombus and residual thrombus after each run. The thrombus extending from the posterior tibial vein through the popliteal and into the femoral vein was treated with ultrasound-accelerated thrombolysis with rt-PA after passing an EKOS catheter from the posterior tibial vein at the ankle into the distal femoral vein. Tissue

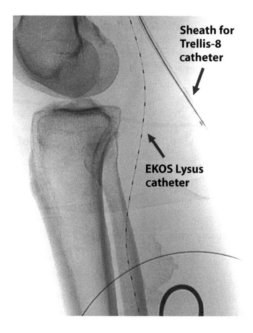

Sheath for Trellis-8 catheter

EKOS Lysus catheter

Figure 10   Both the Trellis and EKOS infusion catheters were used to eliminate clot as part of a strategy of thrombus removal. The Trellis catheter was used on thrombus in the femoral and iliac veins, and the EKOS catheter-treated clot in the posterior tibial and popliteal veins.

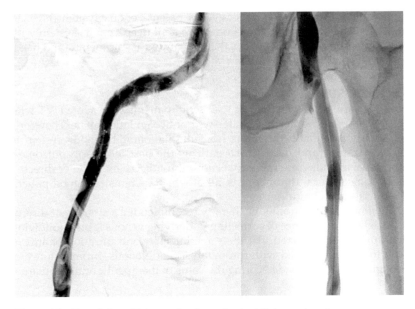

Figure 11 Completion phlebography showed patent iliofemoral system.

plasminogen activator was infused through the EKOS catheter during its activation. Areas of segmentally persistent thrombus were treated with rheolytic thrombectomy using the AngioJet catheter.

Summary
The patient received a minimal amount of tPA systemically. His thrombus rapidly lysed and his symptoms resolved. The external iliac vein was compressed by his pelvic lymphadenopathy

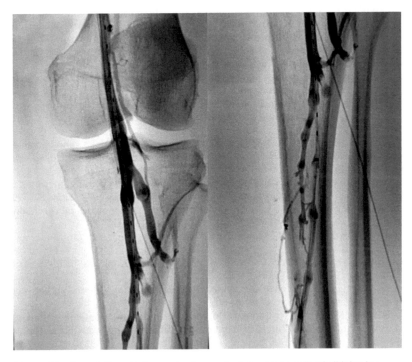

Figure 12 Completion phlebography demonstrated patent popliteal–tibial veins.

and required stenting. Completion phlebography showed a patent venous system (Figs. 11 and 12). Posttreatment, noninvasive studies demonstrated a patent deep venous system with competent venous valves and, at 16-month follow-up, the patient was asymptomatic and had a patent deep venous system with normally functioning valves.

PART 3: SUMMARY OF KEY ISSUES

Patients with iliofemoral DVT are a clinically relevant subset of patients with acute DVT who suffer the most severe postthrombotic morbidity if treated with anticoagulation alone. Therefore, aggressive therapy designed to eliminate thrombus from the iliofemoral venous system is the preferred management strategy and offers these patients the best long-term outcomes. Strategies of thrombus removal include contemporary venous thrombectomy, catheter-directed thrombolysis, and pharmacomechanical thrombolysis, all of which demonstrate good patient outcomes via randomized trials and clinical series.

The 2008 ACCP guidelines on antithrombotic therapy recommended a strategy of thrombus removal and emphasized the importance of correcting underlying venous lesions following thrombus removal. They further emphasized that the same intensity and duration of anticoagulant therapy be given to patients treated with thrombolysis and venous thrombectomy as those treated with anticoagulation alone, underscoring the value of therapeutic anticoagulation to prevent rethrombosis.

REFERENCES

1. Kearon C, Kahn SR, Agnelli G, et al. Antithrombotic therapy for venous thromboembolic disease: ACCP evidence-based clinical practice guidelines (8th ed). Chest 2008; 133(6):454S–545S.
2. Kahn SR, Kearon C, Julian JA, et al. Predictors of the post-thrombotic syndrome during long-term treatment of proximal deep vein thrombosis. J Thromb Haemost 2005; 3(4):718–723.
3. Kahn SR, Hirsch A, Shrier I. Effect of postthrombotic syndrome on health-related quality of life after deep venous thrombosis. Arch Intern Med 2002; 162(10):1144–1148.
4. O'Donnell TF, Browse NL, Burnand KG, et al. The socioeconomic effects of an iliofemoral venous thrombosis. J Surg Res 1977; 22(5):483–488.
5. Delis KT, Bountouroglou D, Mansfield AO. Venous claudication in iliofemoral thrombosis: long-term effects on venous hemodynamics, clinical status, and quality of life. Ann Surg 2004; 239(1):118–126.
6. Akesson H, Brudin L, Dahlstrom JA, et al. Venous function assessed during a 5 year period after acute ilio-femoral venous thrombosis treated with anticoagulation. Eur J Vasc Surg 1990; 4(1):43–48.
7. Comerota AJ, Throm RC, Mathias SD, et al. Catheter-directed thrombolysis for iliofemoral deep venous thrombosis improves health-related quality of life. J Vasc Surg 2000; 32(1):130–137.
8. Shull KC, Nicolaides AN, Fernandes e Fernandes J, et al. Significance of popliteal reflux in relation to ambulatory venous pressure and ulceration. Arch Surg 1979; 114(11):1304–1346.
9. Nicolaides AN, Schull K, Fernandes E. Ambulatory venous pressure: new information. In: Nicolaides AN, Yao JS, eds. Investigation of Vascular Disorders. New York: Churchill Livingstone, 1981: 488–494.
10. Johnson BF, Manzo RA, Bergelin RO, et al. Relationship between changes in the deep venous system and the development of the postthrombotic syndrome after an acute episode of lower limb deep vein thrombosis: a one- to six-year follow-up. J Vasc Surg 1995; 21(2):307–312.
11. Cho JS, Martelli E, Mozes G, et al. Effects of thrombolysis and venous thrombectomy on valvular competence, thrombogenicity, venous wall morphology, and function. J Vasc Surg 1998; 28(5):787–799.
12. Rhodes JM, Cho JS, Gloviczki P, et al. Thrombolysis for experimental deep venous thrombosis maintains valvular competence and vasoreactivity. J Vasc Surg 2000; 31(6):1193–1205.
13. Killewich LA, Bedford GR, Beach KW, et al. Spontaneous lysis of deep venous thrombi: rate and outcome. J Vasc Surg 1989; 9(1):89–97.
14. Markel A, Manzo RA, Bergelin RO, et al. Valvular reflux after deep vein thrombosis: incidence and time of occurrence. J Vasc Surg 1992; 15(2):377–382.
15. Meissner MH, Manzo RA, Bergelin RO, et al. Deep venous insufficiency: the relationship between lysis and subsequent reflux. J Vasc Surg 1993; 18(4):596–605.
16. Monreal M, Rey-Joly BC, Ruiz MJ, et al. Asymptomatic pulmonary embolism in patients with deep vein thrombosis. Is it useful to take a lung scan to rule out this condition? J Cardiovasc Surg (Torino) 1989; 30(1):104–107.
17. Martinez J, Comerota AJ, Kazanjian S, et al. The quantitative benefit of isolated, segmental, pharmacomechanical thrombolysis for iliofemoral DVT. J Vasc Surg 2008; 48(6):1532–1537.

18. Goldhaber SZ, Buring JE, Lipnick RJ, et al. Pooled analyses of randomized trials of streptokinase and heparin in phlebographically documented acute deep venous thrombosis. Am J Med 1984; 76(3):393–397.
19. Comerota AJ, Aldridge SC, Cohen G, et al. A strategy of aggressive regional therapy for acute iliofemoral venous thrombosis with contemporary venous thrombectomy or catheter-directed thrombolysis. J Vasc Surg 1994; 20(2):244–254.
20. Alkjaersig N, Fletcher AP, Sherry S. The mechanism of clot dissolution by plasmin. J Clin Invest 1959; 38(7):1086–1095.
21. Vedantham S, Vesely TM, Parti N, et al. Lower extremity venous thrombolysis with adjunctive mechanical thrombectomy. J Vasc Interv Radiol 2002; 13(10):1001–1008.
22. Lin PH, Zhou W, Dardik A, et al. Catheter-direct thrombolysis versus pharmacomechanical thrombectomy for treatment of symptomatic lower extremity deep venous thrombosis. Am J Surg 2006; 192(6):782–788.
23. Kasirajan K, Gray B, Ouriel K. Percutaneous AngioJet thrombectomy in the management of extensive deep venous thrombosis. J Vasc Interv Radiol 2001; 12(2):179–185.
24. Parikh S, Motarjeme A, McNamara T, et al. Ultrasound-accelerated thrombolysis for the treatment of deep vein thrombosis: initial clinical experience. J Vasc Interv Radiol 2008; 19(4):521–528.
25. Plate G, Einarsson E, Ohlin P, et al. Thrombectomy with temporary arteriovenous fistula: the treatment of choice in acute iliofemoral venous thrombosis. J Vasc Surg 1984; 1(6):867–876.
26. Einarsson E, Albrechtsson U, Eklof B. Thrombectomy and temporary AV-fistula in iliofemoral vein thrombosis. Technical considerations and early results. Int Angiol 1986; 5(2):65–72.
27. Ganger KH, Nachbur BH, Ris HB, et al. Surgical thrombectomy versus conservative treatment for deep venous thrombosis; functional comparison of long-term results. Eur J Vasc Surg 1989; 3(6):529–538.
28. Neglen P, al-Hassan HK, Endrys J, et al. Iliofemoral venous thrombectomy followed by percutaneous closure of the temporary arteriovenous fistula. Surgery 1991; 110(3):493–499.
29. Kniemeyer HW, Sandmann W, Schwindt C, et al. Thrombectomy with arteriovenous fistula for embolizing deep venous thrombosis: an alternative therapy for prevention of recurrent pulmonary embolism. Clin Investig 1993; 72(1):40–45.
30. Juhan C, Alimi Y, Di Mauro P, et al. Surgical venous thrombectomy. Cardiovasc Surg 1999; 7(6):586–590.
31. Meissner AJ, Huszcza S. Surgical strategy for management of deep venous thrombosis of the lower extremities. World J Surg 1996; 20(9):1149–1155.
32. Comerota AJ, Gravett MH. Iliofemoral venous thrombosis. J Vasc Surg 2007; 46(5):1065–1076.
33. Bjarnason H, Kruse JR, Asinger DA, et al. Iliofemoral deep venous thrombosis: safety and efficacy outcome during 5 years of catheter-directed thrombolytic therapy. J Vasc Interv Radiol 1997; 8(3):405–418.
34. Mewissen MW, Seabrook GR, Meissner MH, et al. Catheter-directed thrombolysis for lower extremity deep venous thrombosis: report of a national multicenter registry. Radiology 1999; 211(1):39–49.
35. Comerota AJ, Kagan SA. Catheter-directed thrombolysis for the treatment of acute iliofemoral deep venous thrombosis. Phlebology 2000; 15:149–155.

19 | The Complex Patient with Multivessel Disease

N. Diehm

Swiss Cardiovascular Center, Clinical and Interventional Angiology, Inselspital, University Hospital Bern, Bern, Switzerland

Barry Katzen

Baptist Cardiac and Vascular Institute, Miami, Florida, U.S.A.

Jennifer Franke and Horst Sievert*

CardioVascular Center Frankfurt Sankt Katharinen, Frankfurt, Germany

PART 1: INTRODUCTION

Multivessel disease is encountered in up to more than two-thirds of patients with critical limb ischemia (CLI) (1). Especially in the presence of diabetes mellitus and chronic renal insufficiency, CLI is frequently associated with infrapopliteal lesions and extensive calcifications of the arterial media (1–3).

Considering the dismal natural course of CLI (4), there is no doubt that arterial revascularization improves prognosis, even in diabetic patients (5,6). Indeed, current recommendations call for attempts of arterial reconstruction in any patient with CLI if one-year probability of survival and limb salvage can be estimated higher than 25% (7,8). Level-A evidence indicates that an endovascular-first strategy in patients presenting with severe limb ischemia due to infrainguinal disease is preferred over a primary surgical approach since outcomes are comparable to those of bypass surgery (9). Moreover, angioplasty offers advantages such as minimal access trauma, low infection rates, and shorter hospital stays (9).

What Makes a Patient with Multivessel Disease "Complex"?

Patients with multilevel disease and CLI are oftentimes medically frail and many of these patients, for various reasons, cannot tolerate exceedingly endovascular procedures. Thus, besides the technical complexity associated with multilevel revascularization procedures, elaboration of individually tailored treatment strategies oftentimes requires an interdisciplinary approach.

At present it remains unclear, whether a maximum revascularization strategy is necessary or if direct flow to the foot through one patent artery is sufficient to grant relief from CLI symptoms. Given the comparatively high rates of restenosis in patients with multilevel disease and infrageniculate disease involvement, extensive use of below-the-knee angioplasty might be advantageous in CLI patients (10,11) (Table 1).

What Are the Clinical Indications for Endovascular Treatment of Complex Lesions in Patients with Multivessel Disease?

Given limited data on outcomes of complex multilevel revascularization procedures in claudicants, the currently well-accepted indication is acute or chronic CLI.

Hazards and Complications of Endovascular Treatment of Complex Lesions in Patients with Multivessel Disease

A maximum revascularization approach might not be a viable option in a subset of CLI patients for various reasons (Table 2). Individually tailored treatment strategies and multistep revascularization will be required in this challenging patient group.

---

*Complex Case 2 Provided by Drs. Franke and Sievert.

Table 1 Advantages of a Maximum Revascularization Attempt in CLI Patients with Multilevel Disease

→ Optimization of flow to the foot by revascularization of *at least* one straight line
→ Patients may benefit from two or even three patent crural vessels

Interventional Strategies for Endovascular Treatment of Complex Lesions in Patients with Multivessel Disease

Interventional strategies have to be custom-tailored to the very specific needs of each individual patient. In general, we recommend the following strategies:

- Adequate pre and posthydration in patients with impairment of renal function.
- Preprocedural planning using duplex sonography for the aortoiliac and femoropopliteal tract to limit use of contrast agents.
- Antegrade (primary 4-F) puncture in case of femorocrural lesion pattern, retrograde crossover approach in case of iliac artery obstruction.
- In selected cases, pedal puncture of dorsalis pedis artery may be necessary to obtain access to the anterior tibial artery.
- Glycoprotein IIb/IIIa antagonists for multivessel revascularizations of exceeding extent and duration (12).
- Dual platelet therapy for patients undergoing stent placement in the iliac, femoropopliteal or tibial arteries for 28 days (compassionate use despite lack of evidence).

Interventional Tools for Endovascular Treatment of Complex Lesions in Patients with Multivessel Disease

Besides standard interventional tools, our clinical practice involves the following devices:

- CTO devices (such as the Outback® catheter).
- Balloon expandable stents for use in the iliac, common femoral, deep femoral, and proximal superficial arteries.
- Self-expanding nitinol stents for use in the femoropopliteal arteries. In general, the use of nitinol stents in the femoropopliteal segment should become more liberal with increasing lesion lengths and worsening clinical presentation of the patient.
- Long low-profile balloon catheters for extensive obstructions of tibial arteries.
- Drug-eluting coronary stents for complex tibial artery interventions (such as recurrence of CLI in focal lesions or restenosis of bypass anastomoses).

Summary of Outcomes

Clinical outcomes of CLI patients undergoing complex endovascular multilevel revascularization should be judged in the light of its dismal natural course if left untreated. In a series by Lepantalo and colleagues, unreconstructed CLI was associated with a 54% mortality and a 46% amputation rate at one year (4).

Faglia and colleagues analyzed a prospective series of 993 consecutive diabetic patients with CLI undergoing primary endovascular treatment. Two-thirds of these patients had multilevel arterial obstructions (11). Technical success was 83.6% in these patients with severely calcified arteries. During a mean follow-up of 26.2 ± 15.1 months, clinical restenosis rate was 11.3% and major amputations were necessary in 1.7% of patients. Five-year primary patency rate was 88% and mortality rate was 6.7% per year.

According to our own experience with 383 CLI patients undergoing surgical or endovascular revascularization, however, repeated revascularization procedures may be necessary to grant clinical midterm success (6).

Table 2 Hazards of a Maximum Revascularization Attempt in CLI Patients with Multilevel Disease

→ Contrast amount (renal failure)
→ Fluid amount (heart failure)
→ Risk of complications
→ Age—general condition

PART 2: CASE PRESENTATIONS

Complex Case 1: Limb Salvage in a Patient with Critical Limb Ischemia Due to Severely Calcified Multilevel Lower Limb Obstructions

Case Report

What Was the Clinical Indication for Treatment of This Patient?
A 71-year-old male was admitted for limb-threatening ischemia of the left forefoot. He complained about ulceration of the left great toe. His risk factor background contained type II diabetes mellitus, arterial hypertension, hyperlipidemia, and mild renal insufficiency. The patient had undergone coronary artery bypass grafting and percutaneous transluminal angioplasty (PTA) of the left renal artery 10 years ago, and was asymptomatic with regard to cardiac symptoms.

Upon admission, the patients' lower limb distal pulses were not palpable. Ankle brachial index (ABI) could not be measured bilaterally due to arterial incompressibility. Oscillographic reading of the left leg was conspicuous of relevant lesions in the femoral and below-the-knee arteries. Duplex ultrasound revealed an occlusion of the left distal superficial femoral artery. The patient was scheduled for a diagnostic angiogram and an endovascular revascularization in the same session.

What Made the Case "Complex"?
The case was considered complex for the presence of multilevel disease, presence of severely calcified arteries due to medial arterial calcinosis and considering the limited amount of contrast medium that could be used in this patient with impaired renal function.

Which Interventional Strategies Were Considered?
Access was gained in the right common femoral artery using fluoroscopic guidance and a single-wall 18-gauge needle. A 5-French pigtail catheter was advanced into the abdominal aorta and an abdominal aortic angiogram and peripheral runoff was performed. Digital subtraction angiography of the left leg revealed significant atherosclerotic changes including an occlusion of the superficial femoral artery within the distal adductor canal (Fig. 1) and a high-grade, severely calcified stenosis in the tibiofibular trunk (Fig. 2).

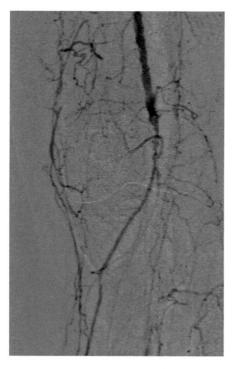

Figure 1 Angiographic image of the distal superficial femoral artery.

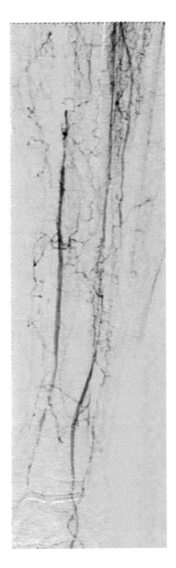

Figure 2 Angiographic image of diffusely stenosed tibiofibular trunk.

The patient was repositioned and a left antegrade approach was performed with fluoro-scopic guidance and a single-wall 18-gauge needle (Table 3). Dense calcification was noted in the common femoral artery as well as the profunda and superficial femoral arteries.

The access was upsized for a 6-French Terumo vascular sheath. The proximal calcified superficial femoral artery (SFA) stenoses were crossed with a Wholey torque wire, followed by balloon angioplasty of the left superficial femoral artery at the level of the adductor canal using a 6 mm Ultrathin (Boston Scientific) balloon. Attention was then directed to the occluded popliteal artery with only single vessel runoff. Initial attempts were made to recanalize the popliteal artery with a multipurpose-shaped catheter and straight wire both intraluminal and then subintimal. While subintimal passage was obtained to the level of the distal popliteal artery, re-entry could not be achieved. The 0.035″ guidewire was exchanged for a 0.014″ BMW wire, placed into the tibioperoneal trunk. An Outback Re-entry Device (Cordis, Johnson & Johnson) was used for successful re-entry, and progressive dilation of the tract was accomplished. The guidewire was placed in the peroneal artery. A critical proximal, calcified peroneal artery was dilated to 10 atm pressure with a conventional angioplasty balloon (3 × 100 mm, Invatec Amphirion) without effect. No change in the waist of the balloon was noted due to the extensive calcification (Fig. 3). A 3 × 20 mm Angiosculpt scoring balloon was inserted and the lesion was successfully angioplastied (Fig. 4) before a 3.5 × 33 mm Taxus stent could be deployed, which

Table 3 List of Equipment Used in this Case

→ 6-French vascular sheath (Terumo)
→ 3 × 20 mm Angiosculpt scoring balloon (AngioScore)
→ 6 mm Ultrathin balloon (Boston Scientific)
→ 5 FMPA catheter (Cook Medical)
→ LLT wire (Cook Medical)
→ 6 × 80 mm LifeStent (Edwards Life Sciences)
→ 6 × 4 mm balloon (Boston Scientific)
→ 0.014″ BMW wire (Abbott Vascular)
→ 3 × 100 mm balloon (Amphirion, Invatec)
→ Angiosculpt balloon 3.0 × 20 mm (Angioscore)
→ 3.5 × 33 mm Taxus Stent (Boston Scientific)

was postdilated to 3.5 mm at 10 atm (Fig. 5). Following treatment of the outflow, a 6 × 80 mm LifeStent (Edwards Life Sciences) was deployed in the popliteal artery and postdilated to 6 mm.

The completion angiogram demonstrated excellent flow across the distal left superficial femoral artery stent and the stent in the left tibioperoneal trunk. There was inline flow via the peroneal artery to the foot (Fig. 6).

What Were the Potential Hazards of Treating This Patient and Anatomy?
Potential treatment hazards for these lesions included dissections of these rigid vessels as well as embolization with subsequent clinical deterioration.

Summary: How Was the Case Managed, Is there Anything That Could Have Been Improved, What Was the Immediate and Long-Term Outcome?
Technical and clinical success in complex multivessel endovascular revascularization may be dependent on dedicated interventional devices facilitating lesion success in highly calcified

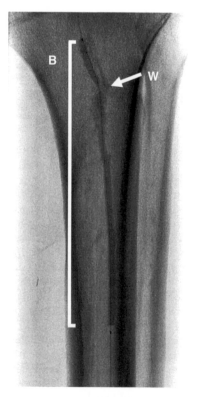

Figure 3 Unability to fully expand a 3/100 "0.014 low profile balloon (B) due to severe calcification of tibifibular trunk resulting in a waist (W) of the balloon.

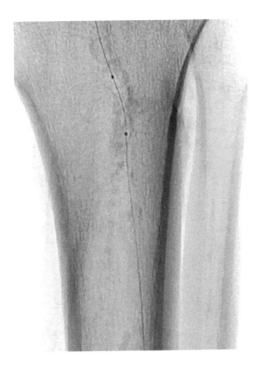

Figure 4 Balloon angioplasty with a 3/20 Angiosculpt scoring balloon.

obstructions. Although level-A evidence on the primary use of drug-eluting stents in tibial arteries is currently lacking, use of this technology can be associated with favorable clinical outcomes.

Four months postprocedurally, the patients' ulcers were healed and oscillographic reading significantly improved on the left side. Duplex ultrasound showed wide patency of the treated femoral and infrapopliteal segments.

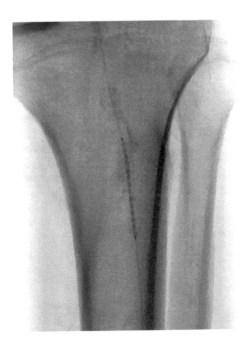

Figure 5 Deployment of a 3.5/33 drug eluting stent.

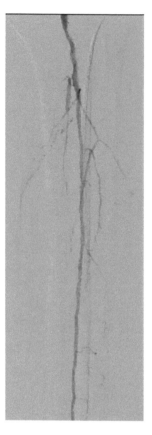

Figure 6 Final angiogram showing straight flow after recanalisation of the distal femoral artery and tibiofibular trunk.

Complex Case 2: Catheter Treatment in Complex Supra-Aortic Disease

Clinical Summary

A 68-year-old woman was referred by her general practitioner with pain in her right shoulder and paresthesia of her right hand. Blood pressure measured 81/56 mm Hg on the right and 113/68 mm Hg on the left side. MR-Angio showed an aortic arch type III, an ostial stenosis of the left common carotid artery, a 2-cm long occlusion of the brachiocephalic trunk, retrograde flow in the right common and internal carotid artery as well as bilateral inverse flow of the ophthalmic arteries.

First Procedure: Recanalization/Stenting of the Brachiocephalic Trunk

Angiographic imaging confirmed the occlusion of the brachiocephalic trunk (Fig. 7). Recanalization was performed via right radial access. Femoral access was challenging due to an acute-angled takeoff of the brachiocephalic trunk as showed in Figure 8. An 8 mm Dynamic Biotronic stent was implanted. Figure 9 demonstrates the final angiographic result. After postdilatation of the stent, the patient developed paresthesia of her left hand and rapidly lost consciousness. The intracranial runs revealed embolic occlusions of middle cerebral artery side branches. By using microcatheters, urokinase, and tirofiban, the occluded intracerebral arteries were successively reopened [Fig. 10(A) and 10(B)]. The patient regained consciousness during the process of intracranial rescue, and suffered no residual neurological sequelae.

Interventional Tools

0.035″ Emerald Guidewire (Cordis)
Radiofocus stiff Guidewire (Terumo)
5-French radial sheath (Terumo)
4-French radial sheath (Terumo)

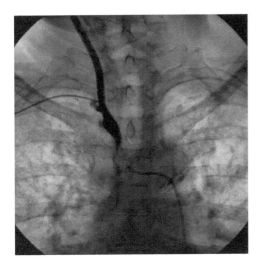

Figure 7 Occlusion of the brachiocephalic trunk.

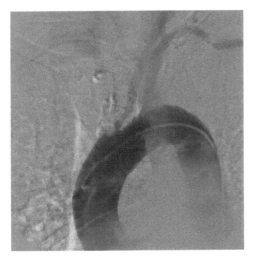

Figure 8 Type III aortic arch.

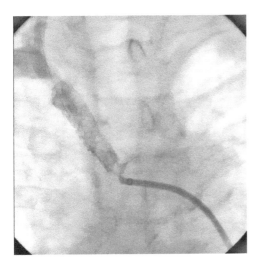

Figure 9 Result after stent implantation.

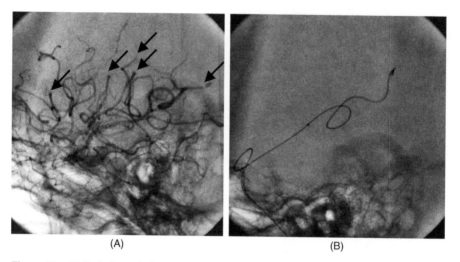

Figure 10   (A) Embolic occlusions of middle cerebral artery side branches. (B) Intracranial rescue.

8/40/130 Sailor plus balloon catheter (Krauth/Invatec)
6 mm/40 mm Submarine balloon catheter (Krauth/Invatec)
8 mm/25 mm Dynamic stent (Biotronic)
0.014″ Transcend Guidewire (Boston Scientific)
0.035 Amplatz extra stiff wire (Cook)
Taper 14-Flex Guidewire (Boston Scientific)
V-18 Control wire (Boston Scientific)

Second Procedure: High-Grade Restenosis of the Brachiocephalic Trunk

Two months after the initial procedure, the patient was admitted with a suspected restenosis of the brachiocephalic trunk. The angiogram (Fig. 11) revealed severe stent compression at the ostium. The guide that was initially introduced via femoral access was caught between the proximal stent struts. A second access via the right brachial artery was established to perform retrograde crossing of the stent. The wire was then directed out of femoral access and a long sheath was placed via the femoral access (Fig. 12). During these maneuvers, embolic protection was performed by intermittent manual compression of the right common carotid artery. Angioplasty was performed with an 8-mm balloon and a second stent (9 mm/19 mm

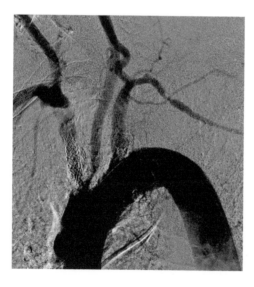

Figure 11   Restenosis due to stent compression.

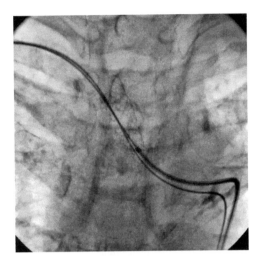

Figure 12 Wire directed out of femoral access.

Onda Stent, Krauth/Invatec) was implanted at the ostium of the brachiocephalic trunk. After attending the brachiocephalic trunk, a third stent (8 mm/5 mm Dynamic stent, Biotronic) was placed in the right subclavian artery (Fig. 13). The final result indicated no measurable pressure gradient (Fig. 14).

Interventional Tools
4-French radial sheath (Terumo)
5-French radial sheath (Terumo)
0.035″ Emerald Guidewire (Cordis)
V-18 Control wire (Boston Scientific)
8 mm/15 mm Dynamic stent (Biotronic)
Radiofocus stiff Guidewire (Terumo)
Iron Man wire (Terumo)
Admiral Xtreme Balloon catheter (Krauth/Invatec)
9 mm/19 mm Onda Stent (Krauth/Invatec)

Third Procedure: Stenosis of the Left Subclavian and Common Carotid Artery
A third procedure was scheduled four months later to treat the stenosis of the left subclavian artery and left common carotid artery (Fig. 15). Angioplasty of the left subclavian artery was performed via a femoral access. A retrograde approach was attempted with a wire crossing from

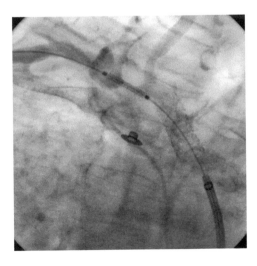

Figure 13 Stent implantation in the right subclavian artery.

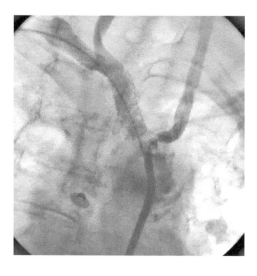

Figure 14   Final result. No measurable pressure gradient.

the right brachial artery to the left femoral artery (Fig. 16). A third access was gained via the right femoral artery. This enabled crossing of the left common carotid artery with two coronary wires. Balloon angioplasty was done with a 4-mm coronary balloon (Fig. 17). The final result after balloon angioplasty is shown in Figure 18.

Interventional Tools
V-18 Control wire (Boston Scientific)
Iron Man wire (Terumo)
0.035″ Emerald Guidewire (Cordis)
Balance Middleweight wire (Abbott Vascular)
5-French diagnostic catheter (Cordis)
5 mm/20 mm Avion plus Balloon catheter (Krauth/Invatec)
8-French femoral Sheath (Terumo)

Key Learning Issues
As demonstrated in this patient, embolic events can occur during angioplasty of the brachio-cephalic trunk. However, in this challenging scenario, establishing embolic protection is quite difficult. Intermittent manual compression of the common carotid artery during the most dangerous steps of the procedure is an alternative.

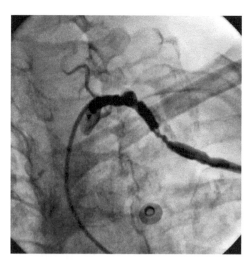

Figure 15   Stenosis of the left subclavian artery.

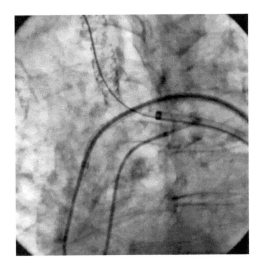

Figure 16 Wire crossed from the right brachial artery to the left femoral artery.

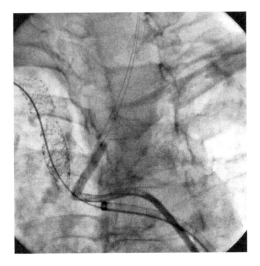

Figure 17 Access via the right femoral artery, crossing with 2 coronary wires, balloon angioplasty.

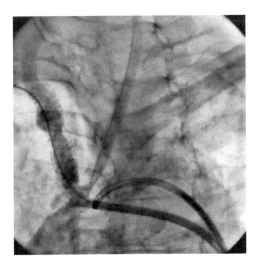

Figure 18 Final result.

Table 4 Equipment Checklist for Complex Interventions in Patients with Multivessel Disease

- CTO devices (such as the Outback® catheter)
- Balloon expandable stents for use in the iliac, common femoral, deep femoral, and proximal superficial arteries
- Self-expanding nitinol stents for use in the femoropopliteal arteries. In general, the use of nitinol stents in the femoropopliteal segment should become more liberal with increasing lesion lengths and worsening clinical presentation of the patient
- Low-profile (0.018″ and 0.014″) wires and long low-profile balloon catheters for obstructions of tibial arteries
- Drug-eluting coronary stents for complex tibial artery interventions (such as recurrence of CLI in focal lesions or restenosis of bypass anastomoses)

Table 5 Key Learning Issues

→ Patients with CLI frequently present with multilevel disease
→ Presence of diabetes mellitus and renal insufficiency is associated with severe arterial calcifications that might preclude technical success of plain balloon angioplasty
→ Therefore, the interventionist treating patients with complex multilevel disease should be aware and experienced using an advanced endovascular armamentarium
→ Utilization of a scoring balloon allows for a controlled disruption of fibrocalcific lesions

SUMMARY

In recent years, technical improvements (Table 4) have substantially facilitated endovascular treatment of CLI. Thus, endovascular treatment is increasingly considered to be the primary treatment approach in CLI patients (Table 5) (9,13).

The present case highlights that the interventional management of patients with CLI and multilevel disease may require advanced endovascular techniques such as the use of balloons with a more aggressive outward luminal expansion or bare metal or drug-eluting stents. Endovascular treatment using a standard PTA balloon might be limited in highly calcified arteries and diffuse disease in patients with diabetes mellitus and renal insufficiency (14).

The patient treated in the present case clearly benefited from the use of the scoring balloon since the use of a conventional balloon did not allow for a recanalization of this heavily calcified lesion. Initial results from a prospective study assessing the AngioSculpt scoring balloon in CLI patients indicate that use of the this device can be applied with a high technical success rate (14). Endovascular technology is unfolding more rapidly than it can be assessed in a scientific setting (15). Thus, in contrast to the femoropopliteal segment (16–21), no level-A data supporting the preferential use of various devices such as scoring or cutting balloons, bare metal or drug-eluting stents, etc. are currently available in the infrapopliteal segment.

Alternative treatment options in this patient would have been conservative treatment alone. However, it has recently been shown that diabetics with CLI clearly benefit from endovascular as well as from surgical revascularization approaches (6).

Clearly, patency rates were reported to be substantially lower as compared to clinical success rates (22). However, once ulcer healing has occurred, less perfusion is required to maintain stable skin conditions (tide-over concept) (22). Thus, aggressive invasive follow-up strategies and repeated endovascular procedures are mandatory in CLI patients with infrapopliteal disease (3,6).

REFERENCES

1. Graziani L, Silvestro A, Bertone V, et al. Vascular involvement in diabetic subjects with ischemic foot ulcer: a new morphologic categorization of disease severity. Eur J Vasc Endovasc Surg 2007; 33(4):453–460.

2. Diehm N, Shang A, Silvestro A, et al. Association of cardiovascular risk factors with pattern of lower limb atherosclerosis in 2659 patients undergoing angioplasty. Eur J Vasc Endovasc Surg 2006; 31(1): 59–63.

3. Brosi P, Baumgartner I, Silvestro A, et al. Below-the-knee angioplasty in patients with end-stage renal disease. J Endovasc Ther 2005; 12(6):704–713.

4. Lepantalo M, Matzke S. Outcome of unreconstructed chronic critical leg ischaemia. Eur J Vasc Endovasc Surg 1996; 11(2):153–157.

5. Ebskov LB, Schroeder TV, Holstein PE. Epidemiology of leg amputation: the influence of vascular surgery. Br J Surg 1994; 81(11):1600–1603.

6. Dick F, Diehm N, Galimanis A, et al. Surgical or endovascular revascularization in patients with critical limb ischemia: influence of diabetes mellitus on clinical outcome. J Vasc Surg 2007; 45(4):751–761.

7. Nasr MK, McCarthy RJ, Hardman J, et al. The increasing role of percutaneous transluminal angioplasty in the primary management of critical limb ischaemia. Eur J Vasc Endovasc Surg 2002; 23(5):398–403.

8. Norgren L, Hiatt WR, Dormandy JA, et al. Inter-society consensus for the management of peripheral arterial disease (TASC II). J Vasc Surg 2007; 45(suppl 1):S5–S67.

9. Adam DJ, Beard JD, Cleveland T, et al. Bypass versus angioplasty in severe ischaemia of the leg (BASIL): multicentre, randomised controlled trial. Lancet 2005; 366(9501):1925–1934.

10. Faglia E, Mantero M, Caminiti M, et al. Extensive use of peripheral angioplasty, particularly infrapopliteal, in the treatment of ischaemic diabetic foot ulcers: clinical results of a multicentric study of 221 consecutive diabetic subjects. J Intern Med 2002; 252(3):225–232.

11. Faglia E, Dalla Paola L, Clerici G, et al. Peripheral angioplasty as the first-choice revascularization procedure in diabetic patients with critical limb ischemia: prospective study of 993 consecutive patients hospitalized and followed between 1999 and 2003. Eur J Vasc Endovasc Surg 2005; 29(6):620–627.

12. Keo H, Diehm N, Baumgartner R, et al. Single center experience with provisional abciximab therapy in complex lower limb interventions. Vasa 2008; 37(3):257–264.

13. Kudo T, Chandra FA, Kwun WH, et al. Changing pattern of surgical revascularization for critical limb ischemia over 12 years: endovascular vs. open bypass surgery. J Vasc Surg 2006; 44(2):304–313.

14. Bosiers M, Deloose K, Cagiannos C, et al. Use of the angiosculpt scoring balloon for infrapopliteal lesions in patients with critical limb ischemia: 1-year outcome. Vascular 2009; 17(1):29–35.

15. Diehm N, Baumgartner I, Jaff M, et al. A call for uniform reporting standards in studies assessing endovascular treatment for chronic ischaemia of lower limb arteries. Eur Heart J 2007; 28(7):798–805.

16. Schillinger M, Sabeti S, Loewe C, et al. Balloon angioplasty versus implantation of nitinol stents in the superficial femoral artery. N Engl J Med 2006; 354(18):1879–1888.

17. Schillinger M, Sabeti S, Dick P, et al. Sustained benefit at 2 years of primary femoropopliteal stenting compared with balloon angioplasty with optional stenting. Circulation 2007; 115(21):2745–2749.

18. Krankenberg H, Schluter M, Steinkamp HJ, et al. Nitinol stent implantation versus percutaneous transluminal angioplasty in superficial femoral artery lesions up to 10 cm in length: the femoral artery stenting trial (FAST). Circulation 2007; 116(3):285–292.

19. Katzen B. Paper Presented at: International Symposium of Endovascular Therapy; 2008; Miami, FL, USA.

20. Amighi J, Schillinger M, Dick P, et al. De novo superficial femoropopliteal artery lesions: peripheral cutting balloon angioplasty and restenosis rates—randomized controlled trial. Radiology 2008; 247(1):267–272.

21. Diehm N, Silvestro A, Do DD, et al. Endovascular brachytherapy after femoropopliteal balloon angioplasty fails to show robust clinical benefit over time. J Endovasc Ther 2005; 12(6):723–730.

22. Soder HK, Manninen HI, Jaakkola P, et al. Prospective trial of infrapopliteal artery balloon angioplasty for critical limb ischemia: angiographic and clinical results. J Vasc Interv Radiol 2000; 11(8):1021–1031.

Index

T - #0236 - 111024 - C0 - 254/178/15 - PB - 9780367445997 - Gloss Lamination